Sister Mary Daniel Ruffing

Sister M. Sylvia Schwind

Sister M. Rosita Wellinger

Healing Body, Mind, and Spirit

Healing Body, Mind, and Spirit

The History of
the St. Francis Medical Center
Pittsburgh, Pennsylvania

Carolyn Leonard Carson

Carnegie Mellon University Press
Pittsburgh 1995

Library of Congress Catalog Number 95-67955
ISBN 0-88748-201-5

All photographs in this book are reproduced by permission of St. Francis
Hospital Archives.

For Sister Adele

Contents

Foreword

Some eight hundred years ago Francis of Assisi ran away from the world and the world has been running after Francis ever since. Today he is one of the most popular figures in history whose influence continues to be felt all over the globe. The influence of Francis comes from the witness of his life which gives a message ever ancient, ever new. Assisi continues to draw large wondrous spirit that emanated from Francis, the Saint.

Through the centuries, thousands have chosen to follow Francis ever more closely, to join together as brothers or sisters in community and to make his rule of life their own. The world is richer for their lives of service to God's people everywhere! One such group is the Sisters of St. Francis, Millvale, Pennsylvania, who have served the people of Pittsburgh area for 130 years. From the three women tended the sick in a small frame house on Thirty-seventh Street in Lawrenceville, a Franciscan presence in Pittsburgh has flourished.

Challenges to women in healthcare were many and great then as now. Such challenges were like the different pieces of a mosaic which when hewn, polished and placed accurately makes a complete entity. A totality of such as this is the integrated network known today as St. Francis Health System. The building of the present System has been long and arduous at times. With each breakthrough, changes were carefully orchestrated to make the Health System a leader among modern-day healthcare providers.

The pages of this book detail lives and events of courageous, dedicated and determined religious women who sought something much greater than themselves. With Phenomenal leadership skills, the sisters paved the way for others. At a time when women rarely ventured beyond the narrow confines of their homes, these sisters blazed the trail for professional women in the healthcare field. By acting boldly despite momentous opposition, these confident women moved to meet the needs of the poor German immigrant people.

Despite the many advances in society, poverty continues. However, today's poor have a different face from yesterday's. Millvale Franciscans and the St. Francis Health System remain committed in service to the poor. The Boards of Directors and employees of the Health System are the sisters' partners in ministry who carry the spirit of Francis of Assisi and the mission of the Millvale Franciscans to the people of God. The sisters' aim to deepen the Franciscan spirit and mission by working with lay associates who will carry this hallmark to the impoverished into and through the twenty-first century.

Today, many women rightly seek equality and recognition. Carolyn Carson has been tireless in her efforts to identify some of the significant accomplishments women religious, specifically the Sisters of St. Francis of Millvale, have given to healthcare. Achievements listed herein have been duplicated by other women religious across the country. Such efforts have made Catholic Health Care in the United States a giant in this field.

As I reflect on the gifted and selfless service of my Franciscan sisters who have served others these many years with dignity, respect and reverence, I am proud and privileged to be sister to them. I can see clearly that we still run after Francis today. Hopefully, our mark of deep love and concern for people will perdure for years to come.

Joanne Bich, OSF
Community Minister

Preface

Sister M. Adele Meiser OSF devoted her life to the St. Francis Hospital and had always wanted to develop a published history of the institution. Wanting very much to help her fulfill one of her greatest desires, the St. Francis Health Foundation provided funding for the publication of this book. It is with great joy that I am able to offer this completed work to Sister Adele. She died having only seen the first two chapters, but this work will remain as a tribute to her and the hospital for which she worked so diligently.

As I worked on this book, many people offered invaluable assistance. Scholars, whose work I have admired, willingly offered insights and suggested important other works which aided in my understanding of Catholic institutions and psychiatric medicine. Joan E. Lynaugh, of the Center for the Study of the History of Nursing, made many valuable suggestions as to how I could approach my topic when I met with her for the first and only time at the AAHM meeting in Louisville in 1993. Gerald N. Grob suggested key people for me to talk with. I am deeply grateful to Edward C. Atwater for the extensive list of sources which he sent to me, titles otherwise unobtainable. Those texts were invaluable in helping me to place St. Francis in the context of Catholic hospital history.

Staff at Carnegie Mellon University offered much help. I am grateful to Irma Tani, Carnegie Mellon University Press, for gently introducing me to the world of publishing. Clearly historians would accomplish little without the irreplaceable services provided by librarians and archivists. Susan Collins, reference librarian at the Hunt Library, offered her expertise in searching databases. The Hunt Library inter-library loan staff honored my numerous requests with alacrity. I am equally indebted to Rowinea Walker and Gail Dickey of the Carnegie Mellon University History Department.

They helped more than they'll ever know, always cheerfully assisting me as I attempted to unravel the mysteries of the copying machines.

Many individuals at St. Francis Hospital readily offered assistance and guidance. I am grateful to the St. Francis Health Foundation for funding this project. David Dombrowiak and his staff introduced me to the complex organization of the hospital. Shirley Freyer, director of the hospital public affairs department, opened their files for me allowing me to search for valuable photographs and articles. Malcolm Berman fortunately saved old material which may otherwise have been lost and willingly made everything available. I would also like to thank the many individuals who took time out of their busy schedules to submit to interviews, frequently helping me to clarify important issues or to solve many unanswered questions regarding the hospital's history.

The Sisters of St. Francis of Millvale profoundly influenced the writing of this book. Sister M. Thomaseta Heller answered many of my questions regarding the history of the Order. Thank you, too, to all of the sisters who carefully reviewed this manuscript and offered constructive criticism, resulting in a more readable text. I offer appreciation also to Sister Joanne Bich and Sister M. Sylvia Schuler who supported this project throughout. Sister M. Adele Meiser, my friend, spent many hours recalling and sharing her past experiences in order to make me aware of the sisters' goals and the significance of the St. Francis Hospital to the wider community. Her love for her life's work, her open-mindedness and perpetual belief in the strength of the human spirit were traits which have a positively influenced my life and work. She created the impetus for this work, for this published history was her life-long dream. She lovingly saved valuable written material and kept ongoing notes which proved to be invaluable in the research process. Her enthusiasm for this project was infectious. I will be forever grateful for the experience of having known Sister Adele.

Words simply cannot express how profoundly grateful I am to my adviser and mentor, Peter N. Stearns. He not only offered the project to me, but he has given advice, encouragement and support. His ability to review manuscript material and offer coherent constructive criticism in record time is nothing short of astounding. My understanding of social history and my love of the whole research process has grown under his guidance. The words "thank you," are far from adequate.

In addition to my colleagues and professional associates, friends and family played a key role in the production of this book. My friend, Mary Wolf, not only helped me iron out some grammatical problems, but more importantly, she listened enthusiastically whenever I discussed my work. Ultimately, work such as this would be unimportant without the understanding and support of my family. My husband Don and children, Meredith and Donnie, have always understood how important my work is to me, without questioning why. Their love and inspiration have sustained me throughout this project and all of my endeavors.

Carolyn Carson

Introduction

This book examines the history of one of Pittsburgh's most interesting and varied hospitals, St. Francis. Like any good history, it can be read for several purposes. Many people, attached to St. Francis and its traditions, will look to this book for a careful account of how this particular institution developed and how it has experienced a host of wider changes in the city it serves and in the practice of medicine, while maintaining a recognizable common purpose. Other readers will find in this book a significant contribution to an understanding of what modern hospitals are all about, as they have evolved over more than a century. For the sponsors of this project, though eager for a record of their own institution, have consistently supported a serious, analytical effort to make this study speak to a larger need to gain fuller historical perspective on how hospitals have gained a growing place in American society and how they have changed and adapted in the process.

The importance of hospitals in modern American history is undeniable. From the late nineteenth century onward hospitals have formed one of the most rapidly-growing institutional sectors of American society. They have become, clearly, one of the institutions that touches almost everyone's life, in most cases frequently, intimately and unto death itself. Given their significance, it is surprising that more hospital histories are not available. This book adds a major case study to what is in fact a rather slender shelf.

Several important hospital histories have been generated over the past two decades, seeking to go beyond a simple descriptive account or panegyric to an analysis of some of the major changes over the past century that have brought hospitals to their present place in American life. Attention has focused on the early decades of the modern hospital, with examples from Boston, Philadelphia and a few other cities. Changes in hospital policy, as what had been initially charitable resources for people both poor and sick turned into medical recourses for a wider population, have held pride of place. Several accounts see a growing influence of business criteria supplanting earlier motives of charity as hospitals grew and became more complex in the initial decades of the twentieth century. A second major historical vantagepoint, focused not on individual hospitals but on larger policy dimensions, looks to more recent shifts in hospital administration. The role of the federal government in hospital construction and, with the Great Society programs of the 1960s, in the financing but also the management of medical care for the poor and the elderly necessarily receives attention. So, in a vital study of American medicine by Paul Starr, does the growing replacement of doctors with businessmen in the determination of hospital policy, again in very recent decades.

This historical literature (though generated by sociologists as well as professional historians) has responded to wider trends in the historical discipline, that see serious purpose in the treatment of topics once outside the mainstream. Hospitals and their roles in society both have histories; they both have changed, which means that understanding even their present situations requires a perspective from the past. Currently, hospitals are caught up in political history itself, as medical costs and alternative health proposals become a major factor in political life. But even before hospitals and federal politics intertwined, it is obviously important to know how these institutions responded to changes in the American population, in medical care and technology, and in the nature of the leading diseases. Hospitals connect closely to the range of subjects historians now consider, from the response to new sources of immigration to American cities to definitions of sickness and health. The importance of the subject in modern history is undeniable; what is needed is more serious historical work.

Historians also, as they have widened their historical net, have discovered the necessity of maintaining a tension between generalizations about major trends and developing individual case studies. Over a decade ago, several historians ventured models of modern institutional development that emphasized how new social controls were extended over ordinary people, often amid proclamations filled with humanitarian rhetoric. Thus, it was claimed, doctors and early psychiatrists (called alienists, in the nineteenth century) defined illness and mental disturbance more rigorously, encouraging the placement of more people in hospitals and asylums. These generalizations offered important insights, but a more recent generation of scholars has argued that they were overdrawn and that they failed to note the important differences from one institution to the next, depending on particular goals, administration and context. In portraying a major but distinctive urban hospital amid awareness of larger trends in medicine and hospital administration, this book advances this more subtle, ultimately more realistic kind of social history.

The study of St. Francis Hospital in Pittsburgh offers an important addition to the available literature. It examines the evolution of a major hospital in what was long one of the nation's leading industrial centers. Pittsburgh hospital history extends the urban cases, providing not only a distinctively industrial, heavily immigrant setting but also an example of a city that did not develop a single municipally-supported hospital designed to take on a disproportionate share of those both sick and poor. St. Francis also adds to the literature the case of a major Catholic institution, a clearly understudied sector of hospital history more generally. Available historiography has oddly neglected the role of Catholic sisters in hospital development, focusing instead on lying-in hospitals or major teaching centers. The study of St. Francis helps repair this omission, which strangely ignores the involvement of organized religions in the evolution of health care institutions. It also reveals, as a good case study should, how religious governance and motivations force some changes in the standard model of hospital history, particularly in terms of the ongoing concern for the poor and the tensions this concern created with changes in medical goals, government policies and available resources.

The experience of St. Francis also spans an extended time period, allowing consideration of the turn-of-the-century decades that have been highlighted by other hospital histories, but also the more recent decades singled out in policy research, and previous and intervening periods as well. The hospital records have permitted reasonably extensive and consistent treatment of a number of aspects of hospital evolution over a longer timespan than most historians in this field have been able to embrace. The result, in turn, provides a number of opportunities to determine what the experience of St. Francis contributes to our understanding of how modern hospitals have operated and what impact they have had. It also allows more consideration of continuities, from founding goals to recent implementation, than has been common in this field—a vital aspect for St. Francis, as Carolyn Carson shows, but also a spur to further attention to this historical ingredient in future studies of other institutions.

St. Francis, like any major hospital, has displayed some unique characteristics. This book makes no effort to establish St. Francis as fully typical of any pattern. It is not even a clearly representative Catholic hospital, though its founding and early history resemble those of other Catholic centers. St. Francis was not the favored institution of the Pittsburgh diocese and had from its inception to make a number of significant adjustments and to display interesting kinds of flexibility as a result. Yet the size and range of services St. Francis has offered makes it a significant case in the wider consideration of hospital history. Whether because of its special characteristics or its wider Catholic sponsorship, the historical experience of St. Francis partially differentiates this hospital from others that historians have considered in that the movement away from charitable motivation toward business accountability was less pronounced. This book demonstrates that the sisters' role is responsible for this divergence, and for the opportunities and problems that resulted for the hospital in the twentieth century. Despite important changes over time, St. Francis seems to display more persistence in style and values than historians dealing with other hospitals have found in their bailiwicks. This continuity embraces not only the religious and charitable focus, but also a kind of eclectic entrepreneurship, an eagerness to explore additional forms of service and support, that was built into the hospital's early history and has continued into the later twentieth century.

The alertness of St. Francis' administrators to new needs and opportunities adds to the historical connections this study serves. While functioning as a general hospital with particular attention to immigrant and, more recently, African American populations, the experience of St. Francis also touches on other aspects of the history of health and medicine. The hospital, like many of its Catholic counterparts, developed an early role in nursing training. The history of nursing has its own literature, increasingly rich, which this study has utilized and to which it in turn contributes. While several features of nursing training at St. Francis illustrate trends already established in accounts of nursing, the special focus on community services brings out a distinctive point.

The hospital early developed psychiatric services, and from this base introduced treatments for alcohol and drug addiction. While an unusual feature of general hospitals for many decades, these facets allow the history of St. Francis to add to our understanding of the evolution of mental health treatments—again a field with its own historiography, but benefiting from a chapter derived from general hospital experience. Here too, existing historical work on mental illness and its treatment—in one of the most exciting branches of social history in recent decades—has largely neglected the role played by religious orders, while also downplaying twentieth-century developments in favor of a fascination with nineteenth-century trends. The history of St. Francis Hospital demonstrates the dilemmas inherent in a struggle to maintain a strong mental health facility initially devoted to providing rest and treatment superior to what was available in asylums amid recurrent upheaval in mental health theory, practice and policy. Tensions between the sisters' assessments of patients' unmet needs and their desire to provide what was perceived to be modern mental health care services and to comply with government mandates describe an important part of St. Francis' twentieth-century history.

The St. Francis record also allows consideration of the relationship between hospitals and state, rather than simply federal, policy, another underexplored facet in the juncture of medical and political history. Here, particularly after 1920, historians must take up policy developments from a hospital, as well as a government, point of view, and the St. Francis experience adds to our understanding in this regard.

Historical analysis of voluminous, generously open records of an important urban institution should produce varied fruit, and this study lives up to expectations in this regard. The specifics are clear enough: the book contributes to hospital history, but also to the history of medical training, psychiatry and the treatment of addiction and to the history of government policy. But the study serves other audiences as well. The experience of St. Francis sheds light on the history of Pittsburgh and of urban society generally. And of course it also illumines the history of American Catholicism in practice. Just as Catholic hospitals loom large in the study of American medicine, as this book demonstrates, so the hospital outreach plays a major role in understanding the impact and adaptations of the American Church. Here too, the focus on the varied experience of a single institution provides insights well beyond the expanding confines of the hospital walls.

The story of St. Francis offers a number of dramas and conflicts, of interest to readers devoted to this particular hospital and to those concerned with more general findings alike. Charles Rosenberg, one of the deans of American medical history, has noted that the "decisions that shaped the modern hospital have been consistently guided by the world of medical ideas and values . . . the attitudes and aspirations that gave the profession its peculiar identity." But neither doctors, nor more recently business administrators, have fully ruled St. Francis. The sisters who founded and directed the hospital made concessions to a number of forces, within their hospital and without, even diluting, surprisingly early on, the exclusive effort to woo a Catholic patient population and to maintain a full range of symbols and nomenclature derived from the Church. But they did maintain control, and the analysis of what this meant for a hospital, and how religious control meshed with some of the more familiar facets of hospital history, advances our understanding of this important branch of modern medical and institutional history.

Peter N. Stearns

Healing Body, Mind, and Spirit

Chapter One

Early History

Early History—Lawrenceville

St. Francis Hospital was first established in the Lawrenceville section of the city of Pittsburgh where it remains to this day. In 1724, the section was known as Shannopintown, named for Chief Shannopin of the Delaware Indians. The village was originally on the east side of the Allegheny River, two miles above the Point in the area now between Twenty-seventh and Thirtieth Streets, between Penn Avenue and the river. The first white settler known to have existed in the area was George Croghan. An Indian trader known for his knowledge of Indian life, he was appointed by the British Colonial government as deputy superintendent of Indian affairs. He was invaluable when the Indians threatened to turn to the French. As a result of the 1749 Purchase Treaty in Logstown (Ambridge), Croghan acquired 1,600,000 acres from six Indian nations. Later, at a Fort Stanwix meeting, the chiefs of six nations also deeded 40,000 acres to Croghan including 1,352 acres in what is now Lawrenceville.[1]

Croghan settled in the area and built his first home there in 1762. It was burned by warring Indians on June 16, 1763, but was rebuilt as 'Croghan Hall' and became the center of social, military and political activities. Being suspected of having British sympathies, he was replaced as local Indian agent by the Continental Congress. His fall from favor extended to the Indians, who raided his plantation in 1777. The area at that time became known as Bayardstown and Croghansville.[2]

More white settlers continued to arrive, and by 1790 there were 377 residents who were predominantly Scotch-Irish, English and German. Immi-

[1] Joseph A. Borkowski, "Lawrenceville: An Historical Profile," (Lawrenceville branch of the Carnegie Library: manuscript, 1977), p. 6.
[2] Borkowski.

1

grants continued to populate the area after the completion of the Allegheny Arsenal, which was built in 1814 as a result of the War of 1812. Most of them shared the same ethnic origins as the earlier settlers. William B. Foster, Stephen Foster's father, bought land in the vicinity of the arsenal in 1814 and laid out the town of Lawrenceville. The town was named for Captain James Lawrence who died a hero's death in a naval engagement in Boston harbor during the War of 1812. The borough was incorporated on February 18, 1834, and was annexed by the city of Pittsburgh on June 6, 1868.[3]

After Lawrenceville was first established, additional industries developed and the population grew with the demand for labor. The onset of the Mexican War in 1846 resulted in a need for more employees to work in the artillery manufacturing plants. Skilled laborers, many of them German, were recruited from eastern shores where there was a preponderance of skilled workers. German immigrants were the second largest segment of Pittsburgh's foreign-born population between 1850 and 1870. They comprised between 10 and 15 percent of the residents of both Pittsburgh and Allegheny at that time, and resided primarily in 'Dutchtown' in Allegheny, the lower Strip district and Lawrenceville along the Allegheny River.[4] It is important to note that the Germans of Pittsburgh, although they shared a language and culture, were a very diverse religious group, belonging to several branches of the Lutheran Church and the Roman Catholic Church. By the 1860s, when St. Francis Hospital was first built, it developed in a community dominated by German speaking people. The streets were paved with cobblestones or wooden blocks, as was the case of Penn Avenue, then known as 'the Pike' (Greensburg Pike). The air was filled with dense smoke from the iron and steel mills and the Pennsylvania Railroad Twenty-eighth Street engine yards. This was a thriving community in need of a hospital.[5]

German Immigration and Separatism

In order to comprehend why St. Francis Hospital was organized, it is imperative to understand the attitudes of German Americans as well as sentiments directed toward them. German immigration to the United States had increased markedly after the Civil War because of economic and political in-

[3] Borkowski; "St. Francis Hospital, 1865," manuscript, n.d., St. Francis Hospital Archives.
[4] Nora Faires, "Immigrants and Industry," in *City at the Point, Essays on the Social History of Pittsburgh*, ed. Samuel P. Hays, (Pittsburgh: University of Pittsburgh Press, 1989), p. 7.
[5] Borkowski; "St. Francis Hospital, 1865," manuscript, n.d., St. Francis Hospital Archives.

stability in Europe. In addition, the '*Kulturkampf*' prompted many Catholics to seek homes elsewhere. *Kulturkampf* was the term applied to the struggle between the Roman Catholic Church and the German government chiefly over the latter's efforts to control educational and ecclesiastical appointments. The May Laws of 1873 practically annulled papal jurisdiction over German Catholics by abolishing religious orders and imposing fines on resisting German bishops. German Catholic immigration, therefore, increased. Catholics made up over 35 percent of the total German immigration to the United States after the Civil War; and Germans became the largest Catholic immigrant group arriving in the United States before the Italian immigration. The Germans, in Pittsburgh as well as in other cities, generally settled in the same regions as earlier German immigrants.[6]

Native-born Americans often held the Germans in contempt. During the middle of the nineteenth century, anti-Catholicism as well as nativism flourished in the form of Know-Nothingism. Pittsburgh's Catholic immigrants would have felt this even more strongly; the mayor of Pittsburgh, Joe Barker, was elected as the "People's and Anti-Catholic" candidate in 1850 while jailed for inciting anti-Catholic demonstrations in Market Square. His name did not even appear on the ballot.[7] He served for only one year, but the fact that he was elected at all is indicative of the strong and pervasive anti-Catholic sentiment that prevailed at that time.[8]

Studies have suggested that German Catholics had different political views from their Protestant counterparts. German Protestants, in 1860, identified the Republican party with anti-Catholicism and tended to support Republican candidates, whereas the German Catholics clung to the Democratic party.[9] Because of this pervasive anti-Catholic sentiment, German Catholics did not associate regularly with German Protestants.

Not only were the Roman Catholic Germans victims of nativism and anti-Catholicism, but prejudice toward them from other immigrant groups within their own church resulted in neglect of their spiritual and social needs, and a separation from other Catholic immigrant groups. Evidence seems to suggest that the ethnic background of the local bishop or priest determined

[6]Colman J. Barry O.S.B., *The Catholic Church and German Americans*, (Milwaukee: Bruce Publishing Co., 1953), pp. 5–7.

[7]Linda K. Pritchard, "Religion in Pittsburgh," and Nora Faires, "Immigrants and Industry," in *City at the Point, Essays on the Social History of Pittsburgh*, ed. Samuel P. Hays, (Pittsburgh: University of Pittsburgh Press, 1989), pp. 9, 337; Unpublished manuscript in the Lawrenceville branch of the Carnegie Library, history of Lawrenceville, no date but c. 1965–1980, no author.

[8]Stefan Lorant, *Pittsburgh, The Story of an American City*, (Lenox, Mass.: Authors Edition, Inc., revised edition 1975), p. 120.

[9]Nora Faires, "Immigrants and Industry," in *City at the Point, Essays on the Social History of Pittsburgh*, ed. Samuel P. Hays, (Pittsburgh: University of Pittsburgh Press, 1989), p. 8.

which immigrant group received the most attention. They generally assisted those with whom they shared ethnicity. Mother Theresa of the Poor School Sisters of Notre Dame noted in the 1840s that entire German families were growing up and dying without ever being baptized or instructed in their religion. English-speaking institutions received assistance in abundance, but the poor Germans were left unattended. "The German priests receive no support for their churches, schools, and parishes. Anything German is an object of contempt to the British, and is suppressed, even by the Bishops."[10]

The issue of favoritism shown by the bishop for one ethnic group over another was evident in Pittsburgh prior to the Civil War. The Redemptorist Father John Neumann welcomed the Bavarian order, the Poor School Sisters of Notre Dame, to Pittsburgh in 1847 and took great interest in their affairs. But Bishop O'Connor saw them in a less than favorable light. Mother Theresa wrote to Father Siegert in Munich, "Germans are not liked here. It is openly stated that German schools should close, so that the Germans can be assimilated into the English-speaking nation, and become one with her. The superior here ... spoke emphatically against this when he discussed with the Most Reverend Bishop the establishment of a branch house of our order here at Pittsburgh. The latter did not even state whether he would permit us to be here. He is afraid of jealousy and disharmony on the part of the sisters he requested from Ireland. Since he himself is Irish, these sisters are his favorites and darlings. He has entrusted the hospital, the orphanage and the English-speaking schools to them."[11] Mother Theresa was referring to Bishop O'Connor and his relationship to the Sisters of Mercy. They had strong ties with the bishop because of their shared ethnicity and were commonly known as "the bishop's nuns."[12] Bishop O'Connor referred to his German constituents as "those people," who "do not wish to adapt to the customs of the nations to which they have come."[13] Obviously, even though immigrants may have had religion in common, different language and customs did not allow for any kind of cooperative efforts in the establishment of Catholic

[10] *The North American Foundations: Letters of Mother M. Theresa Garhardinger, School Sister of Notre Dame,* (Winona, Minn.: St. Mary's College, 1977), quoted in Mary Ewens, OP, "Removing the Veil: The Liberated American Nun," in *Women of Spirit,* eds. Rosemary Ruether and Eleanor McLaughlin, (New York: Simon and Schuster, 1970), p. 263.

[11] *The North American Foundations: Letters of Mother M. Theresa Garhardinger, School Sister of Notre Dame* (Winona, Minn.: St. Mary's College, 1977), quoted in Mary Ewens, OP, "Removing the Veil: The Liberated American Nun," in *Women of Spirit,* eds. Rosemary Ruether and Eleanor McLaughlin, (New York: Simon and Schuster, 1970), p. 263.

[12] Patricia Mary Tarbox, "The Origins of Nursing by the Sisters of Mercy in the United States, 1843–1910," (Ed.D. dissertation, Columbia University Teachers College, 1986), p. 107.

[13] Linda K. Pritchard, "Religion in Pittsburgh," in *City at the Point, Essays on the Social History of Pittsburgh,* ed. Samuel P. Hays, (Pittsburgh: University of Pittsburgh Press, 1989), p. 335.

institutions, and so a kind of separatism prevailed in Pittsburgh, which was strengthened by the attitudes of Catholic clergy.

Given the sentiment of the Catholic Church hierarchy in Pittsburgh, it is not surprising that, from the outset after their arrival, the German immigrants, as well as religious leaders, insisted that separate churches be established for them. They wanted churches of their own in which traditional religious observances and customs would be carried out, and where their mother tongue was spoken. German spiritual leaders in the United States were supportive of the immigrants' desires because they had witnessed immigrants turning to non-Catholic churches, especially Lutheran, where they felt more at home with their own language. Priests were often sent to areas specifically to serve the growing immigrant Catholic population.

The Redemptorist priests, who played a prominent role in the development of St. Francis Hospital, first arrived in the United States in 1832 to work with the German immigrants. The church felt that the German immigrants were in danger of losing their Catholic faith because there was no one to instruct them in their own language.[14] The Rev. Joseph Prost founded the Redemptorist congregation in Pittsburgh in 1839. The Bishop gave them the responsibility of caring for the German parishioners of the city. Father Prost united various sectional elements and prepared to build St. Philomena's Church, which was dedicated by Bishop O'Connor in 1846.[15] The Catholic Church addressed the issue of Catholic immigrants in the United States by providing priests for them, and by supporting their desires for separate churches, which helped them preserve their culture and language in a foreign country. The editors of the German American press, liberals and influential German societies sharing church leaders' views, all led a concerted campaign to preserve the German language and culture in the New World.[16]

This separatism, based on ethnicity, was common. In Philadelphia, for example, intradenominational squabbles began as early as 1788. Germans organized a separate congregation, establishing a trend towards separatism which continued as more Germans arrived in the United States. Two separate hospitals were established in that city, one for the Irish and one for the Germans. Clergy throughout the United States encouraged this separatism

[14] Mary Ewens OP, "Removing the Veil: The Liberated American Nun," in *Women of Spirit* eds. Rosemary Ruether and Eleanor McLaughlin, (New York: Simon and Schuster, 1970), pp. 262; *The Redemptorists in Pittsburgh, Pa.*, *One Hundred Years*, Jubilee souvenir booklet, 1939, p. 12.

[15] Catholic Historical Society of Western Pennsylvania, *Catholic Pittsburgh's First One Hundred Years 1843–1943*, (Chicago: Loyola University Press, 1943), p. 124.

[16] Colman J. Barry O.S.B., *The Catholic Church and German Americans*, (Milwaukee: Bruce Publishing Co., 1953), pp. 9–11.

as the best means of keeping Germans firm in their faith. It is not surprising that separatism would be extended to other institutions such as hospitals.[17]

Early History—Origins of the Franciscan Sisters

The establishment of the Franciscan Order in Pittsburgh, and the resultant development of a hospital, serves as a striking example of Catholic hospital growth in the United States. Many orders in the United States were established as a result of the local bishops' desire to serve the rapidly growing Catholic immigrant population. Priests and bishops were well aware of the unmet educational and health needs. Clergy commonly solicited help from religious orders, sometimes from their own country of origin, and sometimes from other orders already established in the United States. They sought assistance from religious orders which would be compatible with the specific ethnic group of immediate concern to the bishop.[18] Numerous examples support this. Bishop Henni invited the Sisters of Charity to the diocese of Milwaukee in the 1840s, to establish schools and a hospital.[19] In 1847, the Redemptorist priests (German) requested the Poor School Sisters of Notre Dame to come to America to teach.[20] Many bishops solicited help from sisters primarily to educate parishioners, but sisters were frequently called upon by the community to aid in caring for the sick.[21] Bishop Lefevre obtained the Daughters of Charity to assist him in caring for the needs of the poor in Detroit.[22] In the 1840s Bishop O'Connor of the Pittsburgh diocese specifically asked for the Sisters of Mercy to come to Pittsburgh from Ireland to assist him in meeting the needs of the diocese's poor.[23] Subsequently, the Right Rev. William Quarter invited some of the sisters from Pittsburgh to help him meet educational

---

[17]Gail Farr Casterline, "St. Joseph's and St. Mary's: The Origins of Catholic Hospitals in Philadelphia," *Pennsylvania Magazine of History and Biography* (July 1984): 305.

[18]Patricia Mary Tarbox, "The Origins of Nursing by the Sisters of Mercy in the United States, 1843–1910," (Ed.D. dissertation, Columbia University Teachers College, 1986), p. 246.

[19]Timothy Walch, "Catholic Social Institutions and Urban Development: The View from Nineteenth Century Chicago and Milwaukee," *Catholic Historical Review* 64 (January 1978): 16–32.

[20]Mary Ewens, OP, "Removing the Veil: The Liberated American Nun," in *Women of Spirit* eds. Rosemary Ruether and Eleanor McLaughlin, (New York: Simon and Schuster, 1970), pp. 262.

[21]Judith Cetina, "In Times of Immigration," in *Pioneer Healers: The History of Women Religious in American Health Care*, eds. Ursula Stepsis, CSA, and Dolores Liptak, RSM, (New York: Crossroad Publishing Co., 1989), p. 90.

[22]Edward G. Martin, M.D., *Early Detroit: St. Mary's Hospital 1845–1945*, (Detroit: Baring Press, Inc., 1945), p. 42.

[23]Patricia Mary Tarbox, "The Origins of Nursing by the Sisters of Mercy in the United States, 1843–1910," (Ed.D. dissertation, Columbia University Teachers College, 1986), p. 113.

and health needs in Chicago.[24] The clergy's solicitation of help from religious orders was not true only of the Roman Catholic faith, although it may have been more prevalent. William Passavant, an ordained Lutheran pastor, invited Lutheran deaconesses from Kaiserwerth in the Austro-Hungarian empire to come to Pittsburgh to help staff the Pittsburgh Infirmary, which he established in 1849.[25] Similarly, the Sisters of St. Francis of Millvale were established as a result of priests' and bishops' desires to assist the German Catholics.[26]

The history of the Sisters of St. Francis of Millvale began in 1854 when the first German speaking bishop to govern an eastern diocese, John N. Neumann (who had earlier worked in Pittsburgh), the fourth Bishop of Philadelphia, needed sisters to care for the sick poor. He had initially planned to establish a community of Dominicans, but Pope Pius IX directed the bishop to form a community of Franciscans instead.[27]

The first American Franciscans had been born in Europe. Anna Marie Boll was born in Bavaria, and married Anthony Bachmann in 1846 at the age of twenty-two. In 1847, they emigrated to Philadelphia, and in the following year her younger sister, Barbara Boll, and widowed mother also emigrated to the United States. Anthony was injured in the quarry where he worked and was taken to St. Joseph's Hospital, which served primarily the Irish. Only 1 percent of the patients admitted there that year were German born.[28] He subsequently died on September 14, 1851, leaving Anna Marie pregnant and with three children. Barbara and her mother came to live with Anna Marie, and in 1854, Anna Dorn, a friend of the Boll sisters, arrived from Germany. After Mrs. Boll's death, at the suggestion of the Rev. John B. Hespelein, pastor of St. Peter's (German Catholic) Church, the three younger women shared their home with poor, single, immigrant girls who had no homes of their own. Father Hespelein, under Bishop Neumann's guidance, organized the Sisters of

[24]Joy Clough, RSM, *In Service to Chicago: The History of Mercy Hospital*, (Chicago: Mercy Hospital and Medical Center, 1979), p. 9; There are numerous other examples of this. See also: Sister Mary Carol Conroy, "The Historical Development of the Health Care Ministry of the Sisters of Charity of Leavenworth," (Ph.D. dissertation, Kansas State University, 1984).

[25]Carlan Kraman, OSF, "Women Religious in Health Care: The Early Years," in *Pioneer Healers: The History of Women Religious in American Health Care*, eds. Ursula Stepsis, CSA, and Dolores Liptak, RSM, (New York: Crossroad Publishing Co., 1989), p. 36.

[26]For additional discussion of the roles of the bishops, see Edward C. Atwater, "Women, Surgeons, and a Worthy Enterprise: The General Hospital Comes to Upper New York State," in *The American General Hospital, Communities and Social Contexts*, eds. Diana Elizabeth Long and Janet Golden, (Ithaca: Cornell University Press, 1989), p. 49.

[27]*100 Years of Franciscan Spirit, 1866–1966*, (Seniors of 1966, Mt. Alvernia H.S., 1966) Motherhouse Archives.

[28]Gail Farr Casterline, "St. Joseph's and St. Mary's: The Origins of Catholic Hospitals in Philadelphia," *Pennsylvania Magazine of History and Biography* 108 (July 1984): 304.

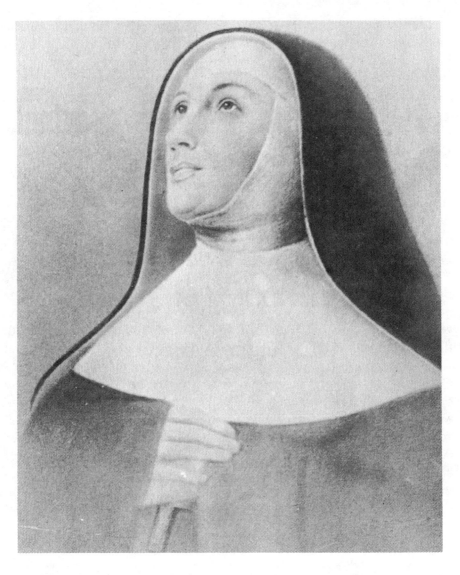

Reverand Mother Mary Francis Bachmann

the Third Order of St. Francis. On April 9, 1855, the three women were given new names and were received into the Third Order of St. Francis by Bishop John Neumann at St. Peter's Church in Philadelphia. They pronounced their vows on May 26, 1856. Anna Marie Bachmann worked closely with the priests to build the order into a multipurpose social agency for German newcomers.[29]

Mrs. Bachmann's children were cared for by relatives until they were old enough to devote their lives to the Roman Catholic faith, following in their mother's footsteps. Johanna subsequently joined her mother. Anna Marie's youngest children, Aloysius and Cunigunda, were cared for by Anna Marie's aunt, Mrs. Bielefeld. In later years, Cunigunda became a member in her mother's community, and Aloysius became a secular priest serving the Buffalo diocese as pastor of St. Francis of Assisi Church in Tonawanda, New York. Anna Marie's other son, Frederick, died in the Civil War on January 16, 1864.[30]

This new congregation of sisters was the first American Franciscan community. There were other Franciscans in the United States, but they had emigrated from European communities.[31] Bishop Neumann established the order for the express purpose of being attentive to the needs of the German sick poor, orphans and the elderly in the Philadelphia diocese. The order supported themselves by sewing, but most of their time was taken up by responding to calls from the community for help in caring for the sick in their homes.[32]

Word of their work with the sick poor in Philadelphia became known, and in 1860, Rev. Robert Kleineidam C.S.S.R., rector of St. Mary's Church in Buffalo, requested sisters to establish a similar community. Anna Marie, who became Mother M. Francis, sent Sister Mary Margaret (Barbara Boll), Sister M. Elizabeth and Sister M. Bonaventure along with her own daughter, Johanna Bachmann (who became Sister Mary Robertine), a postulant, to the Buffalo mission, where Sister M. Margaret became superior. A year later,

---

[29]*High Road to Happiness*, (Millvale: Sisters of St. Francis of the Immaculate Virgin Mary Mother of God, Mt. Alvernia, c. 1950); Gail Farr Casterline, "St. Joseph's and St. Mary's: The Origins of Catholic Hospitals in Philadelphia," *Pennsylvania Magazine of History and Biography* (July 1984): 305, 307; *75th Anniversary of Sisters of St. Francis in Buffalo Diocese, 1861–1936*, St. Francis Hospital Archives.

[30]*100 Years of Franciscan Spirit*, pp. 11, 22; *75th Anniversary of Sisters of St. Francis in Buffalo Diocese, 1861–1936*, St. Francis Hospital Archives.

[31]"Foundation of the Sisters of the Third Order of St. Francis of the Immaculate Virgin Mary Mother of God, Mt. Alvernia," Motherhouse Archives.

[32]Carlan Kraman, OSF, "Women Religious in Health Care: The Early Years," and Judith Cetina, "In Times of Immigration,"in *Pioneer Healers: The History of Women Religious in American Health Care*, eds. Ursula Stepsis, CSA, and Dolores Liptak, RSM, (New York: Crossroad Publishing Co., 1989), pp. 36, 93.

they were joined by Sister M. Johanna Boll, Sister M. Magdalen Hess and five postulants. In 1863, due to a misunderstanding after Mother M. Francis's death, the Buffalo community separated from Philadelphia.[33]

The First Hospital—1865

As noted earlier, immigrants of the Roman Catholic faith strove to maintain their own cultural identity. Religion did not unite the immigrants who differed markedly in customs as well as language. The Germans' desire to maintain their cultural identity, along with the animosity they felt from the local hierarchy, may explain why St. Francis Hospital was established in Pittsburgh; there was already another Catholic hospital (Mercy) in the city, and a private general hospital nearby (West Penn). There was a German hospital in the city, but it was Protestant (Pittsburgh Infirmary, later the Passavant Hospital). German Catholics and Protestants were divided politically, partially due to a pervasive anti-Catholic sentiment; but in addition, American Protestant institutions may not have met the spiritual needs of Roman Catholic immigrants. Catholics, for example, were afraid they would not receive last rites if they were not in a Catholic institution.[34] Although such sentiments were more prevalent during the antebellum period, many believed that Protestant facilities attempted to proselytize the immigrant poor, inculcating Protestant-American values in the hope of separating the immigrant from his traditional religious beliefs. The underlying purposes that motivated the acts of charity of deaconesses and sisters differed considerably. Protestant deaconesses, generally, were much more proselytizing than the Roman Catholic sisters, who simply desired to alleviate suffering of the sick and bring them spiritual consolation. The Protestants often had religious conversion as their primary goal, believing that the basic needs of food, work and family had to be met if spiritual change was to follow. Middle-class Protestants looked to deaconesses as agents of social control.

Roman Catholic clergy recognized the necessity of developing their own network of institutions and social programs to meet the needs of their im-

[33] 100 Years of Franciscan Spirit, pp. 11, 22; 75th Anniversary of Sisters of St. Francis in Buffalo Diocese, 1861–1936, St. Francis Hospital Archives; Judith Cetina, "In Times of Immigration," in Pioneer Healers: The History of 'Women Religious in American Health Care, eds. Ursula Stepsis, CSA, and Dolores Liptak, RSM, (New York: Crossroad Publishing Co., 1989), p. 93.

[34] Paul Starr, The Social Transformation of American Medicine: The Rise of a Sovereign Profession and the Making of a Vast Industry, (New York: Basic Books, Inc., 1982), pp. 173–175.

migrant parishioners.[35] Similar to separate ethnic churches, hospitals were often founded to serve Catholics of a particular ethnic background. A desire for an institution that would meet their spiritual needs encouraged religious leaders to establish their own Catholic hospitals; interestingly, culture was important, too.

The Sisters of St. Francis of Buffalo conducted a home for the aged on Pine Street, known as the St. Francis Asylum.[36] In November 1865, Mother Margaret Boll sent Sisters M. Elizabeth Kaufmann and M. Magdalen Hess to Pittsburgh by train to solicit funds for their home, which was in financial difficulty at that time.[37] The Civil War had just ended, and Pittsburgh was thriving as the emerging steel capital of the world. Because they were German speaking, the sisters went to St. Philomena's Church on Fourteenth Street, where they met Fathers Anwanderer and Tschenhens, Redemptorist priests.[38]

The priests were deeply concerned about the German-speaking Catholics of Pittsburgh, and were responsible for establishing several institutions for the benefit of German Catholics of the diocese. In 1850, they established St. Joseph's Orphan Asylum in Troy Hill; and in 1854, they founded a thrice-weekly German newspaper, the *Pittsburger Repudikaner*. They also opened a German High School in 1863. It was not surprising that they were interested in the development of a new hospital as well.[39]

As noted earlier, bishops and priests often solicited the help of sisters with whom they shared ethnicity. Father Tschenhens, who had known Bishop Neumann when he was a pastor at St. Philomena's in the 1840s, proposed to the sisters from Buffalo that they begin a hospital in Pittsburgh to serve the German Catholics.[40] One historical account states that the two sisters, with Father Tschenhens' help, set up a small temporary hospital before consulting with either the bishop of Pittsburgh or the superiors in Buffalo. When Mother

[35]Judith Cetina, "In Times of Immigration," in *Pioneer Healers: The History of 'Women Religious in American Health Care*, eds. Ursula Stepsis, CSA, and Dolores Liptak, RSM, (New York: Crossroad Publishing Co., 1989), pp. 89, 113.

[36]Letter to Sister M. Adele from Sister Mary Dolores Cook, OSF, Buffalo Diocese, October 9, 1990.

[37]Sister M. Thomasita Heller, "Sisters of St. Francis, Pittsburgh Foundation," Article in manuscript, n.d. Motherhouse Archives; Sister M. Clarissa Popp, *History of the Sisters of St. Francis of the Diocese of Pittsburgh, 1868–1938*, (Millvale: Sisters of St. Francis, 1939), p. 9.

[38]"Foundation of the Sisters of the Third Order of St. Francis of the Immaculate Virgin Mary Mother of God, Mt. Alvernia," Motherhouse Archives.

[39]St. Francis Day Address, April 11, 1953, W. S. McEllroy, M.D.

[40]"From Frame House to Multi-facilities," article in manuscript, n.d., Motherhouse Archives; Judith Cetina, "In Times of Immigration," in *Pioneer Healers: The History of 'Women Religious in American Health Care*, eds. Ursula Stepsis, CSA, and Dolores Liptak, RSM, (New York: Crossroad Publishing Co., 1989), p. 93; *Catholic Historical Society of Western Pennsylvania, Catholic Pittsburgh's First One Hundred Years 1843–1943*, (Chicago: Loyola University Press, 1943), p. 30.

Margaret, Mother Superior of the sisters of Buffalo, heard of the project she called the sisters home.[41]

The members of the "German Catholic St. Franciscus Beneficial Society of Pittsburgh" assisted the priests in their endeavor to establish a hospital. Dr. Philip Weisenberger, one of the society's leaders, wanted to build a hospital because "there was a great need for such an institution for the German people."[42] Benevolent societies among immigrant groups were common. As early as 1840, German Catholic immigrants found expression for their charity through benevolent societies, which had been a part of German tradition for centuries.[43] Benevolent societies frequently assisted in fund raising or in purchasing memberships in the hospital for their members. They bought property for hospitals or assisted in the management of institutions. For example, the Brotherhood of St. Joseph, composed chiefly of members of the congregation of St. Paul's Church, was established to direct fund raising and the initial business operation of Mercy Hospital.[44]

Dr. Weisenberger became an American citizen in 1843, and in the subsequent twenty years he was engaged in contracting and building. He was responsible for the building of St. Joseph's Orphan Asylum in Troy Hill, six churches, one of which was St. Philomena's Catholic Church on Fourteenth Street (1846), and over one hundred houses. His first large contract was for the construction of the main building of St. Vincent's Abbey in Latrobe in 1845. In 1862, Weisenberger purchased a large oil refinery at Twenty-third Street, which he operated until 1878. He lost all of his savings supposedly because he placed too much confidence in others, and retired from the oil business in 1880. As a physician, he had an office on Pearl Street in Bloomfield. It is not clear when he became a physician, or what his training was, but he was noted "for his skill and success in treating patients." He died in 1915 at the age of ninety-nine.[45]

[41] Sister M. Aurelia Arenth, OSF, *As A Living Oak*, *Biography of Mother Baptista Etzel* (Pittsburgh: Sisters of the Third Order of St. Francis, 1956), pp. 47–48.

[42] St. Francis Day Address, April 11, 1953, W.S. McEllroy, M.D.; Popp, p. 121.

[43] John O'Grady, Ph.D., LL.D., *Catholic Charities in the United States: History and Problems*, (Washington D.C.: National conference of Catholic Charities, 1930), p. 333.

[44] Sister M. Jerome McHale, RSM, *On the Wing: The Story of the Pittsburgh Sisters of Mercy, 1843–1968*, (New York: Seabury Press, 1980), p. 57; Patricia Mary Tarbox, "The Origins of Nursing by the Sisters of Mercy in the United States, 1843–1910," (Ed.D. dissertation, Columbia University Teachers College, 1986) p. 118; see also Charles E. Rosenberg, *The Care of Strangers: The Rise of America's Hospital System*, (New York: Basic Books, Inc., 1987), p. 112; Gail Farr Casterline, "St. Joseph's and St. Mary's: The Origins of Catholic Hospitals in Philadelphia," *Pennsylvania Magazine of History and Biography*, (July 1984): 298.

[45] "Dr. Philip Weisenberger, Vigorous at 94 Years," article in manuscript, c. 1910, St. Francis Hospital Archives; "Foundation of the Sisters of the Third Order of St. Francis of the Immaculate Virgin Mary Mother of God, Mt. Alvernia," Motherhouse Archives.

The priests, Dr. Weisenberger, other society members, and influential men in the city encouraged the sisters to seek permission to return to Pittsburgh to set up, or continue with, the hospital. Dr. Weisenberger even traveled to Buffalo to meet with Mother Margaret and Bishop Timon. Within three weeks the two sisters returned with Sister Stephen Winkelman. They established their fifteen bed hospital in a small frame house, previously owned by a Mr. Engol. The hospital was located on a street known as "the alley," which ran parallel to Butler and Penn Avenues, extending from Thirty-sixth to Thirty-ninth Streets; it was later renamed Bank Street and then Bandera Street. The sisters cared for German patients who had been sent to them by pastors of the German parishes. The following year, after the sisters had moved, that first hospital became a tenement, housing a number of families until it was torn down in later years.[46]

It was not long before a larger facility was obviously necessary. Weisenberger approached the Episcopal Residence and requested the Bishop to establish a hospital. Bishop Right Reverend Michael Domenec, D.D., did not have the financial resources to do so, but agreed that Weisenberger could take the work upon himself. Mercy Hospital was already part of the diocese and the Bishop felt the diocese could not afford to operate two hospitals. On May 22, 1866, for $25,000.00, Dr. Weisenberger purchased a plot of six acres and thirty-three perches on Forty-fourth Street, with a dwelling to accommodate thirty beds. The deed was made in his name and the contract required five payments of $5,000.00 each. A small chapel was built, and the hospital was dedicated on Thanksgiving Day, November 26, 1866.[47]

From its inception, the day-to-day administration of the hospital was under the direction of one of the sisters assigned as superintendent, although the Mother Superior also actively participated in decision making. Sister Elizabeth Kaufmann, Sister M. Euphrosine Koehler, Sister M. Magdalen Hess, Sister M. Paschala Kiefer and Sister M. Angela Endres functioned as superintendents of the hospital during the first twelve years. Sister M. Seraphine Farrell, the first administrator in the position for more than three years, was in charge from 1877 to 1892, when Sister M. Francis Hensler succeeded her for

[46]Sister M. Thomasita Heller, "Sisters of St. Francis, Pittsburgh Foundation," Article in manuscript; n.d., Motherhouse Archives; "St. Francis Hospital," article in manuscript, c. 1940, St. Francis Hospital Archives; "Foundation of the Sisters of the Third Order of St. Francis of the Immaculate Virgin Mary Mother of God, Mt. Alvernia," Motherhouse Archives; Popp p. 9.

[47]Sister M. Thomasita Heller, "Sisters of St. Francis, Pittsburgh Foundation," article in manuscript, n.d., Motherhouse Archives; "St. Francis Hospital," article in Manuscript, c. 1940, St. Francis Hospital Archives; "Foundation of the Sisters of the Third Order of St. Francis of the Immaculate Virgin Mary Mother of God, Mt. Alvernia," Motherhouse Archives; Popp p. 9.

one year. Sister Seraphine was reassigned to the position again the following year until 1904.[48]

Although the sisters managed the daily routine within the facility, they were assisted by physicians and priests as well. Because hospital care primarily meant nursing care, doctors were not in regular attendance at first. When the sisters needed a physician, they merely called on one of the doctors in the neighborhood.[49] By April of 1867, however, Dr. G. T. Jacobi was the hospital's regular physician, although he was not paid.[50] In meeting the patients' spiritual needs, the sisters were assisted by the first hospital chaplains, priests from St. Augustine's Church, organized in 1860. Reverend Philip Schmidt, and later the Reverend John T. Tomchina, sent assistants regularly to perform religious services and to minister to the sick. By 1874, however, St. Augustine's parish passed to the Capuchin fathers who then held the chaplaincy at the hospital.[51]

Household management and nursing was to be "done only and solely by the ordained sisters of the Third Order of St. Franciscus taken from the Motherhouse at Buffalo." The sisters' responsibilities were varied. They not only nursed patients, but they also scrubbed floors, prepared meals and raised funds. Every morning, two sisters went forth begging for the necessities for the day. They would go to the butcher, for example, and beg for leftover bones from which they would make soup for themselves and their patients. People of the community objected and suggested that the sisters charge patients. The sisters, however, were "determined to follow the ideals of St. Francis" and refused to change their policy. The community pleaded with the Bishop to intervene. He advised the sisters to formulate a system of rates. Before the hospital was chartered in 1868, they began to charge three dollars per patient per week.[52] Historian Charles Rosenberg suggests that a great majority of the early Catholic hospitals did charge their patients, although the rates were low, allowing the working class to avoid the stigma of receiving charity.[53] It is not clear if the residents of Lawrenceville objected to the sisters begging or if

---

[48]*Seventy-fifth Anniversary 1901–1976,* (Pittsburgh: St. Francis General Hospital School of Nursing, 1976,) p. 7.

[49]"For All of Us," building campaign brochure, 1927.

[50]Second Annual Report of St. Francis Hospital in Pittsburg, 4/23/67–3/14/68, translated from article which appeared in "Freiheits Freund," 3/26/68, a secular German newspaper, manuscript, n.d., in St. Francis Hospital Archives.

[51]Charter, 1868, Article XI, Sections 5 and 6; Popp, p. 136.

[52]St. Francis Day Address, April 11, 1953, W. S. McEllroy, M.D.; "From Frame House to Multi-Facilities," manuscript, n.d., in Motherhouse Archives, Millvale; Charter, 1868, Article XI, Sections 5 and 6; Popp, p. 136.

[53]Charles E. Rosenberg, *The Care of Strangers: The Rise of America's Hospital System,* (New York: Basic Books, Inc., 1987), p. 111.

they preferred that the hospital charge its patients in order that the patients could maintain some sense of dignity.

It was not unusual for sisters to go forth into the community to beg for money in order to support themselves and their charitable works, although bishops, apparently, did not condone the activity. At the Third Plenary Council of Baltimore in 1884, bishops took note of the growing importance of begging as a way of solving financial needs of religious communities. They warned that in some parts of the country it had become an "intolerable abuse that needed to be checked with an iron hand."[54]

The early hospital, under the management of a board of directors, clearly suffered from financial difficulties. Dr. Philip Weisenberger was president and The Rev. John Michael Bierl, pastor of Saints Peter and Paul Church, East Liberty, was the secretary. Although the second annual report showed a clear profit of $4,667.23, that was misleading. The only way the hospital was able to remain open was by taking out three short term loans of $4,400.00 each. One was due in forty days, the second in thirty days and the third in twenty-one days. In addition, Sister Elizabeth loaned $400.00. Almost 50 percent of the hospital's receipts came from contributions through collections. The German parishes contributed $9,005.21 for the care of their parishioners, and $2,029.10 was donated to the sisters. A picnic in July netted $1,273.48, dues collected added up to $547.10 and patient billing supplied $1,810.60 of income. Unfortunately, however, $10,190.00 came from the sale of property, probably the Thirty-seventh Street site, and that would not have been an annual source of income. Three societies, in addition to the German Beneficial Society, paid a flat sum for the care of members. The Pittsburgher Society, Lawrenceville Society and the Birmingham Society contributed a total of $466.67.[55]

In spite of the difficulties, the hospital remained financially solvent because labor and medical supply costs were minimal. The hospital paid $1,846.83 for the maintenance of the sisters' living quarters and their salaries ($200.00 annually per sister). Household expenses alone ($3,735.73), which included $65.00 for the purchase of a new cow and $6.25 for shoeing a horse, were more than double the fees for the sisters' maintenance. The cost for medicine suggests, not surprisingly, that the cost of medical care was minimal ($521.82). Hospital care primarily meant nursing care.[56]

During the second year of operation, the hospital cared for 201 patients.

[54]Mary Ewens, OP, "The Role of the Nun in Nineteenth Century America: Variation on the International Theme," (Ph.D. dissertation, University of Minnesota, 1971), p. 253.

[55]Second Annual Report of St. Francis Hospital in Pittsburg, 4/23/67–3/14/68.

[56]Second Annual Report of St. Francis Hospital in Pittsburg, 4/23/67–3/14/68.

One hundred sixty-five of those were discharged cured, twelve patients died and twenty-four patients remained hospitalized. Eighty patients paid and 121 were charity patients. That number is misleading, however, because it includes all of the patients that were supported by the German parishes or other German societies. A donation from a parish or society assured free care for their members. In October of 1867, the hospital began to issue pass-books, which entitled patients who were otherwise not cared for by a parish or a society to receive free hospitalization. The fee charged was "a mere trifle," and most of the holders were non-Catholics. There were some real charity patients cared for, however, and the board was appropriately grateful and thanked the sisters publicly for caring for the sick and poor. The hospital even paid $65.00 for a patient's funeral, and paid for three coffins for other patients.[57]

In the hospital's first two years, despite its Catholic commitment, it served patients regardless of their religious affiliation. However, what is more evident was that it specifically served the German people. The Franciscans were a German order and spoke the language of that ethnic group. Several of the sisters, in fact, had been born in Germany. The hospital was advertised in the local German newspaper, which also ran articles requesting support from the community for the institution. The hospital "extends its blessings to all suffering regardless of creed, is a benefactor to every community and as such desires the support of every man, no matter to what religious denomination he belongs." This newspaper, although written in the German language was a secular paper which largely ignored religion.[58]

On June 20, 1868, an application for a charter was made to the state in the name of the German Catholic St. Franciscus Beneficial Society of Pittsburgh. After a comprehensive inspection, the Commonwealth of Pennsylvania granted the charter on July 20, 1868, and congratulated the board, administration, doctors and nurses.[59] The purpose of the society was "for purpose of raising funds to be used in supporting poor German people and sick and helpless persons generally."[60] The name of the hospital was "The German Franciscus Hospital."[61]

Membership in the German Catholic St. Franciscus Beneficial Society of Pittsburgh was open to any male sixteen years or older. He was to pay one dollar upon admission to the society, and then ten cents or more per

---

[57]Second Annual Report of St. Francis Hospital in Pittsburg, 4/23/67–3/14/68.

[58]Second Annual Report of St. Francis Hospital in Pittsburg, 4/23/67–3/14/68; *100 Years of Franciscan Spirit*.

[59]Sister M. Adele Meiser, "History of St. Francis Medical Center," paper given at Lawrenceville Historical Meeting, June 1985; Popp, p. 119.

[60]St. Francis Day Address, April 11, 1953, W. S. McEllroy, M.D., excerpt from application.

[61]Charter, 1868, Article IX.

month. Only those who contributed their $1.20 annually were eligible to vote. Members were dropped if they failed to pay for six months. Women were admitted as honorary members only; "they shall choose from their own number, special collectors, who shall collect their monthly contributions and transmit the same to the Treasurer of the Society."[62]

A Board of Managers was chosen to govern the society. Twenty-four members were chosen by and from the membership. Every year, twelve of those would retire and twelve new managers would be elected. Retiring members could be reelected. A president, vice president, secretary and treasurer were chosen from the membership. Managers were required to contribute $12.00 annually, and anyone contributing $1,000.00 became a life board member. Standing committees of three members each were appointed by the president. The building committee was responsible for ordering necessary repairs, and the committee on Wills and Testaments had the duty of seeing that the wills of hospital patients "were drawn up in legal form and in all litigations to defend the interests of the Society." A finance committee was selected to raise funds for support of the hospital by subscriptions and collections. In addition, the Board of Managers annually appointed a committee to inspect the hospital.[63]

Branch societies were established in various German Catholic communities and congregations in Allegheny County. Whenever a church or organization supported a branch society, they had the benefit of hospital accommodations for their sick and destitute. No Catholic community or congregation that did not aid the Beneficial Society by establishing branch societies or by paying regular contributions received such a benefit.[64]

Admission to the hospital was controlled by the Committee on Admissions. "All destitute persons soliciting reception and entertainment in said hospital, must report themselves to the Committee on Admissions and the said committee, after having made the necessary inquiry relative to the worthiness of the applicant, shall give due notice to them as to whether they will be received or not within three days after their application shall have been made." No one was admitted into the hospital without producing a certificate issued by the committee and signed by the president.[65] Rules were established whereby disobedient, offensive or discourteous patients could be expelled from the hospital. The charter explicitly stated also that the poor or sick "suffering with diseases past cure or recovery and are bereft of all support will be received and treated as other persons free of charge." Those who

[62]Charter, 1868, Articles III and VII.
[63]Charter, 1868, Articles IV and V.
[64]Charter, 1868, Article X, Sections 1 and 2.
[65]Charter, 1868, Article IX, Sections 2 and 3.

could, paid five dollars per week for room, board, nursing and medical attention.[66]

In spite of the fact that a committee had to approve an application for
admission, it appears that the hospital did not discriminate based on gender,
age, diagnosis, socioeconomic class or religion. This exemplifies how Catholic
hospitals' admission policies differed from those of other private hospitals
of the period. Private hospitals strove to distinguish between sickness and
dependency. They generally refused to accept contagious or incurable cases
as free patients. Patients with venereal disease or alcoholism were also usually
admitted on a pay basis only. Private hospital boards were unwilling to provide
care to the unworthy who they viewed would be better served at the local alms
house. The worthy patient was the hard working individual who was doing
his/her best to live respectably, "whose dwellings, though humble, are neat and
orderly; who have a laudable desire to rise out of their present condition."[67]
Catholic and ethnic hospitals, conversely, accepted patients with chronic or
contagious illnesses such as tuberculosis. They regularly found beds for the
aged. Although patients were required to seek permission for admission from
the committee on admissions who inquired regarding their 'worthiness,' it
seems apparent from the language in other portions of the charter that the
definition of 'worthiness' is not what historians have so frequently suggested.
Implicit in the charter is the belief that all were accepted unless their day-to-
day behavior was deemed to be unacceptable. The St. Francis Hospital records
indicate that no distinction was made between the worthy and unworthy poor,
except in cases where the board wanted to carefully determine if a patient
was unable to pay.[68]

Although the sisters had managed the hospital since it first opened, they
did not own it. Dr. Weisenberger, who had been instrumental in the founding
of the institution, never intended to retain ownership of the facility or the
property. After buying the Forty-fourth Street property in 1866, he subsequently succeeded in interesting others in the hospital and paid off his debt.
In April 1867, Dr. Weisenberger offered the deed to the hospital to Bishop
Domenec as a gift to the diocese. The Bishop felt that at that time the diocese
could not undertake the supervision of the work at the hospital, and suggested
that the deed be turned over to the sisters. On January 21, 1869, an agreement
was drawn whereby Philip Weissenberger, Gabriel Weisser, Andrew Koman,

---

[66]Charter, 1868, Article XI, Sections 1–3.
[67]Charles E. Rosenberg, "And Heal the Sick: The Hospital and the Patient in 19th Century America,"
Journal of Social History 10 (Summer 1977): 430–431.
[68]Charles E. Rosenberg, *The Care of Strangers: The Rise of American's Hospital System* (New York: Basic
Books, 1987) p. 113; Interview with Sister Adele, 1993.

Joseph Meyer, John Kleinhenz, survivors of the deceased Francis Felix and Trustees of the German Catholic St. Franciscus Beneficial Society of Pittsburgh sold the hospital and property to Sister Elizabeth Kaufman for one dollar. The indenture contained several conditions by which Sister Elizabeth was bound. The said property was intended "for the uses and purposes of a Hospital for the accommodation of German and persons of German origin and for no other uses and purposes whatsoever ... " In addition, Sister Elizabeth was "subject to such rules and regulations and management as shall or may from time to time be imposed, laid down or prescribed for the government thereof by the Right Rev. Michael Dominec, Roman Catholic Bishop of Pittsburgh." The property was not to be disposed of without the approval and consent of the Bishop. If the sister violated any of these conditions, then the Bishop was to gain control of the property.[69]

The property did not remain in the sisters' possession, however. Sister Elizabeth Kaufman sold the property to the Bishop on November 7, 1871. She granted and conveyed said lot to Right Reverend Michael Domenec, Bishop of Pittsburgh.[70] It is quite likely that the sisters were unable to manage financially and sought the assistance of the bishop.[71] The property was subsequently held by Bishops John Twigg and Richard Phelan, who succeeded Bishop Domenec. More than two decades passed before the sisters again held title to the hospital and property. Bishop Richard Phelan sold the property to the Sisters of the Third Order of St. Francis on April 6, 1895, again for one dollar.[72] On December 1, 1908, the Right Reverend J. F. Regis Canevin again granted the title to the property to the sisters because of some doubt regarding the earlier transaction.[73] There were no stipulations or conditions attached to these last transactions. The bishops clearly intended for the sisters to maintain complete interest in, and control over, the hospital and property.

On September 9, 1871, a new, much larger facility was opened and dedicated by the Right Reverend Bishop Domenec. The three-story brick building, measuring 120 by 52 feet with a wing extending from the center for a chapel, sat on top of the hill in Lawrenceville overlooking the city. At the time,

---

[69] Deed book Volume 242, p. 110.

[70] Recorder's Office, Deed book, Vol. 282, p. 33.

[71] Sister M. Thomasita Heller, "Sisters of St. Francis, Pittsburgh Foundation," article in manuscript, n.d., Motherhouse Archives; "St. Francis Hospital," article in Manuscript, c. 1940, St. Francis Hospital Archives; "Foundation of the Sisters of the Third Order of St. Francis of the Immaculate Virgin Mary Mother of God, Mt. Alvernia," Motherhouse Archives; Popp, p. 118; "Dr. Philip Weisenberger, Vigorous at 94 Years;" Sister M. Aurelia Arenth, OSF, *As A Living Oak, Biography of Mother Baptista Etzel,* (Milwaukee: Bruce Press, 1956), p. 50.

[72] Deed book, Vol. 900, p. 328.

[73] Record of litigation between Constitutional Defense League and St. Francis Hospital, May 1932, Plaintiff's exhibit #4, p. 113a.

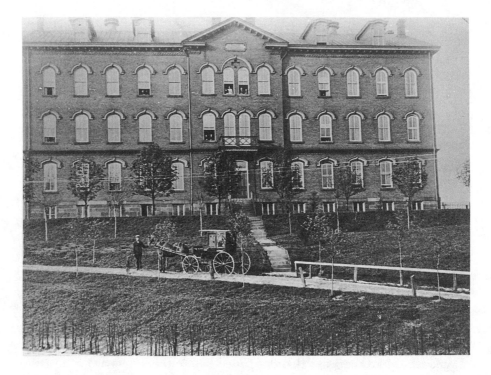

The New Hospital, 1871

the location was considered to be ideal because the area was free from at peren-
nial cloud of smoke that covered the city. It was "very healthfully situated"
on high ground in the outskirts of the city. Its situation gave "every assurance
for highest sanitary influences, as its elevated position, commanding a broad
sweep of comparatively unoccupied country, allows more air and sunshine
than a city hospital can usually enjoy."[74] The pleasant porches allowed the
patients to exercise without weariness; and the surrounding gardens also provided quiet space for walks. In addition, there was a constant supply of fresh
vegetables.[75] The building itself, however, had one serious flaw. There was
only one central staircase and no fire escape. The Board of Commissioners of
Public Charities viewed this "as a most serious omission, and in the event of
a fire occurring would be likely to cause terrible consequences. It can not be

[74] *Annual Report of the Board of Commissioners of Public Charities of the Commonwealth of Pennsylvania*
for 1886, pp. lxxix, clxxxv.
[75] *Annual Report of the Board of Commissioners of Public Charities of the Commonwealth of Pennsylvania*
for 1887, p. cxcviii.

too soon provided."[76] The hospital continued for a number of years without remedying the situation. The first floor housed private rooms, a reception room and the dispensary. Wards and private rooms for women were on the second floor with similar facilities for men on the third floor. The hospital, with a capacity for one hundred beds, was placed under the patronage of St. Francis. The old frame building was reserved for patients with contagious diseases. The cost of the new facility was $49,209.57. At least $11,000.00 for the construction of the institution had been raised the previous winter during a fair, and additional funds had been raised by Catholic churches.[77]

In 1872, the first gratuitous professional staff was appointed. Dr. Jacobi, a friend of Dr. Weisenberger, was the first attending physician, as previously noted. The new members of the staff were Dr. John Perchman, president of the medical staff, Dr. P. Perchman, Dr. J. M. Stevenson and Dr. John Ahl.[78] Ten years later, Dr. Stevenson became president of the Allegheny County Medical Society, evidence that he was one of the community's leading physicians.[79] Curiously, the Anglican names of the physicians may denote a partial decline in the ethnic characteristics of the hospital at this early date, although, to be sure, it can only be suggestive.

During the 1870s the sisters worked relentlessly administering to the sick of the community, establishing a trend which has lasted until the present day. A smallpox epidemic prevailed in Pittsburgh from 1866 to 1872. The out-buildings on the grounds were used to isolate victims of the disease. The mortality rate of the two hundred smallpox patients was comparatively low. Interestingly, only one of the sisters, a candidate, Miss Bridget Byrns, died of the disease.[80]

Industry, its related accidents and labor unrest, also increased the patient census. During the hospital's first years, there was a stone quarry somewhere between Fifth and Forbes Avenues. Two men were injured and brought into the hospital personally by Dr. Weisenberger.[81] Hospital lore suggests that

---

[76] *Annual Report of the Board of Commissioners of Public Charities of the Commonwealth of Pennsylvania* for 1886, p. lxxix.

[77] Popp, p. 120; "St. Francis Hospital," c. 1940, in St. Francis Hospital Archives; *Annual Report of the Board of Commissioners of Public Charities of the Commonwealth of Pennsylvania, Second Report of the Committee on Lunacy for 1884*, pp. 151a–152a; *Annual Report of the Board of Commissioners of Public Charities of the Commonwealth of Pennsylvania for 1889*, pp. 68, 163.

[78] *Report of the St. Francis Hospital, 1911*, p. 4.

[79] Theodore Diller, *Pioneer Medicine in Western Pennsylvania*, (New York: Paul B. Hoeber Inc., 1927), p. 194.

[80] *Report of the St. Francis Hospital, 1911*, p. 3.

[81] Sister M. Adele Meiser, "History of St. Francis Medical Center," paper given at Lawrenceville Historical Meeting, June 1985.

this may have been the first incident of St. Francis Hospital's long history of involvement with industrial medicine. On August 3, 1877, a devastating accident which occurred at the Lucy furnace of the Carnegie Steel Works resulted in the deaths of four men. A Mr. Davidson offered the use of his sand wagon to transport the injured men to the hospital. Three men spent two months at St. Francis Hospital, where the sisters nursed them and treated their burns. There was a young man who lived in the area who was studying for the priesthood but had developed serious doubts about the commitment. His pastor advised him to visit the victims of the Lucy furnace accident. The work that he did with those men convinced him that the clerical state was the correct choice for him.[82]

The summer of 1877 was obviously a busy one for the community as well as the hospital. The railroad strike affected Pittsburgh adversely when angry and excited mobs burned, pillaged and robbed the city, destroying three million dollars worth of property. The state militia was called in to suppress the rioting. One of those men was a man named Jones who was taken to St. Francis Hospital when he was wounded. He was so affected by the care he received there that he asked to be baptized into the Catholic faith. Years later, when he returned to visit, he continued to credit the sisters with restoring him to life not only physically, but spiritually as well. Twenty-seven people were killed on July twenty-first and twenty-second, and many more who were wounded were taken to St. Francis Hospital.[83]

The tremendous growth of industry is one of the factors which led to the development of hospitals in general. The arrival of immigrants, attracted by industry's need for a labor force, resulted in large numbers of indigent and dependent individuals without family networks in their new country to care for them if they became injured or ill. Secondly, the expansion in manufacturing resulted in an increase in work-related injuries.[84] St. Francis Hospital, located in a working class community near a number of industrial sites, began its role in caring for victims of industrial accidents very early.

The hospital was plagued with monetary problems during the seventies and eighties. Interestingly, toward the end of the seventies, 49 percent of the receipts came from patients with the remainder coming from donations, in spite of the fact that by 1878, there had been 2,000 patients admitted to the hospital. Of those, 1,215 had been unable to pay for their care. Apparently,

---

[82]"St. Francis Hospital," c. 1940, manuscript, St. Francis Hospital Archives; St. Francis Day Address, April 11, 1953, W. S. McEllroy, M.D.

[83]"St. Francis Hospital," manuscript, c. 1940, p. 7, St. Francis Hospital Archives.

[84]This has been widely studied by historians, but for a brief discussion see David Rosner, *A Once Charitable Enterprise: Hospitals and Health Care in Brooklyn and New York, 1885–1915*, (Princeton: Princeton University Press, 1982), p. 27.

most of the patients paid something, but it was frequently less than the actual cost of maintenance. Catholic hospitals, unlike non-denominational institutions, have a long history of supporting themselves primarily with income from patients. It is not clear if congregations and benevolent societies continued to pay flat sums for their members' care. It seems possible that those methods of payment, including the pass books, may no longer have been utilized by that time, as there is no reference to them.[85] The hospital sisters continued to assist in raising funds, but had abandoned their earlier practice of begging. In addition to their duties in the hospital, the sisters gave private lessons and contributed the proceeds for the support of the hospital.[86] The sisters, board of management and physicians also appealed "to the citizens, that they pay a visit to the institution and see for themselves the benevolent service rendered." Presumably, this appeal was made to solicit donations. The appeal was made to the German speaking people; it appeared on the first page of the Saturday edition of the German language daily newspaper, *Der Freiheitsfreund*.[87]

By the mid-1880s, financial difficulties continued in spite of the efforts of the board and sisters to raise funds. A restriction in the Pennsylvania Constitution denied aid to all sectarian hospitals.[88] The corporation, however, applied for state aid in 1886, but their requests were denied. They asked for $23,500.00 to cover indebtedness and $30,000.00 for building purposes. Since most of the patients paid for at least part of their care, the Board of Commissioners of Public Charities for the State refused to grant aid. The State Board of Public Charities did approve Mercy Hospital's request for $30,000.00 even though the sisters, in order to receive state aid, appointed a non-sectarian board, the majority of whom were Catholics and who had "no real control over the hospital.[89]

Adding to the hospital's monetary difficulties was the fact that, during the mid-eighties, the hospital was rarely filled to capacity, unlike Mercy, a similar Catholic institution, and West Penn, located roughly within the same neighborhood. In 1882, for example, only 75 of the hospital's 100 beds were

[85] Annual report of St. Francis Hospital, 1878, taken from *Der Freiheitsfreund*, Saturday, 8 February 1879.

[86] *Second Report of the Committee on Lunacy of the Board of Public Charities of the Commonwealth of Pennsylvania for 1884*, pp. 151a–152a; *Annual Report of the Board of Commissioners of Public Charities of the Commonwealth of Pennsylvania for 1886*, p. lxxix.

[87] Annual report of St. Francis Hospital, 1878, taken from *Der Freiheitsfreund*, Saturday, 8 February 1879, p. 1.

[88] Gail Farr Casterline, "St. Joseph's and St. Mary's: The Origins of Catholic Hospitals in Philadelphia," *Pennsylvania Magazine of History and Biography* (July 1984): 292.

[89] *Annual Report of the Board of Commissioners of Public Charities of the Commonwealth of Pennsylvania for 1886*, p. ccx.

occupied when the Board of Commissioners of Public Charities visited.[90] All of Mercy's 63 beds were occupied and all of West Penn's 106 beds were filled; in addition, there were 50 additional patients on cots in the corridors. For the next few years, the situation remained similar. In 1883, St. Francis increased its bed capacity to 130, but the average daily number occupied was only 100 beds. Again, all of Mercy's 60 beds were occupied and West Penn continued to fill their beds with an average of 50 patients on cots in corridors.[91]

It is difficult to explain why the St. Francis Hospital was having difficulty filling their beds, but several plausible explanations can be ventured. A simple reason may be the fact that the interior was considered unattractive. In 1889, the sisters were advised to remove carpet from the floors and, if possible, to brighten the appearance of the inside. "It had a gloomy and depressing look."[92] In addition, the wards were considered to be too warm because the ventilation was inadequate.[93] It is very doubtful that these reasons alone discouraged patients from seeking help there. Population shifts and ethnic alterations in the community may offer other explanations.

St. Francis Hospital was founded to serve German Catholics, and as the community demographics were altered due to changes in immigration patterns, the sick of the community may have been reluctant to enter a German institution. As the 1878 annual report indicates, the hospital readily accommodated all religions and nationalities, but the German born were still the largest group served. During the year 1878, 222 patients were treated. There were more Protestants (101–24 Lutherans, 23 Methodists, 21 Presbyterians, 14 Baptists, 19 Episcopalians) than Catholics (85) treated at the hospital. Thirty-six patients had no church affiliation. The hospital served primarily an immigrant population and German born patients (64) were more common than members of other ethnic groups, but interestingly, they exceeded those born in Ireland by only two. Fifty-four patients were born in the United States, twenty-nine in England, six in Poland, five in France and

---

[90]The Board of Public Charities was established April 24, 1869, and had the power to supervise "all charitable, reformatory or correctional institutions within the state. Presumably, hospitals were visited on a regular basis and statistics compiled. *Annual Report of the Board of Commissioners of Public Charities of the Commonwealth of Pennsylvania for 1882*, pp. x–xi.

[91] *Annual Reports of the Board of Commissioners of Public Charities of the Commonwealth of Pennsylvania* for the years 1882, 1883, 1884, 1887, p. cxcviii.

[92] *Annual Report of the Board of Commissioners of Public Charities of the Commonwealth of Pennsylvania for 1889*, p. 68.

[93] *Annual Report of the Board of Commissioners of Public Charities of the Commonwealth of Pennsylvania for 1889*, p. 163.

two in Italy. Still, in 1880, the hospital was "commonly regarded as a German hospital.[94]

During its first thirty years the hospital survived with little city-wide publicity, unlike other area hospitals of similar size. There was no reference made to St. Francis Hospital in the city's Catholic newspaper, *The Pittsburgh Catholic*, either when it first opened, or when a new wing or building was dedicated. Nor did the hospital administration solicit funds there. Mercy Hospital, however, was mentioned frequently to advertise its services or request funds. St. Francis Hospital, however, was widely publicized in the local German periodical, *Der Freiheitsfreund*. Interestingly, the same scenario was evident in Philadelphia, where German relief projects centered in the parishes were seldom mentioned in the Catholic press. When the Franciscan sisters opened a hospital there in 1860 for the German Catholic community, no mention was made of it in the *Catholic Herald*.[95] Pittsburgh's St. Francis Hospital was first noted in the city directory in 1884, and the advertisement at that time only gave the address and stated that it was "under the direction of the Sisters of St. Francis."[96] In contrast, the West Penn hospital had a full page advertisement in the directory. Allegheny General Hospital and Mercy Hospital also had extensive ads listing admission policies, visiting hours and doctor's privileges. In 1892, the description of St. Francis Hospital expanded to include a list of physicians on staff and to mention that the hospital had two departments, the medical/surgical department and the department for the treatment of the insane.[97] As their financial resources were consistently and severely limited, the sisters were motivated to solicit patients of other ethnic groups in order to augment their meager revenue.

The sisters were, in fact, making adjustments in response to changing community demographics. Although the community surrounding St. Francis Hospital had largely been comprised of German residents, that began to change after 1880, when southern and eastern Europeans began to immigrate to the United States. Between 1880 and 1900, the population of the city of Pittsburgh nearly doubled. By 1900, the recent arrivals, comprised primarily of Italians and Poles, made up nearly one third of the city's foreign born population. The Polish families displaced many of the older German residents,

[94]Rt. Rev. Msgr. A. A. Lambing, *A History of the Catholic Church in the Diocese of Pittsburgh and Allegheny*, (New York: Benziger Brothers, 1880), p. 496; Annual report of St. Francis Hospital, 1878, taken from *Der Freiheitsfreund*, Saturday, 8 February 1879.

[95]Gail Farr Casterline, "St. Joseph's and St. Mary's: The Origins of Catholic Hospitals in Philadelphia," *Pennsylvania Magazine of History and Biography* (July 1984): 305, 308.

[96]City Directory, 1884, 1892.

[97]City Directory, 1897, p. 98.

and settled in the Strip district along the Allegheny River and Lawrenceville. The Italians settled largely in the Bloomfield area, adjacent to Lawrenceville, and nearby East Liberty.[98]

In 1886, when the St. Franciscus Hospital applied for a certificate of Incorporation, the word "German" was dropped from the institution's name, although the German form of Francis remained. Established as a hospital for the Germans, this suggests that, perhaps, there was an attempt to minimize that distinction. Management reorganization occurred when the hospital was incorporated. A corporation, which was to exist perpetually, was formed "to establish and maintain a hospital in the city of Pittsburgh." The twenty-one corporate members, members of varying religious denominations, intended to maintain the hospital by voluntary contributions which had no capital stock and no subscribers. The corporation chose eleven directors, and said corporation had the power to exclude, expel or suspend any of its directors as provided in the by-laws. The involvement of the German Beneficial Society was no longer evident. They may have relinquished responsibilities when they sold the property to Sister Elizabeth Kaufman in 1869.[99] This new corporation leased the hospital and property from the Order of St. Francis for ten years, during which time it was to be controlled by the corporation. At the end of the lease it was to revert back to the order.[100] In 1900, the sisters again agreed to lease the hospital to the corporation. The hospital was to pay a total of $34,000.00, payable in quarterly installments of $2,000.00 beginning on January 1, 1901, for the next four years.[101]

Early Psychiatric Facilities

St. Francis Hospital's psychiatric facility began in order to fulfill the sisters' needs. Sister Mary Magdalen Hess was born in Wurtemberg, Germany in

---

[98]Nora Faires, "Immigrants and Industry," in City at the Point, Essays on the Social History of Pittsburgh, ed. Samuel P. Hays, (Pittsburgh: University of Pittsburgh Press, 1989), p. 11; John Bodnar, Roger Simon and Michael Weber, Lives of Their Own: Blacks, Italians, and Poles in Pittsburgh, 1900–1960, (Urbana: University of Illinois Press, 1982), pp. 20, 24.

[99]Charter and Certificate of Incorporation of St. Francis Hospital of Pittsburgh, recorded December 13, 1886, Charter Book, vol. 10, p. 43, Court of Common Pleas, No. 2 of Allegheny County, No. 188, January Term, 1887.

[100]Annual Report of the Board of Commissioners of Public Charities of the Commonwealth of Pennsylvania for 1886, p. lxxix.

[101]Record of litigation between the Constitutional Defense League and the St. Francis Hospital, May 1921, Defendant's Exhibit #1, p. 118a.

1837, and in 1861, she helped to found the house in Buffalo. In 1865, she was one of the sisters who came to Pittsburgh to solicit funds for their home for the elderly. She remained in Pittsburgh, but in 1871, she asked and obtained permission to return to Philadelphia. She stayed there for three months and when she returned she "begged to be again admitted to the ranks." Her petition was granted and she was appointed superior to the hospital. She remained in that position until she had what the records refer to as a nervous breakdown in 1875. The sisters sent her to St. Joseph's Retreat in Detroit. Sister Magdalen returned to Pittsburgh in 1880 because the sisters could no longer afford to keep her in the private asylum. She became the first psychiatric patient at St. Francis. The sisters took care of her until her death on March 4, 1884.[102] In that same year, the hospital applied to the state for a license to care for insane females.[103] The Lunacy Law passed on May 8, 1883, gave the Board of Public Charities the power to supervise all houses or places in which any person of unsound mind was detained whenever the occupant of the house or person having charge of a lunatic received any compensation for custody, control, or attendance other than as an attendant or nurse. The Board also supervised all houses or places in which more than one person was detained with or without compensation paid for custody and attendance. The law required the board to appoint a committee of five to serve as the Committee on Lunacy and was to include one physician and one attorney.[104]

The frame building which had been the hospital until the new facility was built in 1871 was used for patients with contagious diseases until 1884, when it became the psychiatric department of the hospital. The psychiatric facility sat on six acres along with the main hospital. Two acres were cultivated for garden purposes, and half of the vegetables used in the hospital were raised there. The one story cottage, which was licensed for sixteen female lunatics, had four rooms, two measuring fifteen by twenty feet, one measuring twelve by ten feet and the last measuring six by eight feet. The ceilings were eleven feet high. There were three water closets, one on the main floor and one each in the attic and basement. The building was heated by a hot air furnace and drainage was provided by a ten inch pipe which drained into the city sewer. Although the building did not have lightning conductors and was not fire-proof, means of egress were ample. Doors all through the house connected

[102] "From Frame House to Multi-facilities;" manuscript, n.d., Motherhouse Archives, Millvale; "Necrology," Volume I, Motherhouse Archives, Millvale.
[103] Popp, p. 122.
[104] *Annual Report of the Board of Commissioners of Public Charities of the Commonwealth of Pennsylvania for 1883*, p. viii.

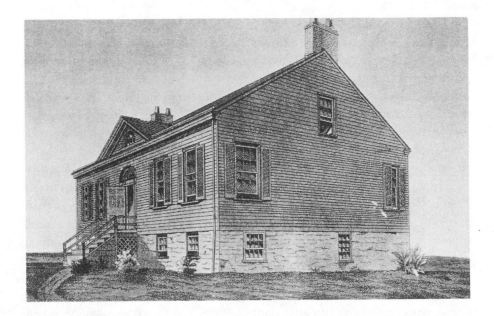

The Insane Department

each room with the passage-way. All doors opened outward and there were three exits.[105]

The Committee on Lunacy gave the hospital a favorable report, describing the apartments as "scrupulously clean, and the patients well-cared for." The beds were made of straw and the pillows of feathers or straw. All beds had sheets which were changed weekly. There were no bath-tubs available, but patients were given "towel baths" every week. Clothing was provided for the patients as well, and was adapted to the season of the year. In winter, the patients had woolen underwear, for example. Patients had Sunday as well as weekday suits, and underwear was changed weekly.[106]

The patients were cared for by two sisters who lived on the premises. Dr. Samuel Ayres was one of the first medical attendants who visited the patients twice every week to care for their mental and physical disorders. He was followed by Drs. David A. Hengst and George W. McNeil who alternated every six months, visiting the patients every other day, also without compensation.[107] Patients were kept fairly busy if possible. They walked all

[105] *Second Annual Report of the Committee on Lunacy of the Board of Public Charities of the Commonwealth of Pennsylvania for 1884*, pp. 151a–152a.

[106] Lunacy Report, 1884, pp. 151a–152a.

[107] *Annual Report of the Board of Commissioners of Public Charities of the Commonwealth of Pennsylvania for 1887*, p. 71.

over the grounds with the sisters for one and a half hours every day. Four of the patients were usefully employed at sewing and house work, reflecting the current trends in psychiatric care, which were based on the belief that inaction and monotony were harmful, and working was therapeutic.[108] Inmates were allowed to wander about the various rooms of their small hospital, and at meal time they all sat down at one table. Each "individual case received all the necessary attention and careful treatment." The hospital "seemed brighter than many of the same class elsewhere."[109] "Their cheerful and contended disposition, the cleanliness of the apartments, the care and attention which the patients receive are unmistakable evidences of the devotion, and conscientious discharge of duty on the part of Mother Superior and the sisters under her charge towards these sadly afflicted beings, and of their high qualifications for the important position to which they have been called."[110] Patients could attend religious services on Sunday, and occasionally clergymen would visit the patients.[111]

All of the patients were quiet, with mild mental illnesses. Others requested admission, but accommodations were limited so they were refused. Of the fifteen patients present on September 30, 1884, nine were natives and six were foreigners. All were private patients. Only one was restrained and none was in seclusion. Two patients had to be fed with a spoon. These types of descriptions of the patients continued in the reports of the Committee on Lunacy for the next decade. The average weekly cost of maintenance was three to five dollars per person.[112]

By the end of the decade, the sisters saw a need for a new psychiatric facility. The Committee on Lunacy, as early as 1886, recommended construction of a large building which provided all the modern appliances. They felt that an "institution of this character is greatly needed in this section of the state, and we believe it would be an important convenience to families of wealth, who have relatives afflicted mentally, requiring hospital care and treatment." It was the only private hospital for the insane in the western part of the state.[113] The Committee on Lunacy, which previously had commended the sisters for the cheery atmosphere, was referring to

[108]Gerald N. Grob, *Mental Illness and American Society 1875–1940*, (Princeton: Princeton University Press, 1983), p. 23.

[109]*Annual Report of the Board of Commissioners of Public Charities of the Commonwealth of Pennsylvania for 1886.*

[110]*Sixth Report of the State Committee on Lunacy of Commonwealth of Pennsylvania for 1888*, p. 100.

[111]Lunacy Report, 1884, pp. 151a–152a.

[112]*Annual Report of the Board of Commissioners of Public Charities of the Commonwealth of Pennsylvania for 1886*, p. clxxxv; Lunacy Report, 1884, pp. 151a–152a.

[113]*Third Annual Report of the Committee on Lunacy of the Board of Public Charities of the State of Pennsylvania for 1886*, p. 44.

"the dreary rooms of the little building containing the insane patients" by 1889.[114]

In 1890, plans were submitted and approved by the State Committee of Lunacy for a new psychiatric building designed to accommodate one hundred women and fifty men.[115] Men were not accepted as patients in the psychiatric department until the new facility was built. The 120 by 52 foot brick and iron fire proof building, which cost $78,000.00 to build,[116] was located to the left of the general hospital, and joined by bridges of iron and glass. There were two main inner stairways of iron and stone which lead down from the wards at either end. An ample fire escape of inclines, slopes and landings communicated with each ward as well. There were porches on two sides of the building, and, like the fire escapes, they were enclosed in iron wire netting. Baths and retiring rooms were built outside of the wards. A large tank in the mansard roof supplied water. On the lower floor there were separate facilities for the care and treatment of inebriates. The Committee on Lunacy forbade the use of the third floor by patients. In the summer of 1891, the insane patients were transferred into the new facility.[117]

The new building provided additional comforts and diversions for the psychiatric patients. Some of the patients were employed. Men worked on the grounds while women patients worked in the dining room, on the ward, or were engaged in fancy work and sewing. The new hospital provided a library complete with novels, periodicals and assorted journals. Amusements included vocal and instrumental music, card playing, indoor games, dancing, listening to the phonograph and outdoor exercise.[118]

The Hospital in the 1890s

In 1891, the general hospital area, built twenty years earlier, was remodeled. Modern baths and toilets provided "more complete sanitary arrangements." The hospital's first two interns, graduates of West Penn Medical College, Drs. A. K. Lyon and L. W. Wilson, who entered the hospital in April, solicited

[114]*Annual Report of the Board of Commissioners of Public Charities of the Commonwealth of Pennsylvania for 1889*, p. 163.

[115]Popp, p. 123.

[116]"St. Francis Hospital," manuscript, c. 1940, St. Francis Hospital Archives.

[117]*29th Annual Report of the Board of Commissioners of Public Charities of the Commonwealth of Pennsylvania*, the report of the Committee on Lunacy for year ending 9/30/98, pp. 107–108.

[118]*29th Annual Report of the Board of Commissioners of Public Charities of the Commonwealth of Pennsylvania*, the report of the Committee on Lunacy for year ending 9/30/98.

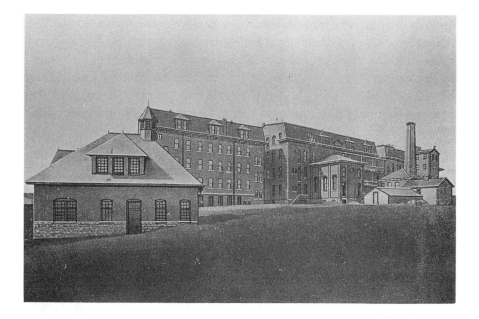

St. Francis Hospital, 1900, from the back

donations from their friends. As a result, the hospital had their first ambulance and horses, and an operating room that was equipped with "all that could be desired at the time to insure efficiency in service."[119]

In 1896, the hospital added another seventy-eight by thirty-five-foot three-story wing for the cost of $42,359.62, and the entire hospital was renovated.[120] A fourth story was added to the general hospital building. Baths and showers were added, steam heating was installed and the bed capacity had increased to 225. A dispensary, physicians' consultation room, reception room and chapel were placed on the first floor. The hospital was modernized according to the standards of the time.[121]

The hospital continued to have financial difficulties. At that time, in Pittsburgh, there existed a Saturday and Sunday Hospital Fund. Donors contributed money, which was to be shared by hospitals in Pittsburgh and Allegheny. Apparently, St. Francis received none of those funds, though the staff was under the impression that funds collected were to be distributed evenly to the hospitals in the two cities. The hospital survived largely because of revenue generated from the insane patients whose care was paid for

[119]"St. Francis Hospital," manuscript, c. 1940, St. Francis Hospital Archives, p. 8.
[120]"St. Francis Hospital," manuscript, c. 1940, St. Francis Hospital Archives.
[121]"St. Francis Hospital," manuscript, c. 1940, St. Francis Hospital Archives, p. 9.

primarily by family and friends. The insane patients were private non-indigent patients.[122] Not only did charitable organizations ignore St. Francis Hospital, but the state neglected to provide aid until 1899. In 1898, for example, Mercy Hospital, which had approximately the same number of beds, received $10,000.00 in state aid.[123] In addition, the bishop of the diocese, the Most Reverend Richard Phelan, favored Mercy Hospital by giving it $1,000.00 in 1894, and again in 1899; he gave nothing to St. Francis Hospital.[124] The St. Francis Board of Directors, with the aid of 'influential friends,' however, finally succeeded in obtaining a yearly appropriation of $8,000.00 from the state.[125]

At that time, the hospital was still having difficulty filling its beds, but some sources suggest that the problem had been remedied somewhat. In 1898, it had 225 beds, but the average daily number occupied was 135, a 60 percent occupancy rate. Signs of improvement were noted by 1900, when the average daily number of beds occupied increased to 173, reflecting an 87 percent occupancy rate. Interestingly, Mercy's rate was 88 percent that year, but West Penn's occupancy rate had begun to decline in the late nineties. In 1898, West Penn's occupancy rate had fallen to 59 percent and by 1900, it had only risen to 69 percent.[126] Other records suggest, however, that as early as 1897, St. Francis Hospital was showing signs of improvement in its occupancy rates. The building was described as crowded. In the fall of that year, the Board of Directors elected ten additional physicians and surgeons to assist the regular medical staff in the work of the institution, "which has become so heavy of late that assistance was needed." The staff at that time included: Consulting surgeon, Dr. Hamilton; Consulting physicians, Drs. McKelvey and Miller; Surgeons (two and a half months each), Drs. Johnson, Clark, Cartwright, Espy, Stillwagen; Insane department, Drs. Stamb, Hersman, McKennan, Diller; Assistants, Irish and Moore; Assistant surgeons, Drs. Tufts, Shields; Assistant physician, Dr. Hopkins; Pathologists, Drs. Matson, Shillito; Oculist, Dr. Edsal; Nose and Throat, Dr. E. Day; Consulting gynecologist, Dr. X. O. Werder.[127]

By the turn of the century, St. Francis, like other Catholic hospitals, was filling its beds and outstripping some of the local general hospitals. Histo-

[122] "The Hospital Fund," *The Clipper*, 21 May 1897; *Annual Report of the Board of Commissioners of Public Charities of the Commonwealth of Pennsylvania* for 1885, 1887, 1888, 1889, 1890, 1891, 1892, 1898.

[123] *Annual Report of the Board of Commissioners of Public Charities of the Commonwealth of Pennsylvania for 1898*, p. 333.

[124] *Pillar of Pittsburgh: The History of Mercy Hospital and the City It Serves*, (Pittsburgh: Mercy Hospital, c. 1990), pp. 60–61.

[125] "St. Francis Hospital," manuscript, c. 1940, St. Francis Hospital Archives, p. 9.

[126] *Report of the St. Francis Hospital*, 1911, p. 5.; *Annual Report of the Board of Commissioners of Public Charities of the Commonwealth of Pennsylvania for 1898 and 1900*.

[127] "New Medical Staff," *The Clipper*, 24 September 1897.

rian Charles E. Rosenberg has suggested that religious and ethnic hospitals were more successful in attracting elusive paying patients of modest means because they seemed less impersonal and alien to patients than the general hospitals.[128] They had an atmosphere of care and concern for patients that was sometimes less obvious in secular institutions.[129] The sisters were known for providing tender loving care. In an era where increasing numbers of people were entering hospitals for care, the reputation of Catholic hospitals may have been attractive. Secondly, this was a period of immigration of largely Catholic Italians and Poles, who comprised a large part of the industrial work force. Industrial accidents were frequent, and this may explain why the Catholic hospitals filled their beds more readily than the local general hospital of similar size.

By the turn of the century, the hospital had been renovated and had a larger staff to accommodate the ever increasing numbers of patients. The outlook for the new hospital as the twentieth century began was a positive one.

The Growth and Development of the Order

As the hospital had grown, so too had the Order. It is interesting to note that the Sisters of St. Francis labored in Pittsburgh for two years before they were formally accepted by Bishop Domenec. They had to prove themselves worthy of the faith and confidence of their friends and loyal supporters. On May 6, 1868, Bishop Michael Domenec issued the following authorization: "I do hereby authorize the foundation of the Franciscan Sisters in the Diocese of Pittsburgh, and I do hereby grant them the privileges which their community enjoys wherever it has been canonically established, and I will protect and encourage them in the performance of their works according to the Rule of their Institute."[130]

The sisters became more and more involved in the wider Pittsburgh community. In 1868, Father Frederick Lang, C. P., petitioned Bishop Michael Domenec for permission to obtain sisters from Buffalo for St. Michael's school on the South Side. In May, eleven sisters arrived and taught at St. Michael's,

[128]Charles E. Rosenberg, *The Care of Strangers: The Rise of America's Hospital System*, (New York: Basic Books, Inc. 1987), p. 240.

[129]Edward C. Atwater, "Women, Surgeons, and a Worthy Enterprise: The General Hospital Comes to Upper New York State," in *The American General Hospital, Communities and Social Contexts*, eds. Diana Elizabeth Long and Janet Golden, (Ithaca: Cornell University Press, 1989), p. 49.

[130]Popp, p. 13.

St. John's and St. Malachy's. The convent, on Pius Street in St. Michael's parish in Birmingham, was known as St. Joseph's. It was a small, dilapidated one story frame house which had recently been vacated by the Sisters of Mercy. Sister M. Coletta Farrell was the first superior of the teaching sisters, but was soon replaced by Sister M. Louis Bergem, who had charge of the convent and school.[131]

In 1871, Bishop Domenec decided the community should separate from Buffalo. Bishop Timon of Buffalo released the sisters from his jurisdiction, and the Motherhouse and Novitiate were established at St. Joseph's on the South Side. Sister M. Louis Bergem was elected the first Mother Superior. The new community consisted of twenty-two professed sisters, two novices, and four postulants. The newly constructed Motherhouse on Pius Street, completed in 1875, was a three story brick building, measuring eighty by forty-two feet.[132] Mother M. Louis Bergem wanted very much for the sisters to be a papal, not strictly a diocesan, community. In 1884, with the assistance of the Passionist Fathers, the Rule and Constitutions of the Sisters of the Third Order of Saint Francis were written and sent to Rome for approval. In July 1890, after five years of experiment, the Sisters of St. Francis became an Apostolic Order, granted by Pope Leo XIII. Within five years, the Rule and Constitutions were printed and distributed to the sisters in German and English editions.[133] Thirty years after their arrival in Pittsburgh, there were still German speaking sisters in the Order.

In 1895, the Sisters of the Third Order of St. Francis became incorporated "for the purpose of establishing and maintaining schools for the instruction and education of the young, establishing and maintaining homes for orphan children and establishing and maintaining hospitals for the care of the sick." Sidonia Etzel, Mary Rose, Rose Winter, Anne Farrell and Mary Hessler were the first corporate members. The newly formed Corporation was to be managed by a board of five directors chosen from membership of the corporation.[134]

The community continued to grow, and in 1897, ground was broken for the new Motherhouse in Millvale. Mt. Alvernia, the sisters' new home, had

[131] "Foundation of the Sisters of the Third Order of St. Francis of the Immaculate Virgin Mary Mother of God, Mt. Alvernia," Motherhouse Archives; *100 Years of Franciscan Spirit*, p. 24.; "Sisters of the Third Order of St. Francis in the Diocese of Pittsburgh, 1885–1916," manuscript, Motherhouse Archives.

[132] *100 Years of Franciscan Spirit*, p. 26.; "Foundation of the Sisters of the Third Order of St. Francis of the Immaculate Virgin Mary Mother of God, Mt. Alvernia," Motherhouse Archives; "Sisters of the Third Order of St. Francis in the Diocese of Pittsburgh, 1885–1916," manuscript, Motherhouse Archives.

[133] "History of the Constitutions, The Sisters of Saint Francis of Millvale," manuscript, Motherhouse Archives.

[134] Charter Book, Vol. 21, p. 115.

frontage of 365 feet, was three stories high and had two wings that were 220 and 210 feet in length. On June 12, 1900, the Motherhouse was dedicated.[135] The sisters became more involved in teaching in Western Pennsylvania, and by the end of the century had established approximately a dozen schools in different areas, including Butler, Millvale, Carrick, South Side, Cambria, Johnstown, Mt. Oliver, Manchester and Bloomfield. Today they serve in twenty-seven dioceses in the United States and also in Africa, Japan, Puerto Rico, Guatemala, Dominican Republic and the Virgin Islands.[136]

A New Century

As the new century was dawning, St. Francis was becoming one of the major hospitals serving the Pittsburgh area. Only two other hospitals were larger, Mercy Hospital and Western Pennsylvania Hospital, and they exceeded St. Francis by only a few beds. During the nineteenth century, the sisters resolved important issues which never surfaced again. They were able to establish themselves as permanent owners of the institution, allowing them to direct policy as the hospital underwent change. In addition, the sisters had succeeded in changing the hospital's original purpose of providing care primarily for the German population, and the reputation inherent in that objective, by firmly establishing in the community a hospital serving all ethnic peoples. By 1900, as medical and technological developments set the stage for hospital growth, the sisters were faced with a whole new set of issues. St. Francis Hospital continued to grow in the first few decades of the new century, as did other area hospitals. What is astounding to note is that St. Francis Hospital progressed in spite of its meager financial resources; for this one problem continued unabated for decades.

[135]"Sisters of the Third Order of St. Francis in the Diocese of Pittsburgh, 1855–1916," (Pittsburgh: 1916), Motherhouse archives.
[136]Sister M. Zita Green, *A Chronology of 125 Years—The Sisters of St. Francis of Millvale, 1866–1991,* (Pittsburgh: Typecraft Press, 1991).

Chapter Two

Women Religious in a Secular World

Introduction

The Sisters of St. Francis founded a hospital because of their profound belief that they were to serve the indigent sick. Throughout the twentieth century, they struggled to preserve Roman Catholic, or at least Judeo-Christian, principles which they cherished in a secular world where religious ideals were often viewed with skepticism. Other historians have suggested that the spiritual foundation of the work of women religious was influential in the establishment and operation of sisters' hospitals. However, it will become clear that the effort necessary to maintain those spiritual principles in a secular world directed the growth of hospital development.[1]

The sisters were faced with new and different issues at the dawn of the twentieth century. In the nineteenth century, the sisters' major focus was in serving the German immigrant population, a goal which they achieved, and in the process they established the foundation for a community hospital which served individuals from the city at large. In the twentieth century the sisters were not only confronted with changes in medicine and technology, but also with a society of individuals espousing new attitudes towards science and medicine. New problems arose resulting in a tension between maintaining religious values and striving to develop an up-to-date medical center.

The one problem which did carry over from the early years was that of finances, albeit for different reasons. In the nineteenth century, the sisters struggled to keep their institution open, often because beds were not being filled. As attitudes changed and the community demographics were altered, however, the hospital was regularly filled to capacity. Because of the sisters'

[1] Patricia Mary Tarbox, "The Origins of Nursing by the Sisters of Mercy in the United States," (Ed.D. dissertation, Columbia University Teachers College, 1986).

policies, grounded in religious beliefs, the financial struggles, although occasionally alleviated, never ceased. In order to maintain their hospital founded to serve the sick poor, the sisters had to establish a solid financial foundation, which required great compromise on their part. The sisters were faced with the constant struggle of serving their patients while surviving financially. There were policies, however, on which they continuously refused to compromise. As the struggle between religious principles and a secular world continued unabated throughout the century, the sisters' only recourse was to maintain strict authority within the hospital in order to preserve their fundamental beliefs. Other historians have suggested that conflicts developed between boards, administration and medical staff, and that eventually the medical staff was able to increase their control of other hospitals.[2] In Catholic hospitals, however, the sisters maintained their authority.

The Catholic Hospital Association

This struggle between maintaining an institution with a spiritual foundation, and establishing a progressive medical and scientific hospital, was not unique to St. Francis. Some members of the Catholic hierarchy, in fact, were well aware of the conflict. In 1915, the Catholic Hospital Association (CHA) was established with the help of Father Charles B. Moulinier, S.J., as a response to a standardization movement prevalent at the time. The sisters who managed the Catholic hospitals were often restricted by rules of religious life and, therefore, had limited contact with lay people and various health care organizations. Established as a sisters' organization, the CHA's purpose was to assist sisters in taking more action in the modern health community by providing annual educational conventions, regional meetings and assorted publications in order to place them on a par with other health care administrators. Catholic leaders were concerned that their religious institutions were falling significantly behind prevailing standards of medical, educational and scientific medicine, and were in danger of becoming second class facilities.

The Church was also worried that the Catholic hospitals' commitment to live up to higher standards of medical care might jeopardize their mission as Catholic care givers. The Church wanted to maintain a balance between the need for high quality care and a fulfillment of the Church's mission. The

[2]Charles Rosenberg, *The Care of Strangers; The Rise of America's Hospital System* (New York: Basic Books, Inc., 1987) p. 263.

purpose of the CHA, when it was established, was to help Catholic hospitals maintain their spiritual significance while trying to meet new demands made upon all hospitals.[3] Article II of their Constitution describes their objectives: "the promotion and realization of progressively higher ideals in the religious, moral, medical, nursing, educational, social and all other phases of hospital and nursing endeavor especially in the Catholic hospitals and schools of nursing in the United States and Canada." By 1920, the Catholic Hospital Association was officially recognized by the hierarchy within the Church. The organization, therefore, could operate with the assurance that its work conformed to the directives of the bishops.[4]

The CHA was established in response to the standardization movement being spearheaded by the American College of Surgeons (ACS). In 1913, the American College of Surgeons was established in order to facilitate standardization of medical care. Hospitals at that time were managed rather haphazardly with a wide variety in the quality of care being offered at different facilities. In 1918, the ACS set minimum standards for hospitals which, over the long term, directly affected the setting of policies in hospitals. There were four basic requirements which had to be met in order for a hospital to receive ACS approval. Those included:

- an organized, competent, ethical medical staff which held regular conferences for the review of clinical work
- agreement to forbid fee-splitting,
- accurate and complete clinical records kept on all patients,
- adequate diagnostic and therapeutic facilities, including clinical laboratories and x-ray departments.

Father Charles B. Moulinier, S.J., who was an organizer of the Catholic Hospital Association and its first president, became a member of the standardization committee of ACS in 1917. The purpose of this committee was to serve as counsel and guide in planning hospital standardization. Because of his participation on this committee as a hospital inspector for the ACS, he was able to provide Catholic hospitals with the necessary guidance so that they would remain progressive. Moulinier believed that Catholic institutions

---

[3]*The Past ... A Prologue 1915–1965*, (Ethicon Co., 1965), p. 6; Rosemary Stevens, *In Sickness and in Wealth, American Hospitals in the Twentieth Century*, (New York: Basic Books, 1989), pp. 94, 115; Christopher Kauffman, "The Push for Standardization; Origins of CHA, 1914–1920," *Health Progress* (Jan.–Feb. 1990), p. 57; Robert J. Shanahan, S.J., *The History of the CHA 1915–1965: Fifty Years of Progress*, (St. Louis: CHA, 1965), p. 16.

[4]Robert J. Shanahan, S.J., *The History of the CHA 1915–1965: Fifty Years of Progress*, (St. Louis: CHA, 1965), pp. 79, 93.

were obligated to maintain professional standards on a par with those of any hospital. Catholic hospitals were unique, however, because of their concept of holistic care, which encompassed physical, mental and spiritual care.[5]

Catholic hospitals, and St. Francis serves as a good example, received approval from the American College of Surgeons earlier than other hospitals. St. Francis Hospital was one of the first hospitals to receive approval as a community and teaching facility with the one recommendation that the hospital improve its medical records department. Subsequently, Dr. Cohoe from Johns Hopkins was brought in to be the first chairman of that department.[6] By 1930, of the 641 Catholic hospitals, 364, or 56.7 percent, of the hospitals had gained approval from the ACS, whereas only 25.9 percent of all non-Catholic hospitals had been so approved. Although Catholic hospitals represented only 10 percent of the total number of hospitals at that time, they represented 18.4 percent of the total number of approved hospitals. By 1946, 69.7 percent of all Catholic hospitals received approval compared to 40.4 percent of non-Catholic general hospitals.[7]

It is interesting to note that during the various transitional phases which occurred in all hospitals due to medical and technological innovations, the Catholic Hospitals were able to maintain continuity of purpose. By the 1960s, the CHA continued to encourage Catholic hospitals to provide spiritual as well as medical care. In 1962, the Catholic Hospital Association executive board established their "Philosophy for Catholic Hospitals."[8]

– They are to be an integral part of the work of the Church, an extension of Christ's mission of Mercy.
– It is recognized that man's unique composition is that of body and soul. Their concept of care embraces physical, emotional and spiritual needs.

[5]Rosemary Stevens, In Sickness and in Wealth; American Hospitals in the Twentieth Century, (New York: Basic Books, 1989), p. 115; Robert J. Shanahan, S.J., The History of the Catholic Hospital Association, 1915–1965: Fifty Years of Progress, (St. Louis: CHA, 1965), pp. 32, 44.

[6]Sister M. Adele Meiser, "History of St. Francis Medical Center," paper given at the Lawrenceville Historical Meeting, June 1985, manuscript, St. Francis Hospital Archives; Robert J. Shanahan, S.J., The History of the Catholic Hospital Association, 1915–1965: Fifty Years of Progress, (St. Louis: CHA, 1965), p. 26; Mary Carol Conroy, SCL, "The Transition Years," in Pioneer Healers: The History of Women Religious in American Health Care eds. Ursula Stepsis, CSA, and Dolores Liptak, RSM, (New York: Crossroad Publishing Co., 1989), p. 147.

[7]John O'Grady, Catholic Charities in the United States: History and Problems, (Washington D.C.: National Conference of Catholic Charities, 1930), p. 204; Robert J. Shanahan, S.J., The History of the Catholic Hospital Association, 1915–1965: Fifty Years of Progress, (St. Louis: CHA, 1965), p. 53.

[8]Robert J. Shanahan, S.J., The History of the Catholic Hospital Association, 1915–1965: Fifty Years of Progress, (St. Louis: CHA, 1965), p. 262.

- The primary objective is to maintain and restore health.
- The hospitals must serve all people in charity regardless of race, creed or financial status.
- The hospitals should be formal organizations.
- They are obligated to provide the best possible care.
- They are obligated to provide an adequate staff.
- There should be continued competence of personnel at all levels.
- There should be a program of compensation and working conditions for employees which reflect a spirit of social justice.
- All donations belong to the hospital.
- There should be an obligation to further education and research.
- There should be active community participation and an attempt to meet the needs of the community.

St. Francis Hospital, then, serves as an excellent example of the Catholic hospitals whose needs were recognized by the Catholic Hospital Association. Its struggles to exist amidst the tensions inherent in a society which was so diverse in religion and ethnicity exemplify how Catholic hospitals developed alongside, and in spite of, other non-denominational institutions.

In the twentieth century, the Sisters of St.Francis faced new problems which they were able to resolve, but not always without some controversy. They struggled to maintain their authority within the institution, never relinquishing it to either physicians or board members. This was imperative in order that they continue to provide the holistic or spiritual care for which their hospital was established. The sisters unceasingly provided care to the indigent, regardless of financial crises or disapproval of the medical staff. They solved monetary limitations by acquiescing to State mandates, claiming non-sectarian status, in order to receive funding. They were able to carry out their purpose while striving to develop medical and technological innovations, and improve and enlarge the physical plant. Ultimately, they were able to develop an institution that became the epitome of any highly technological medical complex in the late twentieth century.

Administration and Management

St. Francis Hospital had always been under the management of a lay board since it was first chartered in 1868, but there is little evidence to suggest that those members played much of a role other than in fund raising, especially in the years leading up to the second world war. Amendments to the charter were made in 1937, which provided that a board of twenty-one corporators, elected by themselves, had the power of "making, altering, and amending the by-laws of the corporation." A Board of Managers, composed of fifteen persons elected by the corporation annually for three year terms, governed the hospital's business affairs. The board was arranged in classes of five so that at each annual meeting of the corporators, one class of five directors would be elected.[9] The board had "charge, control and management of the property, affairs and funds of the corporation." They were responsible for appointing the medical staff and, employing the hospital administrator and the comptroller. It is interesting to note that absolutely no mention was made of the sisters in either the amended charter or the by-laws which were approved in 1954.[10]

However, the sisters, from the founding of the hospital until the present, always maintained their authority in the management of the hospital. The autonomy of the Catholic sisters in Roman Catholic institutions stands in sharp contrast to the role played by lay boards or physicians in other institutions. The sisters retained control over internal management, including patient admissions, and restrained efforts on the part of physicians and others to divert them from their goals.[11] This did not go unnoticed by the physicians as recently as 1967. In a discussion regarding how many beds would be allotted to which departments, a member of the medical staff remarked that "we delude ourselves that we feel we govern ourselves." The doctor was referring to the administration at the time.[12]

Although the management of the hospital has always been under the direction of a sister, during the first few years of the new century there was no consistency in the superintendent's office, as someone new filled the role approximately every two years. It was somewhat unusual that the superior of the Order and the superintendent of the hospital were different individuals.[13] Sister M. Adelaide Campbell, OSF, was administrator from 1904 to 1906, Sister M. Cleopha Etzel, OSF, until 1908 and Sister M. Cecilia Maxler, OSF, was in charge until 1913. In that year, Sister M. Thomasine Diemer, OSF, was

[9]"Charter and By-Laws", amendments April 6, 1937, Recorded April 13, 1937, in the office of the Recorder of Deeds of Allegheny County in Charter Book, Vol. 67, p. 67.

[10]By-Laws, St. Francis Hospital of Pittsburgh, adopted and approved June 28, 1954.

[11]Joan Lynaugh, "From Respectable Domesticity to Medical Efficiency: The Changing Kansas City Hospital, 1875–1920," in The American General Hospital, Communities and Social Contexts, eds. Diana Elizabeth Long and Janet Golden, (Ithaca: Cornell University Press, 1989), p. 29.

[12]Minutes, Medical Staff, February 21, 1967.

[13]Talk given by Sister Adele Meiser, manuscript, n.d., St. Francis Hospital Archives.

designated as superintendent in charge of the hospital, a position she held until her retirement in 1959. Sisters were assigned to specific occupations by the Mother Superior. It was not at all unusual for sisters to change roles annually. The fact that Sister Thomasine remained as administrator for so long should be credited to the superiors who recognized the need for consistency in the administration of such a large facility. Not surprisingly, Sister Thomasine believed that sisters should hold the key management positions in the hospital because "their vocation is the best recommendation of their fitness for the responsibility." The superintendent of the hospital, superintendent of nurses and directors of dietary, pharmacy and housekeeping were all to be sisters. This does not imply, however, that the sisters did not need adequate preparation, for Sister Thomasine was adamant that sisters be properly educated for the positions which they held.[14]

Sister M. Thomasine Diemer was born Mathilda Teresa Diemer in Pittsburgh on January 18, 1875. After entering the community, she taught in the grade schools, teaching music after class hours. In 1907, she began to work in the hospital in the bookkeeping department. Six years later she was appointed administrator of the institution.[15] Upon retirement, she served as Consultant to the hospital until her death on April 11, 1964. In 1947, Sister Thomasine celebrated the fiftieth anniversary of her religious life. It is interesting to note that the hospital staff gave her a testimonial dinner honoring her. The "ceremony was well attended, dignified and touching in the tribute paid Sister as administrator and guide of the hospital." The fact that the staff honored her in this way suggests that her role as a spiritual leader was as important to them as her role as an administrator.[16]

Sister M. Adele Meiser, OSF, who had been Sister Thomasine's assistant for many years, became Chief Executive Officer in 1959 and remained until her retirement from the position in 1977.[17] Sister Adele, born Mary Catherine Meiser, on August 15, 1903, attended St. George School in the Allentown section of Pittsburgh. She had wanted to be a nun since the age of seven. Following high school, Sister Adele worked for several years in area firms as a secretary, bookkeeper, and legal stenographer. She entered Mt. Alvernia in 1924 at the age of 21. Sister made her first vows in 1926, and her final vows

---

[14]Sister M. Thomasine, "The Material Welfare of the Hospital," *Hospital Progress*, August 1923.

[15]*Seventy-Fifth Anniversary, 1901–1976*, (Pittsburgh: St. Francis General Hospital School of Nursing, 1976), p. 7; Necrologies, Motherhouse Archives. There are conflicting reports regarding exactly what year Sister Thomasine began her position as chief executive of the hospital, 1913 or 1917.

[16]Minutes, Board of Managers, May 20, 1947; "Sister Thomasine Memorial Fund," *Signs of Life*, n.d.

[17]*Seventy-Fifth Anniversary, 1901–1976*, (Pittsburgh: St. Francis General Hospital School of Nursing, 1976), p. 7.

three years later. Sister Adele attended college during the day and worked in the admitting office of the hospital in the evenings. She received her B.A. and M.A. degrees from Duquesne University, and was one of the first women, and the very first sister, to receive her M.B.A. from the University of Chicago Graduate School of Business Administration with a major in hospital administration in 1940. This program, established in 1934, was the first graduate program in hospital administration in the United States.[18] When she entered the University of Chicago program, she was already a member of the American College of Hospital Administrators. Sister recalled that the program was very experimental, and its faculty was not sure how a nun would fit in. Toward the end of the program, Sister Adele worked as an intern in one of Chicago's sectarian hospitals, at the encouragement of Sister Thomasine, who felt she needed experience in another type of institution. Sister Adele credits the Order with foresight in understanding the need for graduate education for their sisters, reflecting the philosophy of the Order regarding education, which in turn had continuing impact on the development of the hospital.[19]

Sister Adele's concern for people extended beyond the patients in her care. She endeared herself in the hearts of the city's journalists early in her career, long before the establishment of public relations departments (St. Francis' department was established in 1954). When she first came to the hospital, she felt the newspaper reporters were treated very discourteously whenever they came to the hospital to investigate an accident or other similar event. She thought they "were just young men trying to make a living." Sister would gently ask the doctor in charge to let reporters speak with the patients involved. Sister Adele organized a formal press relations code for St. Francis Hospital with the editors of three daily newspapers (*Press, Post-Gazette* and *Sun-Telegraph*).[20]

Sister Adele serves as an excellent example of a sister/administrator whose religious convictions prompted her to direct hospital policy in line with spiritual beliefs. Her leadership, naturally, influenced others in the order. Just as in the early years of the hospital, the indigent were never refused admission. "Sister Adele has been known to wink at hospital regulations and break red tape to get the necessary care for those desperately in need of help." Dr. Abraham

[18]Rosemary Stevens, *In Sickness and in Wealth; American Hospitals in the Twentieth Century*, (New York: Basic Books, 1989), pp. 157–158.

[19]"Hospital Chief a Tough Act to Follow," article in manuscript, n.d. but c. 1977, St. Francis Hospital Archives; Barry Paris, "Profile—Sister Adele, the Gentle Persuader of St. Francis General Hospital," *Pittsburgh Post-Gazette*, 2 July 1983; Interview with Sister M. Adele Meiser, 1993.

[20]Barry Paris, "Profile—Sister Adele, the Gentle Persuader of St. Francis General Hospital," *Pittsburgh Post-Gazette* 2 July 1983.

Twerski once wrote that Sister Adele "has the conviction that Providence placed her in charge of a large hospital to make sure people in need of help receive it with no ifs, ands, or buts."[21] Sister Adele was never interested in the patient's religious affiliation, believing that many people not belonging to a particular denomination are still "holy people," praying and keeping the Commandments. She believed they were people to emulate. The sisters would "never, never proselytize."[22]

It has been noted that sisters' hospitals had an atmosphere of care and concern that was less obvious in secular institutions.[23] Sister Adele believed that the nation's sisters' hospitals have set the pace for others to follow by focusing on the human element in hospitalization. Sister Adele's work exemplifies this concept. When asked to describe St. Francis Hospital's most important contribution to the community, she replied simply, "taking care of people."[24] Even though the position of Executive Director kept her extremely busy, she still attempted to keep in touch with the patients. Every day, she visited on the patient units, and on Sundays she spent five to six hours trying to see every patient.[25] Unlike lay administrators, sisters in that role do not take days off.

Sister Adele received many honors throughout her career. In 1965, she received the Pennsylvania Board of Vocational Rehabilitation Award, and two years later was the recipient of the Goodwill Industries of Pittsburgh Award. Delta Sigma Theta Inc. Religion in Action awarded her with their Social Action Award in 1972, and the following year, the Variety Club of Pittsburgh honored her with their Service Award for her work with the handicapped children in the rehabilitation department. The George Washington Carver Community Leader Award was given to Sister in 1974. In 1976, she received the Virginia Turner Memorial Award from the Grand Auxiliary Fraternal Order of Eagles. In that same year, she also received the Heart Award from the Variety Club of Pittsburgh. Her name is registered in *Who's Who in Health Care*, *Two Thousand Women of Achievement of 1970*, and *The Dictionary of International Biographies*. Duquesne Univer-

---

[21]"Hospital Chief a Tough Act to Follow," article in manuscript, n.d. but c. 1977, St. Francis Hospital Archives.

[22]Interview with Sister M. Adele Meiser, 1993.

[23]Edward C. Atwater, "Women, Surgeons and a Worthy Enterprise: The General Hospital comes to Upper New York State," in *The American General Hospital; Communities and Social Context*, eds. Diana Elizabeth Long and Janet Golden, (Ithaca: Cornell University Press, 1989), p. 49.

[24]Interview with Sister M. Adele Meiser, 9/25/92.

[25]Jerry Vondas, "Nun Cares for Life at St. Francis Hospital," *Pittsburgh Press*, 21 March 1973.

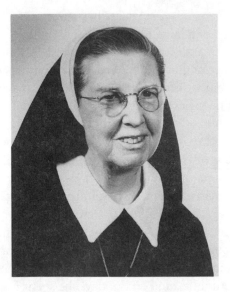

Sister Mary Adele Meiser, OSF

sity honored her by electing her as a member of their Century Club and by awarding her the College of Arts and Sciences Distinguished Alumna Award in 1979.[26]

Sister Adele served in numerous capacities on boards and committees throughout the health care and educational communities. She served as vice president of the Hospital Administrators of Pennsylvania. Sister Adele was the president of the Administrators' Conference of Hospitals in Allegheny County for three terms. Sister served two terms as vice president and declined the nomination of president of the Hospital Association of Pennsylvania. She also served on the committee on administration, and on the nominating committee of the Catholic Hospital Association, which also wanted to nominate her for the presidency; she refused due to a lack of time. She was a trustee of the Hospital Council of Western Pennsylvania, which she had helped to organize, and she served on the board of Point Park College and the Pittsburgh Playhouse. She was also a fellow in the American College of Hospital Administrators. Sister Adele served on the Governor's Committee for the Employment of the Handicapped, the Pennsylvania Citizen's Council and the Western Pennsylvania Association for Women's Deans, Counselors and Personnel Workers. In addition, she was a consultant to the National Center for Health Services Research and Development, and

[26]Jerry Vondas, "Nun Cares for Life at St. Francis Hospital," *Pittsburgh Press*, 21 March 1973; Letter from Malcolm Berman to the Hospital Association of Pennsylvania, 6/7/77; Lettersfrom Duquesne University to Sister Adele, 8/29/79 and 3/1/79; biographical notes, manuscript, St. Francis Hospital Archives.

served on the library committee for the American Hospital Association. She contributed to the literature on the subject of hospital administration by publishing in journals such as *Modern Hospital, News Bulletin, Hospitals* and *Hospital Progress*. Sister led a campaign for building codes to meet the needs of the handicapped in Pittsburgh. She was one of the founders of Gateway Rehabilitation Center, a 150 bed facility providing intensive therapeutic programs for alcoholics and drug abusers.[27] Sister M. Adele Meiser died on March 20, 1994.

During the first half of the twentieth century, evidence suggests that the sisters were directly involved with virtually all departments of the hospital in addition to serving in administrative roles. Their presence permeated every aspect of the hospital. A sister was in charge of the record room in the department of medicine in the early 1920s. This was an important position at the time because the hospital, in order to comply with the new standards set by the American College of Surgeons, had to be responsible for accurate and extensive record keeping. Sisters worked as technicians in the laboratory. Sister M. Laurentine Harrington OSF was in charge of the psychiatric nurses, and later succeeded Sister M. Claudia Evans OSF, R.N. as superintendent of nurses. Another sister was in charge of the obstetrics department. Twenty-four of the thirty-three graduate head nurses were sisters in the early twenties.[28] It is interesting to note that during the late twenties, the Catholic Hospital Association concentrated on the development of hospital personnel specifically in the areas of record keeping, nursing and laboratory technology.[29] St. Francis clearly developed those departments under the leadership of the sisters who functioned as the heads of most of the departments as late as World War II.[30]

Although the sisters may have always maintained authority in the setting of policy and the management of the hospital, they kept a rather low profile publicly. There is very little mention of their activities in the hospital reports, except when a physician praised their work. Oddly, even though medical staff, nursing graduates' and board of directors' names are recorded in the published record, there is no mention of the administrative staff positions which were

---

[27] Jerry Vondas, "Nun Cares for Life at St. Francis Hospital," *Pittsburgh Press,* 21 March 1973; Barry Paris, "Profile—Sister Adele, the Gentle Persuader of St. Francis General Hospital," *Pittsburgh Post-Gazette,* 2 July 1983; letter from Malcolm Berman to the Hospital Association of Pennsylvania, 6/7/77; Shirley Molkenthin, "Sister Adele Meiser," December 13, 1977, manuscript, St. Francis Hospital Archives.

[28] *Report of the St. Francis Hospital,* June 1, 1921–May 31, 1923, pp. 19, 26, 28, 34, 49.

[29] Alphonse M. Schwitalla, S.J., and M. R. Kneifl, "A Survey of the Catholic Hospitals of the United States and Canada," *Hospital Progress,* March 1930, p. 114.

[30] Interview with Dr. George Wright, 10/25/93.

filled by sisters from the Order. Part of this can be explained by the rules of their Order, which prescribed humility and forbade, for example, being the subject of any photograph.[31] This attempt to remain humble probably extended to written reports as well.[32] Interestingly, as noted earlier, the ubiquitous sisters were not mentioned in the charter or articles of incorporation of the hospital. This may have been a result of their desperate need for the state appropriation, which demanded that the hospital be perceived as non-sectarian. This type of compromise must not have come easily. Another explanation for the lack of their presence in the legal documents may be that the sisters did not believe it was necessary. Their presence was known in virtually every department of the hospital, and the sisters filled the chief administrative positions as well as functioning as department heads and supervisors.

Oddly enough, however, although they remained in the background as far as the general public was concerned, they referred to "*their* St. Francis Hospital" within the sphere of the Roman Catholic community. When seeking monetary help from the parishes, the hospital was portrayed as though only the sisters were involved. "Ever true to their vows of charity, the Sisters nursed seventy-seven percent of the number without one penny in payment toward the upkeep of their institution. . . . the gratuitous service of fifty-six of the sisters in positions that would be the most highly paid in other hospitals, has permitted them to continue without once calling upon their Church or the public at large for any financial assistance."[33]

Relationships with the Board and Medical Staff

As the sisters directed their hospital they made every attempt to work with board members and doctors as equals. However, it was, and is, fairly clear that they were the final authorities. Implicit in the forward of the 1923 report, for example, written by the sisters, is an expected deferential behavior towards the sisters. They referred to board members as "ready and willing associates in every enterprise we have contemplated or undertaken." The president of the medical staff was a "ready co-worker and counselor." The sisters were indebted to the staff physicians. "Without their unstinted and unselfish contribution of knowledge and effort our accomplishments would be little indeed." They

[31] Interview with Sister M. Thomasita Heller, Motherhouse, October 25, 1993.

[32] Apparently it was not unusual for boards to publish reports instead of sisters, noted by Mary Patricia Tarbox, "The Origins of Nursing by the Sisters of Mercy in the U.S., 1843–1910," (Ed.D. dissertation, Columbia University Teacher's College, 1986), p. 127.

[33] *That They May do More*, campaign brochure, n.d. but c. 1927, St. Francis Hospital Archives.

praised the loyalty, interest and "splendid spirit of cooperation" of the interns and resident physicians.[34] Sister Thomasine recognized that physicians' "timely advice and suggestion are of inestimable assistance in promoting a good working balance in the organization; this, of course, provided the staff is the right type, and if it is not, why have it?"[35] In other words, physicians were necessary and valuable, provided they were also cooperative and supportive. Implicit in Sister Thomasine's words also is the suggestion that the sisters would not tolerate uncooperative physicians, who would be asked to seek privileges in another institution. The sisters collaborated with medical professionals and board members, and respected their advice and knowledge, but they clearly envisioned the hospital as under their control and authority, a pattern which continues to this day.

This does not mean the sisters did not acquiesce to the suggestions of the physicians or board when necessary for the sake of the growth and development of the hospital. They valued their advice enormously, but ultimately, the sisters made the decisions. As the hospital became reliant on new scientific developments, so, too, the medical staff desired to professionalize the nursing staff. Dr. R. R. Huggins, chief surgeon, was a devoted friend of Mother M. Baptista Etzel, OSF, (superior of the Order 1892–1901, 1904–1910, 1922–1925). He proved to her the necessity of a professional nursing staff. At that time the relationships were similar to those in a closely knit family. "The sisters looked upon the doctors as their particular charges, while the members of the medical staff revered and cherished the sisters, treating them with the greatest deference and respect." The family spirit, however, was not practical in a large institution with lay nurses, sisters and a large mixed medical staff. Dr. Huggins valued a more formal attitude on everyone's part. Mother Baptista was convinced that a change in the general relations between medical staff and hospital personnel was imperative. She began to place graduate nurses from other well-known hospitals in supervisory positions, removing lay nurses and sisters from those roles. The sisters, whose practical experience surpassed any theoretical knowledge of a graduate nurse, were outraged. The hospital's own lay nurses resented the intrusion of strangers. It was months before the furor abated.[36]

Mother Baptista continued to heed Dr. Huggins' advice on other occasions, as well. In May 1910, Mother Baptista, Sister M. Aurelia Arenth, OSF, Dr. and Mrs. Huggins and Mr. and Mrs. S. Heckert visited St. Mary's Hospital

---

[34]*Report of the St. Francis Hospital,* June 1, 1921–May 31, 1923, pp. 7, 8.

[35]Sister M. Thomasine, "The Material Welfare of the Hospital," *Hospital Progress,* August 1923.

[36]Sister M. Aurelia Arenth, OSF, *As a Living Oak, Biography of Mother Baptista Etzel* (Pittsburgh: Sisters of the Third Order of St. Francis, 1956), pp. 119–120.

in Rochester, Minnesota, the site of the work of Drs. Will and Charles Mayo. The two sisters also visited the Sacred Heart Sanitarium in Milwaukee and Mercy Hospital in Chicago.[37] Clearly, the sisters were intent upon educating themselves in the best interest of the hospital. Professionalization of the nursing staff is just one example of their attitudes toward education and their willingness to professionalize their staff for the sake of the improvement of the hospital.

Implicit in these anecdotes is the notion that the Mother Superior of the community was fairly active in the management of the hospital during the first decade of the twentieth century. As noted earlier, there was little consistency in the direct management, as superintendents were appointed every few years. When Sister Thomasine was appointed in 1913, administration of the hospital became consistent, and the Mother Superior was able to attend to other matters.

The shifts in nursing personnel attest to the fact that the sisters, aware of changes in hospital development nationally and cognizant of new advancements in medicine, directed their hospital at the beginning of the twentieth century so that it met the standards of the best institutions of that time. At the forefront of change in hospital standardization and professionalization, they sought to educate themselves and kept an open mind regarding scientific improvements. The medical staff praised the sisters, stating that their "generous and progressive point of view and their cooperation in every step likely to be of benefit to patients is a constant stimulus to every one who comes in contact with them."[38]

In a day when women had few options, the sisters emphasized the need for pursuing intellectual endeavors, as evidenced by Sister Adele. Sister Laurentine Harrington believed that women's progress was slower because others were reluctant to accept the judgment of women, especially women physicians. People were accustomed to hearing diagnoses and treatment plans from men. Sister Laurentine felt that this was unjust. The nursing school director's attitude in 1929 is indicative of views held by many of the sisters of the Order. She believed that treating women differently, or denying them credibility because of their gender, was unfair. These two factors, the need for education for advancement and the unjust attitudes toward women, prompted the sisters to seek college degrees, a view shared by some Catholic Orders, but not all.[39] Sister M. Laurentine Harrington had studied nursing at Mercy Hospital in

[37]Sister M. Aurelia Arenth, pp. 121–122.
[38]*Report of the St. Francis Hospital*, June 1, 1921–May 31, 1923, p. 13.
[39]Sister M. Laurentine, "Women in Medicine," *The Courier of the I.C.F.N.*, Nov.–Dec. 1929.

Baltimore, attended Duquesne University and received her Bachelors degree in nursing from the Catholic University of America. This education allowed her to function well as supervisor of obstetrics and gynecology, supervisor of psychiatry, director of nursing service and director of the nursing school.[40]

1900 to World War II—The Hospital and Its Patients

As the demographics within the community changed, the ethnicity of the patients also changed, as well as the community's perceptions about the hospital. The hospital had been founded to serve the German Catholics, and therefore had a German name. In the twentieth century, people of various ethnic backgrounds were served. In order to eliminate the reputation that the hospital was erected to serve a distinctive group, an amendment was added to the hospital charter in 1933, which formally changed the name of the facility from the St. Franciscus Hospital of Pittsburgh to the St. Francis Hospital of Pittsburgh.[41]

St. Francis Hospital accepted any patient for admission, a policy on which the sisters would not compromise. As the hospital struggled financially, partially due to this policy, the sisters would not alter their deeply held convictions that anyone who was sick and unable to pay was 'worthy' of care. There were no other implied meanings, as historians have so frequently suggested, and which seem to have applied to other kinds of hospitals. According to Sister Adele, who had been affiliated with the hospital since the mid-twenties, any patient who required gratuitous care was deemed worthy. "They were worthy, because they were poor." It is this policy, often difficult to maintain throughout the years, which determined the characteristics of the hospital and the people which it served.

The hospital's admission policies were unlike those of other institutions. Historian Charles Rosenberg has suggested that private hospitals were disinterested in the chronically ill and the incurables. Diagnosis, rather than dependency, generally determined hospital admission by the 1920s.[42] This was not necessarily true for the Sisters of St. Francis, who willingly admit-

---

[40]Necrology, Motherhouse Archives.

[41]Recorded March 11, 1933 in office of Recorder of Deeds of Allegheny County in Charter Book, vol. 65, p. 108.

[42]Charles Rosenberg, *The Care of Strangers; The Rise of America's Hospital System*, (New York: Basic Books, Inc., 1987), p. 345.

ted anyone in need of care. Their belief in providing holistic care, caring for body, mind and spirit, justified their admission policy. The sisters were adamant that no patient be refused admission because of an inability to pay. Sister M. Thomasine was known among the dispensary physicians as the person to call when they needed assistance in gaining admission to the hospital for the needy cases. Inebriates, those with venereal disease and infectious patients were admitted. In 1911, for example, the department of medicine treated four patients with gonorrhea, three with syphilis and fifty-two with typhoid fever. The children's department admitted a child with pertussis.[43] By 1952, the hospital still recorded that they willingly admitted contagious patients as well as those who were chronically ill.[44]

The hospital continued to accept patients of all religions, not unlike other Catholic institutions. In the mid-twenties, one of the few years for which these data are available, Catholic patients outnumbered the Protestants, but only by a very few. There were 4,991 Catholics admitted, compared to 3,809 Protestants and 204 "Hebrews." One hundred forty-five patients were not affiliated with any church.[45]

The St. Francis Hospital was founded because of a perceived need by the German speaking people of the area, and it always continued to treat foreign born patients; but interestingly, yet not surprisingly, the ethnicity of those foreign patients changed, reflecting changing patterns of immigration to America. In 1895, for example, 40 percent of all of the in-patients treated for the year were foreign born. That percentage remained between 18 and 26 percent until 1904 when it dropped to 15 percent. It peaked again in 1906 at 32 percent, but then dropped to 15 percent again the following year. Statistics are not available following 1907. A breakdown of the various nationalities represented is only available for the psychiatric hospital, which had a bed capacity of 150 beds. From 1891 until 1909, the German and the Irish were the most predominant groups of foreign born patients in the psychiatric hospital. It was not until 1912 that patients from Poland outnumbered them.[46] This reflects the changing demographics of the community surrounding St. Francis Hospital. By 1900, an increasing number of Poles had settled in Lawrenceville. Immigrants, largely from southern and eastern European countries, doubled the Catholic population of the county by 1920. Mills and industries along

---

[43] *Report of the St. Francis Hospital*, 1911, pp. 12, 13, 44.

[44] AMA Council on Medical Education, Annual Census of Hospitals, 1952.

[45] "Taking Stock," campaign booklet, 1927.

[46] *Annual Reports of the Board of Commissioners of Public Charities of the Commonwealth of Pennsylvania* and reports of the Committee on Lunacy for years: 1897, 1898, 1900, 1901, 1902, 1903, 1904, 1905, 1906, 1907, 1908, 1909, 1912.

the Monongahela and Allegheny Rivers attracted the growing immigrant population, many of whom settled in Lawrenceville.[47]

Foreign Born Patients Admitted to St. Francis Psychiatric Department

Year	# Foreign Admissions/ % of Total Admissions	% German	% Irish	% Polish
1892	39/ 33%	41%	38%	8%
1898	29/ 9%	24%	45%	0
1900	41/ 26%	43%	17%	0
1902	40/ 28%	38%	30%	3%
1905	70/ 33%	36%	21%	1%
1906	52/ 26%	40%	31%	6%
1907	56/ 26%	36%	27%	2%
1908	63/ 30%	25%	51%	3%
1909	74/ 31%	27%	26%	1%
1912	65/ 17%	20%	12%	26%

Caring for the foreign populations in Pennsylvania's institutions was of great concern to the Board of Public Charities of the Commonwealth of Pennsylvania. They complained in 1906 that the "invasion of the Commonwealth by foreigners has borne heavily upon our charitable resources ... Allegheny County, in which probably the industrial life is more substantial than at any other point in the state, has had more than its fair share of foreigners to provide for.... foreigners, who when overtaken by misfortune, have been provided for in our charitable institutions, often to the disadvantage of our native born."[48] Foreign patients were blamed for the overcrowding which existed in a number of institutions.[49] Foreigners were viewed as a "conspicuous and unnecessary drain upon the charitable resources of the State ... being often without resources and physically weak, they crowd our large hospitals, when misfortune overtakes them."[50] Locally, in West Penn Hospital, health

---

[47]Nora Faires, "Immigrants and Industry," and Linda K. Pritchard, "The Soul of the City: A Social History of Religion in Pittsburgh," in *City at the Point, Essays on the Social History of Pittsburgh*, ed. Samuel P. Hays, (Pittsburgh: University of Pittsburgh Press, 1989), pp. 7 and 338.

[48]*Annual Report of the Board of Commissioners of Public Charities of the Commonwealth of Pennsylvania*, for year 1906, p. 1.

[49]*Annual Report of the Board of Commissioners of Public Charities of the Commonwealth of Pennsylvania*, for year 1907, p. 1.

[50]*Annual Report of the Board of Commissioners of Public Charities of the Commonwealth of Pennsylvania*, for year 1908, p. 5.

care workers and administrative personnel perceived the immigrant poor as less intelligent, negligent in their personal health habits and, therefore, less deserving of services.[51] This type of nativism did not exist within the Order of the Franciscan Sisters, who initially founded the hospital to care for the foreign-born.

It has already been noted that, in this regard, St. Francis Hospital exemplifies many other Catholic hospitals which were founded to care for newly arrived immigrants. The study of hospitals can serve to reflect values and struggles within society. The hospital can be viewed as a microcosm of the larger society of which it is a part by noting issues of class, ethnicity and race, for example. The evolution of Catholic hospitals mirrors American society's struggles, but from a distinctive vantage point. At least in the nineteenth century, and the first few years of the twentieth century, the study of the Catholic hospital highlights issues of nativism, and portrays one denomination's response to the values of a nativistic and prejudiced society.

1900 to World War II—Indigent Care

By 1921, in spite of increasingly overcrowded conditions and financial instability, the sisters continued to be relentless in their willingness to admit all patients, regardless of their economic circumstances. They described their desire to continue doing the work of their "saintly founder, St. Francis, whose great love for the poor and the sick has been found worthy of emulation throughout the centuries." They absolutely would not "refuse any of the free work for which we are called upon to care."[52] In the 1920s, the only patients not promptly admitted were those who were not in immediate need of hospitalization, or those who could afford to pay and were, therefore, acceptable to any hospital. Paying patients were referred to a less crowded institution for the sake of their own comfort. Their other option was to wait for two to three weeks before admission if they wanted a private room. Private service had been curtailed somewhat in the interest of greater ward facilities.[53] Although the hospital was dependent upon paying patients for their financial

---

[51] Margaret Brindle, "Regardless of the Ability to Pay, The Formation and Limits of Health Care Policy for the Poor, Pittsburgh: 1880–1980," (Ph.D. dissertation, Carnegie Mellon University, 1992), p. 80.

[52] Report of the St. Francis Hospital, June 1, 1921–May 31, 1923, pp. 6, 8, 12.

[53] Workers Confidential Handbook, St. Francis Hospital Campaign, c. 1927.

survival, they were willing to deny them admission in order to have room for the indigent who might not be accepted into other facilities.[54]

The psychiatric patients were less likely to be indigent. All patients were not only committed by themselves or friends, but also were supported by themselves, friends or family until 1906, when the hospital first had to support psychiatric patients. It was not until 1912 that the hospital admitted patients who were supported by the county commissioners, in addition to patients which the hospital supported.

Source of Support for Psychiatric Patients Admitted During the Year.[55]

Year	# Psych. Pts. Admitted	Friends/Self	County Commissioners	Hospital
1906	199	192		7
1907	213	205		8
1909	239	210		29
1912	373	318	4	51
1916	309	265	4	40
1917	283	260	1	22

One plausible reason for the lack of indigent patients in the psychiatric facility may be the existence of a large municipal hospital nearby. In 1909, the Pittsburgh City Home and Hospital at Marshalsea had 623 insane patients, 452 of who were paupers.[56] St. Francis was the only private psychiatric facility in Western Pennsylvania at that time.

St. Francis' general hospital facility provided a far greater percentage of free care than did the psychiatric facility. Although Marshalsea, whose name was changed to the Pittsburgh City Home and Hospital at Mayview in 1916, erected a small building to house a general hospital in 1909, which opened the following year, it was apparently not until the twenties that the general hospital was fully established. In 1917, Pittsburgh's city council passed an ordinance mandating the organization of a visiting staff at Mayview, but it was not until 1923 that the staff was officially appointed. In addition, Mayview

[54]*Workers Confidential Handbook, St. Francis Hospital Campaign,* c. 1927.

[55]*Annual Reports of the Board of Commissioners of Public Charities of the Commonwealth of Pennsylvania* and reports of the Committee on Lunacy for years: 1906, 1907, 1909, 1912, 1916, 1917.

[56]*Annual Reports of the Board of Commissioners of Public Charities of the Commonwealth of Pennsylvania* and reports of the Committee on Lunacy, 1909, p. 21.

was located several miles south of the city, and was not readily accessible. Private hospitals in the city, therefore, provided a fair amount of gratuitous care.[57]

The following tables should give some indication of the service provided to the community. It is interesting to compare St. Francis Hospital with other similar hospitals. Both Mercy and West Penn were similar in size. West Penn and Allegheny General were located fairly close to St. Francis and Mercy was the other large Catholic hospital. St. Francis was a leader in providing free care to the poor of the city, an underlying purpose of the hospital which continued into the post World War II era.

Percentage of Free Care Provided by Area Hospitals[58]

Year	St. Francis	AGH	Mercy	West Penn
1913	46	52	40	37
1914	58		42	38
1915	54	62	46	36

Percentage of Free Care Provided by St. Francis Hospital[59]

Year	Percentage
1916	56.5
1917	49
1918	36
1919	40
1920	30
1921	35
1922	30
1923	37
1926	31[60]

The above figures are calculated by dividing the total number of free days by the total number of patient days. The statistics change somewhat when

[57]R. J. Behan, "History of the Department of Welfare Institutions at Mayview, Especially the General Hospital," 1935; undated history; Both in Mayview State Hospital Archives.

[58]Figures from 1913, 1914, 1915 from _Annual Report of the Board of Commissioners of Public Charities of the Commonwealth of Pennsylvania_, for years 1913, 1914 and 1915; All other figures from _Report of the St. Francis Hospital, June 1, 1921–May 31, 1923_, p. 11.

[59]_Report of the St. Francis Hospital_, June 1, 1921–May 31, 1923, p. 11.

another method is utilized. The percentage of the total number of in-patients who were treated gratuitously was higher for St. Francis Hospital than any of the other three area hospitals for the years 1909, 1913 and 1915 (see table).

Percentage of In-Patients Treated Totally Free[61]

Year	St. Francis	Mercy	West Penn	AGH
1909	60	35	41	51
1913	38	35	38	28
1915	55	48	36	32

St. Francis, as well as the other three area hospitals, accepted patients who were able to pay only part of their fee. St. Francis had a lower percentage of these patients than the other three hospitals, but that can be explained by the fact that they cared for so many patients totally gratuitously.

During the Depression, the sisters continued to care for the indigent. Numerous patients requested that charges be waived.[62] In 1931, 394, or two-thirds of the hospital's 600 beds, were designated as 'public' beds, whereas only 25 percent were private beds and the remaining 10 percent were semi-private. These are astonishing figures in light of the fact that the hospital was so dependent upon paying patients in order to stay solvent. Many of those assigned to public or ward beds were patients who paid minimal rates, however, which suggests that the sisters had made some attempt to make hospitalization affordable during times of economic hardship.[63] By 1935, the hospital provided gratuitous care for 30 percent of their patients. For the quarter ending May 31, 1936, 33 percent of the care the hospital provided was given gratuitously. This was in spite of the fact that the institution's income that year was $128,045.00 and their expenses exceeded $148,668.00.[64] The following year, the percentage of totally free hospital days dropped to 15 percent,[65] but by 1938, that figure had risen to 24.3 percent.[66] The board

---

[61] Statistics from *Annual Report of the Board of Commissioners of Public Charities of the Commonwealth of Pennsylvania*, for years 1909, 1913, 1915.

[62] Minutes, Board of Managers, December 13, 1937.

[63] American College of Surgeons survey 9/31, St. Francis Hospital Archives.

[64] Minutes, Board of Managers, June 26, 1936.

[65] Minutes, Board of Managers, December 31, 1937.

[66] Annual report from St. Francis Hospital to the AMA Council on Medical Education, 2/35 and 2/38, St. Francis Hospital Archives.

noted at the end of the decade that the hospital had lost approximately
$80,000 annually as a result of care given to the indigent.[67]

The sisters were not only insistent that indigent patients be admitted,
but they were adamant about preserving their dignity and their privacy. Few
individuals in the hospital were aware which patients were receiving care
gratuitously. Doctors and nurses were not informed. Only the superintendent and cashier, or perhaps social service workers, knew the charity patients.
Other hospitals run by Franciscan Orders established similar policies. The
sisters felt this would assure that the same attention would be given to all
patients.[68] This stands in sharp contrast to other area hospitals which had
been instituting policies whereby the indigent were separated from paying
patients, and received different forms of care. In other Pittsburgh private
non-sectarian hospitals, the poor were frequently discharged from the hospital earlier than paying patients with similar diagnoses, and were relegated
to the dispensary for care. As a result, in other hospitals, the number of patients seen in the dispensary rose dramatically. It has also been noted that
in other Pittsburgh area hospitals, as the dispensary population rose, the
number of patients admitted dropped accordingly. Implicit in this analysis
is that indigent patients were being cared for in the out-patient department
instead of in the hospitals. For St. Francis Hospital, this does not seem to
have been the case.[69] In fiscal year 1922–1923, the St. Francis dispensary
treated a total of 15,623 patients. In 1934, it treated 12,699, and in 1935,
14,818.[70]

No emergency patient was ever denied immediate treatment, but as soon
as possible an investigation was made which determined whether the patient
would be rated as full-pay, part pay, or a free patient. The credit department
thoroughly investigated "all free cases to see whether they are worthy cases."
Once again, the hospital utilized the term 'worthy' to designate someone without financial means to pay for care.[71] The costs for caring for free patients
were absorbed by the hospital, being paid for by voluntary contributions,

[67]Minutes, Board of Corporators, June 12, 1939.

[68]*Weighing the Evidence*, campaign brochure, 1927; *Workers Confidential Handbook*, St. Francis Hospital
Campaign, c. 1927; See also Sister Francis Cooke, OSF, "History of the Hospital Sisters of the Third Order
of St. Francis," (Ph.D. dissertation, Marquette University, 1943), p. 159, Note: this is a Franciscan Order,
but not of the same origins as the Sisters of St. Francis of Millvale.

[69]Margaret Brindle, "Regardless of Ability to Pay; The Formation and Limits of Health Care Policy for
the Poor, Pittsburgh: 1880–1980," (Ph.D. dissertation, Carnegie Mellon University, 1992), pp. 99–102.

[70]Annual report to the AMA Council on Medical Education, 2/34, 2/35; Annual Report of the St.
Francis Hospital, June 1, 1921–May 31, 1923, p. 24.

[71]Minutes, Board of Managers, December 13, 1937; Interview with Sister M. Adele Meiser, 1993.

state appropriations and the money returned to the hospital due to the gratuitous service of the sisters. The hospital wanted to make it clear to paying patients that they were not being charged extra in order to cover the costs of the gratuitous care provided by the hospital. Paying patients paid for only what they received. Special charges were not absorbed in the basic bed rate with the "consequent injustice to those whose care is relatively simple and inexpensive."[72]

The hospital served the indigent in ways other than in providing health care. During the late twenties, even before the pronounced impact of the Depression, a line of hungry individuals formed daily at the entrance to the hospital's kitchen. The hospital served the poor who were not in need of health services simply by providing them with sustenance.[73] St. John's Hospital in Springfield, Illinois, provided a similar service during the Depression.[74] It seems likely that Catholic hospitals, like St. Francis, were less reluctant to provide such services their inclination to serve the indigent of the community due to their religious beliefs.

1900 to World War II—New Facilities

As the new century progressed, the surrounding community fully utilized the sisters' hospital. This reflects a general trend which was occurring in hospitals across the nation. As medical science was making new discoveries, and as new preventive public health measures were proven to practically eliminate previously common diseases, Americans' attitudes towards hospitals began to change. Patients of all socioeconomic levels began to utilize hospital services, due partially to changes in the industrialized urban environment.[75] Although the hospital records refer to overcrowding in the 1890's, which necessitated the appointment of additional staff, the hospital occupancy rates did not reach over eighty percent until the new century had begun. The average percentage

---

[72]*Weighing the Evidence*, campaign brochure, 1927; *Workers Confidential Handbook*, *St. Francis Hospital Campaign*, c. 1927.

[73]*Weighing the Evidence*, campaign brochure, 1927.

[74]Sister Francis Cooke, OSF, "History of the Hospital Sisters of the Third Order of St. Francis," (Ph.D. Dissertation, Marquette University, 1943), pp. 161–162.

[75]Charles Rosenberg, *The Care of Strangers; The Rise of America's Hospital System*, (New York: Basic Books, Inc., 1987), pp. 342–343; Morris J. Vogel, *The Invention of the Modern Hospital; Boston, 1870–1930*, (Chicago: University of Chicago Press, 1980), p. 119.

of beds occupied on any given day within the year ranged from 83 percent to 96 percent for the first ten years of the new century. This trend characterized the twentieth century. New facilities became a necessity.

The Catholic hospitals of the area continued to be more successful than other hospitals in attracting patients during the first fifteen years of the new century, a crucial period in the development of the hospital as a permanent fixture in American society. Mercy Hospital, for example, maintained an occupancy rate of 88 percent or over for the entire period 1883–1917. It is interesting to note that the Catholic hospitals were able to maintain reasonably successful occupancy rates, whereas the two general hospitals of similar size were not so fortunate. West Penn, which was overcrowded in the latter part of the nineteenth century, suffered a decline in occupancy rates in the twentieth century. It ranged from 57 to 69 percent from 1900 to 1915 (with the exception of 1904 when the occupancy rate was 80 percent). By 1916, West Penn's occupancy rates rose to 95 percent, partially due to the impact of the World War. Allegheny General Hospital followed a similar pattern to that of West Penn with occupancy rates ranging from 40 to 69 percent for the first fifteen years of the century. As noted earlier, the presence of the sisters may have lent some respectability to the institution, which attracted the Catholic working classes. In addition, the non-sectarian hospitals had much stricter admission policies.

As a result of the overcrowding, the sisters obtained funds to build a new wing. Additional property was purchased for $3,850.00 on Forty-fifth Street. The new facility, which cost $900,000.00 to build and was designed by architect Sidney F. Heckert, was blessed by the Rt. Rev. Bishop John Francis Regis Canevin on April 3, 1910. Open house was held the following day from 8:00 A.M. until 9:00 P.M. Approximately three thousand people took advantage of the opportunity to inspect the new hospital.[76] The new wing increased the bed capacity by about 600 beds. With 850 beds, the hospital was one of the largest in the country, aside from state institutions. Big porches and sun parlors were added for convalescing patients. Patients' rooms were furnished with beech furniture, including surgical beds on wheels with telescoping legs. The emergency and operating rooms were furnished in Italian marble. The hospital also boasted having its own power plant, ice plant and disinfecting plant. Seven years later, a roof garden was added for the patients' benefit.[77]

[76]Sister M. Clarissa Popp, History of the Sisters of St. Francis of the Diocese of Pittsburgh, 1868–1938, (Millvale: Sisters of St. Francis, 1939), p. 123.; Sister M. Aurelia Arenth, OSF, p. 121.

[77]"Bishop Will Bless New Hospital Today," Post, 3 April 1910; "Hospital Addition is Ready for Inspection and Use," unknown local newspaper, clipping found in Pennsylvania Room files, Carnegie Library, c.

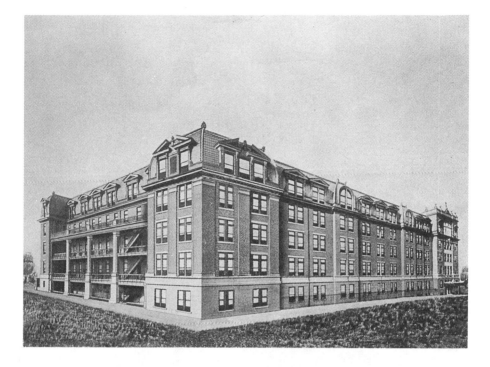

New Addition, Forty-fifth Street Front, 1911

For the first few years after the new building was opened, the occupancy rates dropped to the mid-fifties, but by 1914, the figure once again reached 80 percent. Bed capacity for the general hospital had increased by three hundred beds, which probably accounts for the decline in occupancy rates. By World War I, the rates once again ranged from 87 percent to 89 percent, and by 1920, the hospital was a permanent fixture within the community of Lawrenceville and the surrounding area.[78]

By the early 1920s, St. Francis was established as a thriving hospital in the city, and was generally overcrowded. In order to increase the bed capacity, the sisters enclosed all of the porches and installed a heating system to permit use of the porches during the winter months. In 1915, the hospital had treated 4,008 patients, but by 1923, that number had risen to 7,421. Hospital days

3 April 1910; written history, "St. Francis Hospital," manuscript, n.d., St. Francis Hospital Archives. It is interesting to note that the Annual Report of the Board of Public Charities lists 560 as the total number of beds in 1912. It is not clear why this discrepancy exists.

[78] *Annual Report of the Board of Commissioners of Public Charities of the Commonwealth of Pennsylvania,* for years 1904–1909, 1912–1917.

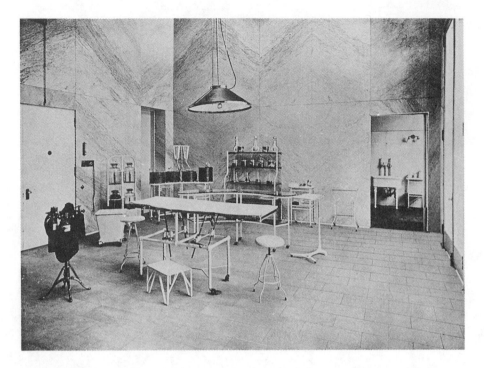

Operating Room, 1913

had also increased from 131,722 in 1915 to 193,694 in 1923. Patients were sometimes given a bed behind a screen in a hallway. It was not unusual for there to be over fifty beds in a ward designed to accommodate thirty patients. Cots were sometimes placed in ward aisles. The hospital which had 600 beds had 709 patients at one time. There was a three week delay for non-emergency private admissions. In contrast, the West Penn and South Side hospitals only maintained occupancy rates of 65 to 70 percent throughout the twenties.[79] Partly as a result of the sister's flexible admission policies, their financial struggles continued unabated.[80]

In response to, and in spite of, these financial difficulties, the sisters were determined to build a new wing to house private and semi-private rooms. They stated this was necessary to continue "to serve the needs of our growing community," as private rooms had been in demand, but clearly this would

[79]Margaret Brindle, "Regardless of Ability to Pay, The Formation and Limits of Health Care Policy for the Poor, Pittsburgh: 1880–1980," (Ph.D. dissertation, Carnegie Mellon University, 1992), p. 78n163.

[80]*Annual Report of the Board of Commissioners of Public Charities of the Commonwealth of Pennsylvania,* for year 1917; *Report of the St. Francis Hospital,* June 1, 1921–May 31, 1923, pp. 6, 8, 12; "For all of Us," building campaign brochure, c. 1927; *Weighing the Evidence,* campaign brochure, c. 1927.

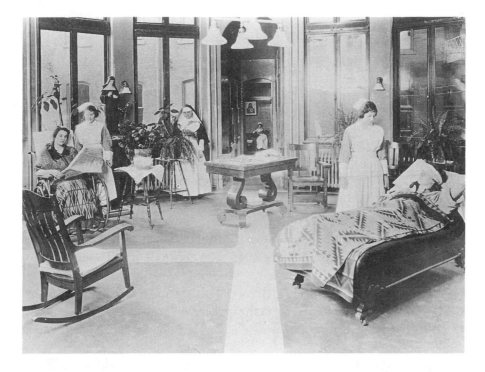

Sun Parlor, 1923

solve some of the monetary problems.[81] At that point, only 150 of 600 beds were in private rooms.[82] Unable to rely on income from investments or large donations, St. Francis relied heavily on income from patients in order to survive. Attracting paying patients was the sisters' primary method of achieving financial solvency.[83]

The physicians, too, felt that additional facilities were imperative in order that the hospital continue to progress. Some of the physicians responded to the problem of overcrowding by discharging their patients as promptly as possible, and then having dispensary physicians supervise their care. Not only was the hospital crowded with in-patients, but the dispensary was not large enough to allow all departments to function at one time. The doctors wanted this because it would have facilitated consultations from one part of the dispensary to another. A rearrangement of hours would also have eliminated the long waits and return visits for patients, often representing a real economic hardship for

[81] *Report of the St. Francis Hospital,* June 1, 1921–May 31, 1923, p. 7.
[82] *For all of Us,* building campaign brochure, c. 1927.
[83] *Report of the St. Francis Hospital,* June 1, 1921–May 31, 1923, p. 12.

them. The Record Room and Department of Physio and Hydrotherapy were in need of larger quarters as well.[84]

Inspectors from the state Department of Welfare also suggested that the board of directors consider an addition to the facility. Following an inspection in 1926 in which the hospital was found to be functioning efficiently, the Secretary of Welfare suggested that an "effort be made to secure active cooperation throughout your community with the ultimate purpose in view for the erection of another unit and a nurses' home."[85]

The need for a nurses' home had been recognized by the sisters even before the Secretary of Welfare's letter. At that time, there were 100 to 150 nurses housed in the hospital. The rest of the nurses were scattered about the district in private homes. At least seventy-five nurses were housed in buildings outside the hospital, making it impossible for the sisters to adequately supervise them. Not only was space needed for housing, but classrooms and demonstration rooms were necessary as well. The sisters wanted to build a nurses' home, but apparently had difficulty locating the necessary lot and felt that an addition to the hospital would alleviate some of the problems. It was evidently anticipated that part of that wing was to be used as either housing for nurses or classroom facilities.[86]

A major building campaign, then, was begun in 1927. Plans called for the erection of a $1.5 million dollar six story building which would add 250 beds. Enlarged industrial wards and new private and semi-private rooms were also planned. There were to be additional ward beds in order to provide more beds at moderate rates. Industrial leaders in the district, business and professional men, former patients and friends of the hospital organized into groups to implement the campaign. At least eight different fund-raising divisions were established, headed by doctors, their wives, industrial leaders and Lawrenceville businessmen. The particular divisions included women's, men's, staff, industrial, church, Lawrenceville business, special gifts and community divisions.

Campaigners appealed to the Roman Catholic community members by focusing on the sacrifices of the sisters, who were "doing in Pittsburgh as did Christ and the Saint under whose name they carry on. They are ... Carrying

[84]*Report of the St. Francis Hospital*, June 1, 1921–May 31, 1923, pp. 14, 23.

[85]Letter from Pennsylvania Department of Welfare Secretary, Ellen C. Potter, M.D., to Charles Muehlbronner, board president, 12/9/26, St. Francis Hospital Archives.

[86]*Report of the St. Francis Hospital*, June 1, 1921–May 31, 1923, p. 50; letter from the Sisters of St. Francis to Cardinal Camillus Laurenti, January 29, 1927; letter from the Sisters of St. Francis to Bishop Boyle, n.d. but c. spring, 1927; *Workers Confidential Handbook, St. Francis Hospital Campaign*, 1927.

forward the banner of the Church, and bringing health and peace to the pain-torn bodies that seek relief at the doors of their St. Francis Hospital. . . . A crisis is upon the Sisters and their hospital. They can do no more. . . . No one knows how soon he will need the Sisters and their hospital—badly."[87] Interestingly, these tactics were only applied within the parish system. Appeals to the public at large downplayed the sisters' roles.

A special appeal was made to the public on May 10–20, 1927, with the goal of raising one million dollars.[88] Donors were assured that none of the money collected would be used to meet campaign expenses or pay hospital debts. Nor would any of the funds collected be used to meet deficiencies created by gratuitous service. Campaigners had been instructed to tell prospective donors that the management felt that the sick should be cared for before the nurses. Although the hospital management wanted to build a nurses' home in the future, they alleged that the 1927 funds would not be used for that purpose.[89] All money was to go into the new building. One of the methods utilized was to offer the opportunity to construct rooms or buy equipment as lasting memorials dedicated to loved ones. Portions of the building could be dedicated and marked with bronze tablets if the donation were appropriate.

The hospital made a clear attempt to appeal to private patients, as it was the income from those patients which supported the hospital. This was a tactic relied on by many hospitals during this period.[90] Appeals were made to the public by emphasizing the hospital's hotel-like atmosphere. Each patient had the same tray, set of dishes and silverware as long as he was in the hospital. The china was dainty, each set different. The rooms were not furnished with typical white enameled beds or stark white curtains. "All was carefully studied color."[91]

The final campaign report, issued in June 1927, noted that approximately $300,000.00 was raised. The nurses division contributed much more than expected with their donations of $33,990.00, and other hospital employees also contributed a substantial amount. Apparently, the returns from the medical staff as well as from local churches were disappointing. Failure to raise adequate funds was attributed to the fact that a suburban hospital had recently

---

[87] *That They May do More*, campaign brochure, n.d. but c. 1927, St. Francis Hospital Archives.

[88] "St. Francis Hospital," history, no author, manuscript, n.d. but c. 1930s, St. Francis Hospital Archives.

[89] *Workers Confidential Handbook, St. Francis Hospital Campaign*, 1927.

[90] Charles Rosenberg, *The Care of Strangers; The Rise of America's Hospital System*, (New York: Basic Books, Inc., 1987), p. 343.

[91] *For all of Us*, building campaign brochure, c. 1927; *The Weekly News of St. Francis Hospital*, V. 1, #2, 4/8/27; *Weighing the Evidence*, campaign brochure, 1927.

had a fund raising drive and, in addition, there was labor unrest in some of the local manufacturing plants.[92]

In the wake of the disappointing campaign, the sisters continued to seek some way to alleviate the overcrowding in the facility. Although the donors had been told that money would not be used to build a home for the nurses, it seemed to be the only solution to the problems, as the erection of such a facility would free up 150 beds in the hospital. In the summer of the following year, land was finally purchased for the erection of a nurses' home. The sisters mortgaged some of their properties, and subsequently planned and built the new residence. Understandably, the new nurses' residence was not erected without some anger and animosity on the part of donors, but the sisters continued undaunted in their mission to serve the sick and the poor. It is worth noting that there were no known resultant lawsuits, which again suggests that sisters often commanded a certain authority just by virtue of their religious calling, and, too, the community must have been aware of the sisters' ultimate goal of providing for the ill and indigent.[93]

The nurses' residence, Mary Immaculate Hall, was formally blessed and dedicated on February 2, 1931. State accreditation for the nursing school had required that nurses' quarters were to be consolidated under one roof. The new twelve story residence, designed by Schmidt, Garden and Erikson, an architectural firm from Chicago, contained about four hundred bedrooms, separate reception and living rooms for students and graduate nurses as well as classrooms, laboratories, a library and school offices. The new residence and property also had an infirmary, courtyard, roof garden, bowling alley, tennis court, swimming pool, skating rink and gymnasium. A tunnel connected the home with the hospital.

Its Gothic design was considered to be an architectural masterpiece. The American Institute of Architects was requested by the Royal Institute of British Architects to prepare an exhibit of "representative and distinguished buildings" to be exhibited in Great Britain. The A. I. A. then decided to prepare a similar and identical exhibit for use throughout the United States. The exhibit, comprised of only one hundred buildings, included the new nurses' residence. The exhibits were to be in circulation for about two and one half years.[94]

---

[92] "Tomorrow ... In Retrospect," printed bulletin, n.d. but c. 1966; "St. Francis Hospital," history, no author, manuscript, n.d. but c. 1930s, Sister Francis Hospital Archives, p. 12.

[93] "Final Report of Campaign," 6/29/27; Letters from Sisters of St. Francis to Bishop Boyle, July 25, 1928 and August 24, 1928; Interview, anonymous.

[94] "Tomorrow ... In Retrospect," printed bulletin, n.d. but c. 1966; Letter from Carl A. Erikson to Sister M. Thomasine, February 24, 1938, St. Francis Hospital archives; *Seventy-fifth Anniversary 1901–1976* (Pittsburgh: St. Francis General Hospital School of Nursing, 1976), p. 8.

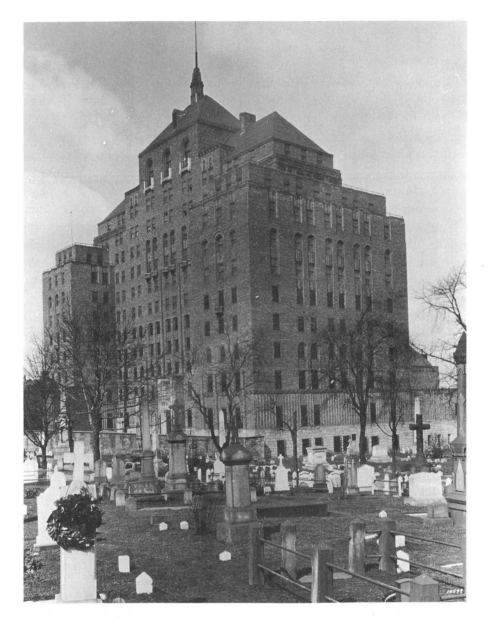

St. Francis Hospital School of Nursing, Mary Immaculate Hall

The average monthly population of the nurses' home suggests that it was not utilized to full capacity, at least in the thirties. In 1935, for example, the building housed 131 students and 53 graduate nurses. The living quarters were also offered to 14 employees as well as to 20 tenants. In 1936, there were 242 people living there, and in 1937, only 221 individuals resided in Mary Immaculate Hall.[95]

The building of the nurses' residence, though oblique in terms of the goals of the capital campaign, did alleviate some of the problems of overcrowding in the hospital. The number of beds for patients was increased as the nurses vacated the main hospital building for Mary Immaculate Hall.[96] Repairs and renovations were made to the main hospital building. The general kitchen was enlarged and a new stove, as well as other up-to-date equipment, was installed. New rubber tile flooring was also added in some areas.[97] A year after the opening of the nurses' home, three wings of the fifth floor were renovated. Other areas were vacated by the nurses and remodeled for patients.[98] It was many years before a building campaign was undertaken again.

During the Depression, Pittsburgh area hospitals were not being utilized to their fullest capacity and, although this was also true of St. Francis Hospital, in light of the overcrowding of the 1920s, the utilization of the facility contrasts markedly with other area hospitals. The social study of Pittsburgh discovered that the average occupancy rates in 1928, 1933 and 1934 for twenty-five voluntary general hospitals in Pittsburgh and Allegheny County were 72 percent, 55 percent and 56 percent respectively.[99] Occupancy rates in the state-supported public hospitals offering free care had occupancy rates of 91 percent. West Penn and South Side Hospitals averaged 55 to 60 percent occupancy rates during the Depression.[100] These figures are explained by the fact that due to financial hardships, paying patients were reluctant to enter the hospital, and hospitals were somewhat resistant to accepting too many free patients; many of them had overbuilt in the twenties, incurring enormous debts.[101] In contrast, in fiscal year June 1930 to May 1931, the St. Francis

[95]Minutes, Board of Managers, December 13, 1937.

[96]Written History, "St. Francis Hospital," manuscript, n.d. but c. 1940, St. Francis Hospital Archives.

[97]Written History, "St. Francis Hospital," manuscript, n.d. but c. 1940, St. Francis Hospital Archives, pp. 13–15.

[98]Popp, p. 134.

[99]Philip Klein, A Social Study of Pittsburgh, Community Problems and Social Services of Allegheny County, (New York: Columbia University Press, 1938), pp. 744–745.

[100]Margaret Brindle, "Regardless of Ability to Pay, The Formation and Limits of Health Care Policy for the Poor, Pittsburgh: 1880–1980," (Ph.D. dissertation, Carnegie Mellon University, 1992), p. 78n163.

[101]Philip Klein, A Social Study of Pittsburgh, Community Problems and Social Services of Allegheny County, (New York: Columbia University Press, 1938), p. 758; Margaret C. Albert, A Practical Vision: The Story of

Hospital boasted an 84 percent occupancy rate.[102] There is some indication that, like local hospitals, occupancy dropped in the early thirties, but the change was less pronounced and existed for a shorter period of time than for other local area hospitals. The number of hospital days recorded in fiscal year 1931 was 184,083, compared to 130,381 in 1936.[103] By 1938, however, the average occupancy rate in the hospital was 89 percent.[104] The contrasting figures shown by St. Francis Hospital reflect the sisters' flexible admission policy. St. Francis Hospital, unlike many other church affiliated institutions, however, was able to remain financially solvent, at least enough to remain open. Between 1928 and 1936, 11 percent of all church sponsored hospitals closed, primarily due to economic hardships.[105]

1900 to World War II—Revenue and Expenditures

In order for the sisters to develop their hospital so that they could carry on their mission, they had to consider financial matters which sometimes forced them to compromise their Catholic beliefs. In some instances, the fact that women religious managed the hospital worked to the benefit of the hospital financially. St. Francis Hospital, representative of other Catholic hospitals, often did not have the revenue of some of the private general hospitals, and were forced to find other non-traditional ways to supplement their income. Seemingly, too, their expenditures were lower than other private hospitals for reasons not yet understood, except that private hospitals were able to invest part of their revenue. In light of these differences between Catholic and private non-sectarian hospitals, St. Francis serves as a striking example of how Catholic hospitals developed quite differently from the private and public general hospitals which have previously been studied. The following table of number of beds in each hospital will be helpful in understanding tables further on in this chapter.

Blue Cross of Western Pennsylvania, 1937–1987, (Pittsburgh: Blue Cross of Western Pennsylvania, 1987), p. 2.

[102] American College of Surgeons, survey form, St. Francis Hospital Archives.

[103] American College of Surgeons, survey form; Annual report to the AMA Council on Medical Education, 2/36, St. Francis Hospital Archives.

[104] Minutes, Board of Managers, September 12, 1938.

[105] Christopher Kauffman, "Church and Society: Developments During the Schwitalla Years, 1928–1947," *Health Progress* 71 (May 1990): 34.

Total Number of Beds[106]

Year	St. Francis	Mercy	West Penn	AGH
1883	130	60	106	
1898	200	208	250	
1899	200	208	225	120
1900	200	242	275	
1901	215	245	300	120
1903	189	275	350	120
1904	187	315	275	
1905	206	320	312	350
1906	236	359	312	
1907	236	359	312	350
1908	250	362	314	
1909	250	370	312	350
1912	560	360	400	
1913	560	376	450	420
1915	450	375	450	432
1916	450	375	450	
1917	485	375	460	

Compared to private general hospitals, St. Francis Hospital, like other Catholic hospitals, was reliant on different sources of revenue in order to maintain its institution. Both Mercy Hospital and St. Francis Hospital received a far greater percentage of their income from patients than did either West Penn or Allegheny General Hospital from 1895 until approximately 1913. Although typical of Catholic hospitals, this is a startling fact when considering the amount of gratuitous care which the hospitals provided.[107] The non-sectarian general hospitals were much more successful in supplementing their patient income with money from investments, donations and state and municipal funding. By 1913, however, the Catholic hospitals began to receive an equitable portion of their revenue from the state, and the general hospitals began to receive a greater portion of their revenue from patients.

---

[106] Annual Report of the Board of Commissioners of Public Charities of the Commonwealth of Pennsylvania, for years 1883, 1898, 1899, 1900, 1901, 1903, 1904, 1905, 1906, 1907, 1908, 1909, 1912, 1913, 1915, 1916, 1917.

[107] Gail Farr Casterline, "St. Joseph's and St. Mary's: The Origins of Catholic Hospitals in Philadelphia," Pennsylvania Magazine of History and Biography (July 1984): 292.

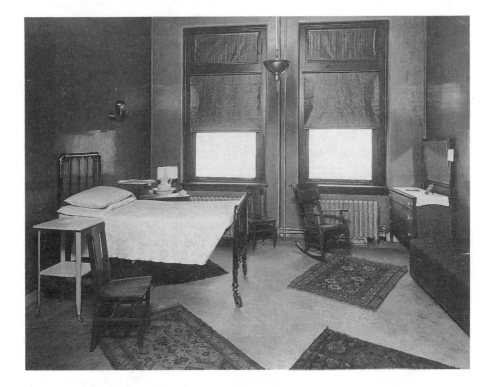

Private Patient Room, 1913

Percentage of Revenue from Patients[108]

Year	St. Francis	Mercy	West Penn	AGH
1895	94	51	27	
1897	99	73	15	
1898	95	76	31	
1899	98	70	30	31
1901	92	66	43	28
1903	90	29	46	42
1905	88	22	39	49
1907	89	64	31	49
1909	68	53	41	43
1912	40	70	53	
1913	50	67	58	44
1914	40	65	58	
1915	45	62	60	37
1917	56	44	55	

In the early twenties, St. Francis continued to rely on patient income. In the year June 1, 1921, to May 31, 1922, the income from full pay patients represented 51 percent of the total receipts. The income from partial pay patients represented an additional 34 percent of the revenue.[109]

The two Catholic hospitals, unlike West Penn and Allegheny General, throughout the period 1899–1915 received very little financial reward from investments or donations. St. Francis and Mercy both credited investments with only 1 percent or less of their revenue for the period. Investments were responsible for 6 to 23 percent of West Penn's revenue, and 1 to 10 percent of Allegheny General's revenue. Donations for the general operating expenses of the hospitals were minimal for all four institutions, but represented a higher portion of operating revenue for the general hospitals. Donations to St. Francis were never higher than 3 percent of its income. Donations to Mercy were similar with the exception of 1901, when 7 percent of its operating revenue was due to donations. Donations to the other institutions generally ranged from 3 to 8 percent, but going as high as 31 percent (Allegheny General, 1901) and 23 percent (West Penn). By 1940, St. Francis continued to receive minimal amounts in the form of donations and contributions from outside sources.[110] Other historians have noted that Catholic hospitals did not fare as well in donations as other hospitals because they often were established to serve working class immigrant populations who received low wages and were unable to contribute very much. In addition, Catholics were often required to support parish priests and schools as well.[111]

Percentage of Revenue from Donations[112]

Year	St. Francis	Mercy	West Penn	AGH
1899	1	0	2	4
1901	0	7	2	31
1903	0	3	4	7
1905	3	1	8	6
1907	0	0.3	23	0.4

[108]Statistics from *Annual Report of the Board of Commissioners of Public Charities of the Commonwealth of Pennsylvania*, for years 1895, 1897, 1898, 1899, 1901, 1903, 1905, 1907, 1909, 1912, 1913, 1915, 1917. Note: between 1902 and 1905 Mercy hospital had a capital fund raising campaign in order to erect a new East wing in 1903 and St. Anne's Hall in 1905. This helps to explain the decrease in percentage of income due to patient fees in 1903 and 1905. The actual monetary amount in 1903 was $64,509.00, and in 1901 it was $64,811.00. They reported that 49 percent of revenue in 1903 and 52 percent of revenue in 1905 came from outside sources.

[109]*Report of the St. Francis Hospital*, June 1, 1921–May 31, 1923, p. 12.

[110]Minutes, Board of Corporators, June 1940.

Percentage of Income From Investments[113]

Year	St. Francis	Mercy	West Penn	AGH
1899	1	1	23	5
1901	0	1	15	1
1903	0	0	11	10
1905	0	0	13	2
1907	0	0	7	6
1909	0	0.1	8	5
1913	0.1	0	6	3
1915	0.1	0	0	3

The fact that a greater percentage of income came from patients does not suggest that financial concerns were limited. The Catholic hospitals, in fact, were plagued for years with financial difficulties. An analysis of receipts and expenditures per bed shows that the hospital had far fewer financial resources than West Penn, Allegheny General or even Mercy Hospital, although Mercy, too, had financial limitations. The following tables should help to clarify this point. Clearly, deficit spending was a common practice for all of the institutions, but these data should also elucidate the fact that St. Francis was functioning with little financial flexibility.

Income/ Expenditures in Dollars—Per Bed[114]

	St. Francis	Mercy		West Penn	AGH
1899	$181/181	307	/305	555/502	462/454
1901	140/199	401	/418	387/383	485/567
1903	181/256	815	/815	338/392	358/416
1905	204/265	932	/932	368/430	193/258[115]
1907	247/273	40[116]	/357	633/563	476/489
1909	257/348	395	/394	399/411	482/501
1913	300/325	449	/502	543/667	504/555
1915	375/373	420	/531	664/534	481/543

[111]Gail Farr Casterline, "St. Joseph's and St. Mary's: The Origins of Catholic Hospitals in Philadelphia," *Pennsylvania Magazine of History and Biography* (July 1984): 292.

[112]Statistics from *Annual Report of the Board of Commissioners of Public Charities of the Commonwealth of Pennsylvania*, for years 1899, 1901, 1903, 1905, 1907. Donations from 1909–1915 dropped off considerably for all four hospitals.

[113]Statistics from *Annual Report of the Board of Commissioners of Public Charities of the Commonwealth of Pennsylvania*, for years 1899, 1901, 1903, 1905, 1907, 1909, 1913, 1915.

It is difficult to determine how other hospitals were spending accumulated revenue. Clearly, private general hospitals utilized a more sizable operating budget than the Catholic hospitals. Costs per diem or costs per patient per week were sometimes twice as high in the non-sectarian institutions. It was not until 1921 that St. Francis' per diem rates exceeded those of Allegheny General Hospital in 1915. In 1925, the hospital operated at a per diem cost 40 percent lower than the average for all hospitals in the United States.[117]

Average Cost Per Patient Per Week[118]

Year	St. Francis	Mercy	West Penn	AGH
1899	$5.85	$ 4.98	$12.88	$10.95
1901	9.17	7.07	10.16	12.53
1903	5.31	8.45	9.80	13.37
1905	6.54	10.36	13.23	16.72
1907	6.00	9.56	12.74	13.51
1909	6.65	8.33	13.09	14.87
1913	10.22	11.48	11.90	15.68
1915	9.24	10.50	13.16	14.70
1916	8.96			
1917	11.13			
1918	13.65			
1919	13.86			
1920	14.00			
1921	17.92			
1922	15.75			
1923	19.74			

[114]These statistics were compiled by dividing the receipts and expenditures by the number of beds in the institution. Data from the *Annual Report of the Board of Commissioners of Public Charities of the Commonwealth of Pennsylvania*, for years 1899, 1901, 1903, 1905, 1907, 1909, 1913, 1915.

[115]This was the first year following a major addition to the hospital. AGH had 120 beds until 1905 when they had 350 beds.

[116]The total receipts listed for this year were $14,000.00, a figure quite inconsistent with other years. A typographical error is suspected.

[117]"Increased Capacity to Make Institution Largest of Class in Country," *Gazette Times*, 4 April 1927.

[118]*Annual Report of the Board of Commissioners of Public Charities of the Commonwealth of Pennsylvania*, for years 1899, 1901, 1903, 1905, 1907, 1909, 1913, 1915; *Report of the St. Francis Hospital*, June 1, 1921–May 31, 1923, p. 43 (for years 1916–1923).

Even by examining the records of the Board of Public Charities in order to ascertain why the private general hospitals were spending so much more per patient, the question remains unanswerable because there are so many variables to consider. Although these were Pittsburgh's four largest hospitals throughout most of this period, their bed capacities were never exactly the same, so precise comparisons are difficult.[119] In addition, it is not always clear in the records just what the various categories of expenditures meant. For example, in 1913, hospitals reported figures for ordinary and extraordinary expenses separately from patients' provisions, medical-surgical supplies, or ambulance service (which were listed together with expenses for painting, water, printing and telephone). Hospitals may not have followed the same guidelines for recording in the various categories.

The one clear difference does seem to be the expense for salaries. Catholic hospitals were able to conserve some of their revenue by paying the sisters very low salaries, just enough for their own maintenance. Because the sisters performed most of the housekeeping, administrative and nursing duties, St. Francis, similar to other Catholic hospitals, spent a slightly lower percentage of their income on salaries and wages. Mercy Hospital, as well, spent a smaller percentage of their expenditures on salaries and wages.

Percentage of Expenditures Spent on Salaries and Wages[120]

Year	St. Francis	Mercy	West Penn	AGH
1901	27	25	29	23
1903	24	12	27	33
1905	25	10	30	38
1907	24	24	23	36
1909	29	26	34	39
1913	34	31	37	37
1915	29	25	33	35

[119]The Homeopathic Hospital in Shadyside reported 125 beds in 1901, 5 more than Allegheny General, but within four years AGH expanded and reported 350 beds. By 1915, these four hospitals were clearly Pittsburgh's largest.

[120]Statistics from *Annual Report of the Board of Commissioners of Public Charities of the Commonwealth of Pennsylvania*, for years 1901, 1903, 1905, 1907, 1909, 1913, 1915. Note, again, that in 1903 and 1905, the statistics for Mercy hospital were quite low, reflecting expenses incurred while expanding their physical plant.

Salaries and Wages, Actual Cost to Institution[121]

Year	St. Francis	Mercy	West Penn	AGH
1899	$ 6,947	$17,526	$ 30,277	$15,078
1901	11,722	25,445	33,140	15,333
1903	11,645	25,915	36,708	16,751
1905	13,430	30,757	40,930	33,981
1907	15,190	30,939	40,993	61,863
1909	25,506	37,287	43,506	69,129
1913	48,621	48,840	79,123	82,375
1915	61,038	58,839	111,031	85,760

In subsequent years when the hospital was having difficulty making ends meet, it would forego payment to the sisters. In 1939, for example, the Board of Managers delayed payment of the sisters' salaries because of a "low bank balance."[122] At times, however, the sisters had to insist they receive a portion of their salaries in order to maintain the Motherhouse. In 1942, the sisters suggested to the board that the salaries in arrears in the amount of $158,000.00 be reduced to $100,000.00. They negotiated with the board that $25,000.00 be paid immediately. That payment was to be followed by a series of thirty-six thirty day non-interest bearing promissory notes of $2,000.00 each, followed by a note of $3,000.00. They were sympathetic with the hospital board's financial hardships, but they had to "relieve the dire needs of the Motherhouse which have accumulated during the past ten years."[123]

St. Francis apparently was not in any position to make investments in the first ten years of the twentieth century, not a surprising fact as its income was so meager. Mercy Hospital's reports also reflect an inability to invest money, but that was not the case for the two general hospitals. In 1907, West Penn invested $40,000.00, reflecting 23 percent of their expenses. Between 1899 and 1905, Allegheny General Hospital invested regularly, with annual investments ranging from $818.00 to $2,614.00.[124]

---

[121] *Annual Report of the Board of Commissioners of Public Charities of the Commonwealth of Pennsylvania,* for years 1899, 1901, 1903, 1905, 1907, 1909, 1913, 1915.

[122] Minutes, Board of Managers, 3/13/39.

[123] Letter to William Brant from the Sisters of St. Francis of Millvale, November 17, 1942, Motherhouse Archives.

[124] *Annual Report of the Board of Commissioners of Public Charities of the Commonwealth of Pennsylvania,* for years 1899, 1901, 1903, 1905, 1907.

1900 to World War II—State Appropriation and Non-Sectarian Status

St. Francis was, by necessity, reliant on money from the Commonwealth. In the early 1920s, Pennsylvania decreased the hospital's appropriation by 30 percent. In 1917, St. Francis had received $85,000.00 from the Commonwealth, but from June 1921 to June 1922, the state gave the hospital only $63,465.00. More importantly, that figure in 1917 represented 40 percent of the total receipts; but in 1921, it dropped to 15 percent of the total revenue.[125]

Percentage of Revenue From the State or Municipality[126]

Year	St. Francis	Mercy	West Penn	AGH
1899	0	16	35	27
1901	8	10	34	39
1903	10	20	35	41
1905	9	25	36	41
1907	11	34	34	45
1909	31	34	50	52
1912	22	24	35	
1913	30	30	29	40
1915	52	35	28	48
1917	40	34	27	

Regardless of the decrease in the state's appropriation, it was a necessary asset which the sisters could not do without. In 1929, the sum of $160,000.00 was appropriated for the hospital for the two fiscal years beginning June 1, 1929, for the purpose of maintenance of medical and surgical patients who received gratuitous care. Shortly thereafter, The Constitution Defense League brought charges against the hospital, Charles A. Waters, Auditor General of Pennsylvania, and Edward Martin, State Treasurer of Pennsylvania, for violation of Section 18, Article III of the Constitution of Pennsylvania, which

---

[125] *Annual Report of the Board of Commissioners of Public Charities of the Commonwealth of Pennsylvania,* for year 1917; *Report of the St. Francis Hospital,* June 1, 1921–May 31, 1923, pp. 6, 8, 12.

[126] Statistics from *Annual Report of the Board of Commissioners of Public Charities of the Commonwealth of Pennsylvania,* for years 1899, 1901, 1903, 1905, 1907, 1909, 1912, 1913, 1915, 1917.

provides as follows: "No appropriations except for pensions or gratuities for military services, shall be made for charitable, educational or benevolent purposes, to any person or community, nor to any denominational or sectarian institution, corporation or association." Claiming that St. Francis Hospital was a sectarian hospital, the plaintiffs believed the hospital did not have the right to state funds. Testimony was presented in Harrisburg on October 16, 1930. The plaintiffs' attorney argued that the presence of a chapel, statues and crucifixes, as well as the existence of sisters in administrative roles, were ample proof that the hospital was sectarian. The defendants' attorneys responded by suggesting that the hospital had always been non-sectarian in its service, as well as in its management. The board was comprised of lay members of various denominations, and the hospital had a long standing policy of accepting any patient for admission, regardless of religious affiliation. Statistics from the period supported the defendant attorneys' arguments. In 1933, forty-nine of the physicians on staff were Protestant, compared to only thirteen Catholic doctors. Five doctors were Jewish. Of a total of 334 patients in the hospital on June 1, 1933, 138 were Protestant and 188 were Catholic. There is no doubt that the hospital, in reality, was non-sectarian in service.[127] The judge, however, ruled in favor of the plaintiff.[128] Apparently $125,000.00 was finally appropriated in 1934, but the Constitution Defense League once again "endeavored to get the Auditor General and State Treasurer to hold up the appropriations."[129] In July 1937, Judge Frank B. Wickersham, Dauphin county court, finally found the St. Francis Hospital to be a non-sectarian hospital. The hospital was able to receive aid in the amount of $156,250.00 retroactive for the biennium June 1, 1933–May 31, 1935, and also for the biennium June 1, 1935–May 31, 1937.[130] It is important to note that although the sisters received no appropriation from the state for nine years, there is no evidence to suggest that they altered their admission policies.

During this period, the board of managers or the administration made some attempt to alter the sectarian appearance of the hospital by advising the sisters to remove or relocate crucifixes, statues or paintings of a religious

[127]Notes in manuscript, June 1, 1933, St. Francis Hospital Archives.

[128]Record in the Court of Common Pleas of Dauphin County between Constitutional Defense League and Charles A. Waters, Edward Martin and St. Franciscus Hospital of Pittsburgh, St. Francis Hospital Archives.

[129]Letter to "Dear Friend" from the Constitution Defense League, Willis Collins, secretary, dated January 1934, forwarded to the hospital by a satisfied non-Catholic patient who sent a copy of the letter anonymously.

[130]Minutes, Board of Corporators, June 13, 1938; "St. Francis Wins $156,250.00 State Aid," local unidentified newspaper article, July 1937.

nature. Some of the sisters were opposed, so Mother M. Chrysostom sought advice from Bishop Hugh Boyle. He responded by stating that "as the servants of the board of directors at St. Francis Hospital, your sisters will be compelled, of course, to obey whatever directives are given them by the board. If some directives seem to be unreasonable … you are free, upon giving proper notice to the board of directors … to withdraw the sisters, and to allow the board to continue the hospital work as it sees fit. … Your only relief from the exactions of the board is the resignation of your sisters as its servants in the conduct of the hospital."[131] Sister Adele recalled seeing the piles of crucifixes which had been removed. Sister, who was very open minded and enlightened, was supportive of the action. She understood that a Jewish patient, for example, would have no desire to be in a hospital room surrounded by symbols from a different religion. Her patients were always her first concern. Crucifixes were available in patient drawers for those who desired them. Clearly, the sisters were not attempting to proselytize; they merely wanted to provide care.[132]

In 1936, it was deemed advisable to transfer the title of all of the property held by the sisters to the board of directors. Apparently, titles to the nursing home and laboratory were not transferred at that time. In December of that year it was decided to lease those two sites for a period of 99 years for one dollar per year.[133]

In spite of the fact that the sisters were motivated by their religious beliefs, they were willing to transfer the title of their properties, and to declare that their hospital was non-sectarian, in order to receive state aid, so necessary to their day-to-day operation. In the early 1950s, when surveyed, they claimed to be a "corporation, not-for-profit," not a church operation or church affiliated institution.[134]

World War II to 1977

As the nation was thrust into a second world war, the concerns of the hospital board and administration had begun to expand. During the years prior to World War Two, the hospital focused primarily on staying solvent financially.

---

[131]Letter from Bishop Hugh Boyle to Mother M. Chrysostom, January 3, 1930, Motherhouse Archives, Millvale.
[132]Interview with Sister M. Adele Meiser, 10/26/93.
[133]Minutes, Board of Managers, September 4, December 18, 1936, April 12, 1937.
[134]AHA survey, year ending 9/30/50.

Its primary goals of the period were to provide medical care for anyone in need, and to develop educational services for nurses and physicians, a topic which will be addressed later. Following the war, the hospital's financial struggles continued, but were alleviated occasionally. A heightened interest in developing the physical plant characterizes the period from the mid-forties to the late seventies. Characteristic of this period also was the desire on the part of administration, physicians and the board to improve and expand medical care and services. This is not to suggest that improvement in medical services was not a priority before the war. To be sure, the sisters acquired the most up-to-date diagnostic equipment, a subject to be addressed later, but major expenditures were not feasible. Medical technology had expanded dramatically after the war, requiring hospitals to modernize. In addition, the hospital broadened its scope and became much more involved in the community. The sisters were successful in preserving their authority so that the hospital's spiritual mission would continue. The tension inherent in maintaining a balance between developing a modern medical center and continuing to meet spiritual goals persisted.

Management and administration of the hospital continued much as it did before the war. The board continued to leave the daily management of the hospital in the hands of the administration. For example, when the Pennsylvania State Nurses' Association recommended that nurses' salaries be increased and their hours be decreased, they left the matter "to the discretion of administration" even though the board was anxious regarding their payroll, which exceeded $40,000.00 in 1950.[135] The sisters also played another role by directly aiding the board in alleviating financial hardships. The sisters occasionally gave money to the board when they were able. For example, in 1949, the Motherhouse paid $20,000.00 to Mellon National Bank and Trust Company against the mortgage. In 1951, when the board had agreed to curtail all spending, they gave the board an additional $35,000.00.[136]

World War II to 1977—Financial Issues

The board of managers was relatively ineffective as a fund raising body. Historically, soliciting funds had always been difficult. Problems in raising donations earlier in the century have already been cited, and were due primarily to the

[135]Minutes, Board of Managers, 12/11/50.
[136]Minutes, Board of Managers, May 14, July 11 and Nov. 19, 1951; Minutes, Board of Corporators, June 6, 1949.

demographics of the Lawrenceville area. In the fifties, however, the hospital suffered because of weak leadership. Although the board members were fine, respected, successful businessmen they did not "fit into the bracket of top community leadership." The hospital's major problems regarding fund raising were due to "the lack of position, community wide, of the board members."[137]

There were other explanations for the hospital's poor financial situation. The St. Francis Women's auxiliary, traditionally a fund raising organization in many hospitals, was small and "comparatively inactive." The Women's auxiliary had been established by Sister M. Beata, who had been appointed by Sister Thomasine, and her friend Mrs. William C. Eichenlaub in 1937 in an attempt to raise funds in the absence of the expected state appropriation. They recruited friends who were interested in helping the hospital. The auxiliary's primary objective was to raise funds for the building and maintenance of a new children's department.[138] They held only two functions a year. Ordinarily, a hospital the size of St. Francis would have had a strong women's group which could have been used as a nucleus for a public relations and fund raising group. The hospital board was advised to initiate a membership drive to increase the membership from two hundred members to five or six hundred members, and to broaden the services to the hospital. As a result, the auxiliary gradually became more active, establishing a wide range of services including a gift cart, a used clothing shop and the gift shop. Other fund raising activities included a dinner dance, bridge luncheons and auctions. Their methods proved to be fruitful, for in 1955, they pledged $400,000.00 for the development of the new South Wing.[139]

Financial struggles, clearly, characterized St. Francis Hospital's entire history. Interestingly, the hospital's costs per patient continued to be comparatively low, which was felt by the board to be due to the presence of the large psychiatric department. The psychiatric patients required fewer services than general hospital patients.[140] This, however, failed to adequately lessen monetary problems. The sisters continued to rely heavily on patient income to

[137]"Analysis of the Situation," manuscript in 'scrapbook' of campaign material, 1954–60, St. Francis Hospital Archives; Early in the fifties, a survey was done of the hospital, its administrators, board members and representative physicians of the medical staff. Those conducting the survey also met with community leaders, executives of different health and welfare organizations, merchants, industrialists, professional men and representatives of 'many walks of life.' Please note that it is not clear who the individuals were who conducted the survey, but the language of the survey suggests that they were outsiders in relation to the institution. Minutes, Board of Managers, 5/23/55.

[138]*St. Francis* (spring 1950); *Signs of Life* (Summer–Fall 1967).

[139]"Analysis of the Situation," manuscript in 'scrapbook' of campaign material, 1954–60, St. Francis Hospital Archives; "The History of the Auxiliary of St. Francis Health System," (Pittsburgh: St. Francis Health System, c. 1985).

[140]Minutes, Board of Managers, 3/12/51.

make ends meet, as the state appropriation paled in comparison. In 1942, for example, income from in-patients represented 85 percent of the total income, whereas the state appropriation represented 7.7 percent of total income.[141] In 1948 and 1950, state funds only represented 5 percent of the total income.[142] In 1949, 62 percent of the total income was due to room and board fees.[143] A year later, income from patients represented 84 percent of the total income.[144] In 1950, Blue Cross accounted for almost 45 percent of the revenue. Although St. Francis continued to rely on income from patients' room and board for a substantial portion of its income, payments were not necessarily coming directly from patients, but from third party payment systems. The hospital, however, returned much of that income to the community. In the mid-sixties, the hospital's largest expenditure was that of personnel salaries. Over two-thirds of the hospital's income was returned to the community through its payroll, but the remaining one third was often inadequate to meet operating expenses and overhead.[145]

Regardless of the hospital's financial struggles, it never lagged in its goal of serving the community. Maintaining a balance between providing care to the indigent and surviving financially continued. Following the Depression, the amount of gratuitous service provided, the cost of which was absorbed by the hospital, decreased substantially. The board noted in 1943 and 1944 that the cash loss from providing free care had decreased considerably compared to the previous years, due to the increase in employment rates in the area and hospitalization plans. If it were not for those plans and state aid, however, most of the patients would still have fit into the classification of charity.[146]

World War II to 1977—The Public Image

During the post war years, the hospital had other difficulties, including a need for improved public relations. A new generation of patients, backed by insurance coverage, showed signs of being more selective. While Americans were

[141]"Miscellaneous Statistics and Report of Income," St. Francis Hospital Archives.

[142]AHA Survey, year ending 9/30/50.

[143]Minutes, Board of Managers, May 1949.

[144]AHA survey, year ending 9/30/50; St. Francis Hospital Archives.

[145]" St. Francis General Hospital, Renovation Fund Program," public relations dept., manuscript, n.d. but c. 1965, St. Francis Hospital Archives, 1965.

[146]Minutes, Board of Corporators, June 14, 1943, June 12, 1944; Minutes, Board of Managers, 1948.

largely passive in their view of hospitals in general, Pittsburghers were also unaware of the degree or scope of work accomplished in St. Francis Hospital. During the 1950s, the community considered the hospital to be either a psychiatric facility or a "poor man's institution."[147] Many patients were often reluctant to be admitted because of its reputation. In order to clarify the hospital's function to the community,[148] the name of the corporation was formally changed in 1955 to the St. Francis General Hospital and Rehabilitation Institute.[149]

Community members had formed other opinions regarding the hospital. Its financial problems were relatively unknown as many felt the hospital was not in need of monetary assistance because it was a recipient of state aid. Some observed that the hospital stuck too close to tradition and was reluctant to change. These perceptions complicated any kind of fund raising campaign from the start.[150]

These community perceptions regarding the hospital may have been due to the reluctance of the administration to be publicity conscious.[151] It is not surprising that the sisters did not seek publicity for the hospital, for the historical analysis of the hospital's early periods suggests that the sisters themselves chose to maintain a low profile. They did not customarily advertise their hospital. It is conceivable that, to them, publicizing their achievements was suggestive of a lack of humility.

Many physicians within the community may also have had an unfavorable perception of the institution. In the early fifties, the medical staff, although considered to be "top flight," was quite small. A great majority of the patients were cared for by only a few physicians, and most of the doctors had primary affiliations at other area hospitals. In addition, few physicians felt any loyalty toward the hospital. This may reflect a long standing problem, as it was noted after the 1920s building campaign that the medical staff donated a disappointingly small amount of money to the fund. They did, however, pledge $430,000, to the building campaign in 1955.[152] There is some suggestion that the medical staff did not always live up to their responsibilities,

---

[147]Minutes, Board of Managers, 1948.

[148]Campaign material, "Analysis of the situation," 1950's scrapbook, St. Francis Hospital Archives.

[149]Recorded in the office for the recording of Deeds, March 1, 1955, Charter Book Vol. 75, p. 289.

[150]"Analysis of the Situation," manuscript in 'scrapbook' of campaign material, 1954–60, St. Francis Hospital Archives.

[151]"Analysis of the Situation," manuscript in 'scrapbook' of campaign material, 1954–60, St. Francis Hospital Archives.

[152]"Analysis of the Situation," manuscript in 'scrapbook' of campaign material, 1954–60, St. Francis Hospital Archives; Minutes, Board of Managers, 7/25/55.

especially those at the lower end of the hierarchy. For example, the board expressed concern over the fact that there was a lack of attendance of doctors working in the dispensary in 1952 and 1953.[153] The physician's lack of loyalty and dedication, and the limited number of doctors seeking privileges at St. Francis suggests that they, too, shared some of the community's views. To be sure, however, this would not have applied to all members of the medical staff, many of whom were devoted to the institution.

In 1962, the charter was once again amended. Apparently the board and administration felt the need to clarify their changing perception of the hospitals' mission. The name of the corporation was changed to the "St. Francis General Hospital." In addition, paragraph two of the Articles of Incorporation, which stated the purpose of the corporation, was expanded to state that the hospital was to include four branches or divisions. The medical and surgical division was "for the care of persons suffering from illness or disability which requires that the patients receive hospital care, both as inpatients and as outpatients." The Rehabilitation Institute was "for the physical and mental rehabilitation of patients, physical and occupational therapy, both as inpatients and outpatients, and treatment in all branches of physical medicine." The purpose of the third division, the psychiatric hospital, was "the care, treatment and rehabilitation of mental and alcoholic patients." The inclusion of 'alcoholic patients,' is an important point worth noting which will be discussed in greater depth in a later chapter. The fourth branch was the education and research division which included, but was not limited to, the schools for registered and practical nurses. The division's purpose was also to "promote and carry on scientific research; to participate, so far as circumstances may warrant, in any activity designed and carried on to promote the general health and welfare of the community which the Board of Managers may from time to time establish, not inconsistent with this charter ... "[154] These changes reflect the administration's and board's desire to expand the hospital's services within the community. Interestingly, the by-laws, which remained relatively the same as those approved in 1955, again made no mention of the sisters of the Order who had founded and managed the hospital for almost a century.[155]

[153] Minutes, Medical Staff, 3/3/53.
[154] Notice given of intention to apply on March 27, 1962, to the Court of Common Pleas of Allegheny County, copy in St. Francis Hospital Archives.
[155] By-laws adopted and approved February 26, 1962.

World War II to 1977—The Maintenance of Authority

During the fifties, tension arose between the sisters and certain board members who wanted increasing involvement in the administration of the hospital. The sisters, unwilling to tolerate any encroachment upon their authority, were compelled to put into a legal document a policy which had been unwritten, and yet understood, for almost a century. The board had always appointed a sister to be the superintendent of the hospital. The hospital charter, although it made a provision for the establishment of a board, never fully stated who would serve as the administrators or chief executive officers of the hospital, probably because it was not deemed necessary by the sisters who had remained in authority from the earliest days of the institution. This was finally put into writing, however, in May 1959. In a written agreement, the Board of Managers acknowledged the contributions made to the hospital by the sisters, and recognized the fact that "without the financial aid, assistance, support and services" of the sisters, the board would not have been able to pay off their past indebtedness, or to proceed with additional building. The board also acknowledged the fact that the sisters lent their support and financial assistance only with the assurance and understanding that the board would continue the services of said sisters permanently in the chief administrative offices of the hospital. Apparently, the sisters were uncomfortable with this as an unwritten agreement. The board, therefore, resolved "that in the event the Board of Managers attempt to replace the Sisters of the Third Order of St. Francis of the Diocese of Pittsburgh in the Chief Administrative Offices of the Hospital without the consent of the Order, the Sisters shall be entitled to receive a sum equal to the value of the Hospital buildings, to-wit, Twenty Million Dollars, and the said Hospital shall pay said sum to the said Sisters in five equal annual installments beginning five days after the date on which any such change shall be proposed to the said Board of Managers and no resolution or order for any such change shall be effective until said sum shall have been paid in full to said Sisters by said Hospital."[156]

---

[156]Memorandum of Agreement-Resolution dated 5/8/59, Motherhouse Archives; Interview with Sister M. Adele Meiser, December 13, 1993.

World War II to 1977—Renovation and Expansion

In spite of all of these problems, occupancy rates remained high. During the war years, and the years following, the occupancy rate ranged between 92 percent and 99 percent.[157] In 1946, it had risen to 99 percent, and a year later it was recorded as 100 percent.[158] By 1952, it was still 90 percent.[159]

Clearly, the hospital served the community well, and so in order to continue to provide space and to offer up-to-date services, it was imperative that the sisters continue to expand and renovate the institution from time to time. Immediately following the war, the board concerned itself with repairing and maintaining the physical plant. Due to a shortage of materials and manpower during the war, the board was unable to maintain the physical plant adequately, and so for several years after the war the board strove to update the facility.[160]

The need to expand the physical plant, first recognized in the twenties, was not realized until 1960. Early in the fifties, the board acknowledged the fact that its bed capacity was inadequate. The board was concerned because patients were no longer waiting for beds, but were seeking admission in other area hospitals. Early preparations for building were underway when the board bought several properties in the residential area immediately surrounding the institution.[161]

In 1955, a campaign was inaugurated to raise money to construct an 8.5 million dollar addition. A general campaign plan was drawn up, and the fund raising began shortly thereafter. The board hired Arthur Sherman, of the American City Bureau, Chicago, a fund raising organization to conduct the campaign.[162] An attempt to heighten community awareness was central to the campaign. This was done with the development of the film "City Within a City," which was shown to numerous organizations throughout the city. There were also thirty second spot announcements made on the radio, and the inauguration of the Women's Auxiliary volunteer services helped to create a broader understanding of the work of the hospital within the community.

[157] AMA and ACS Census of Hospital and Report on Internships and Residencies, manuscript in St. Francis Hospital Archives.

[158] Minutes, Board of Managers, June 10, 1946, June 9, 1947.

[159] AMA Council on Medical Education, Annual Census of Hospitals, 1952.

[160] Minutes, Board of Managers, 6/12/44.

[161] Minutes, Board of Managers, 4/28/52, 8/25/52, 8/23,54, 1/6/55.

[162] Notes for Carl F. Kirschler, Jr., November 22, 1954, manuscript in 'scrapbook' of campaign material, 1954–60, St. Francis Hospital Archives.

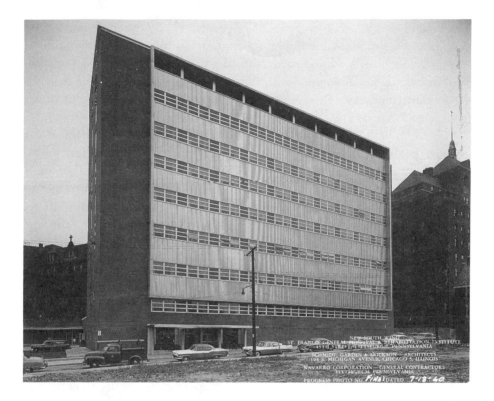

New South Wing, 1960

Funds were received from a number of sources. The Ford Foundation donated $125,000.00 and U.S. Steel provided $350,000.00 in funds for the new buildings. Records suggest that Hill-Burton provided a grant of $359,026.00. Underlying the need for more space was the goal of developing a rehabilitation department. The new south wing, which opened in 1960, raised the hospital's total bed capacity to almost eight hundred beds.[163]

In later years, after 1963, with the advent of increased utilization of out patient facilities, the bed capacity was decreased from 837 to 750 in an effort to reduce health care costs.[164] This was done in spite of the fact that the hospital had an occupancy rate in the mid-sixties of 91 percent, compared to

[163]"Tomorrow ... In Retrospect," printed bulletin, n.d. but c. 1966; Minutes of the Executive Committee of the Board of Managers, May 28, 1956; Letter to Carl Kirschler from Ira J. Mills, Pennsylvania Department of Welfare, Director of Bureau of Homes and Hospitals, 3/2/9/56.

[164]"St. Francis General Hospital—The Groundbreaking 4/5/83," St. Francis Hospital Archives.

a national hospital occupancy rate of 77 percent.[165] By the mid-sixties, 64.3 percent of the hospital's clientele came from the surrounding communities of Arsenal, East Liberty, Homewood, Millvale, Oakland, Sharpsburg, Uptown, Wilkinsburg, Etna, Bloomfield and Blawnox. Of the remaining 35.7 percent, 45 percent came from elsewhere in Allegheny County, and the remainder from outside the county.[166]

In 1973, an 11.8 million dollar addition was opened as a result of the cooperation between the hospital and the Pittsburgh Parking Authority. One of the key players in the development of the parking complex was Gurdon F. Flagg, chairman of the Board of Managers, who urged the administration to pursue the project in spite of opposition from some of the medical staff and sisters. The city built the initial structure, and the hospital rented it. After the building was opened, however, the hospital took over the property by floating a bond issue. Sister Adele influenced the overall design of the project, requesting that the architects plan a building that did not look like a garage. It was also important to her that an underground tunnel be incorporated into the plans so that employees, whose lockers would be housed there, could comfortably walk over to the main hospital building without being exposed to inclement weather. She finally put her foot down against the opposition within the city planners, stating, "no tunnel, no garage." They knew she meant business, and the tunnel was planned.[167] The Medical/Parking complex housed administrative and doctors offices.[168] Physicians' offices, a bank, flower shop, restaurant and gift shop were all located on the main floor. The parking garage added 885 parking spaces on five levels, and the new addition provided facilities for several of the hospital's educational programs. The Professional School of Nursing, the Alvernia School of Practical Nursing and the School of Respiratory Therapy Technicians were all located in the Medical/Parking Complex. In addition, the Community Mental Health/Mental Retardation Center and the Artificial Kidney Center were also housed there.[169]

Two years later, the west wing, which had been built in 1891 for psychiatric patients, was finally demolished. Patients had not used the building since 1965, when it was converted into the nursing school and offices. Known commonly as "high porches," because of its tall open porches, it was the

[165]"Revitalization Plan," manuscript c. 1966, St. Francis Hospital Archives.

[166]" St. Francis General Hospital's Facilities and Plans for the Future," manuscript February 1966, St. Francis Hospital Archives.

[167]Interview with Sister M. Adele Meiser, 1993.

[168]Probe, July/August 1984.

[169]St. Francis General Hospital Medical/Parking Complex, (Pittsburgh: St. Francis General Hospital, c. 1975.)

building which gave the hospital the reputation that St. Francis was a mental institution.[170]

Conclusion

The new additions to the physical plant, and the changes in the charter and articles of incorporation, serve to emphasize how the goals of the hospital had changed. No longer was the primary concern finding an adequate number of beds for in-patients. Instead, there was greater focus on establishing facilities for educational programs and updating medical equipment, as well as on providing space for new medical departments. Scientific research had become a priority. Implicit in the incorporation articles amended in 1962 is an awareness of the surrounding community and the hospital's role in becoming involved. This reflects change in a concept that was developed in the hospital's first years. It had always been concerned with the local community, but only insofar as it could provide care for the sick poor. The new articles of incorporation suggested that the hospital was to be involved in preventive care as well as in other community related issues.

The post-war period, then, is characterized by a tremendous expansion in the physical plant as well as modernization of the facility in order that St. Francis remain competitive in a medical environment that was becoming increasingly technological in nature. The administration focused on providing the most up-to-date equipment, knowledgeable staff and educational services in order to adequately serve Pittsburgh and the surrounding area. Visualizing the hospital in a much broader community and national context, the sisters became involved in local economic and civil rights issues. They were instrumental in the development of cooperative efforts with other area hospitals, sectarian and non-sectarian. The sisters never relinquished their authority, however, and as the hospital developed, it was because of the direction and influence of the Sisters of the Third Order of St. Francis of Millvale.

[170]Caren Marcus, "St. Francis Wing, Image to Fall," *Pittsburgh Press*, 8 August 1975.

Chapter Three

Healing the Body

1900 to World War II

Well established by 1900, St. Francis Hospital introduced a steady series of new departments and services, a sign of the hospital's vitality and the administration's creativity, and an interesting reflection of the challenge hospitals faced in order to remain at the cutting edge. Innovations mirrored changes in technology and doctors' specializations, and also ongoing efforts by the administration to adapt the hospital as a service organization. Some of the experiments had greater impact than others. On the whole, World War II served as something of a dividing line. During the decades before the war, St. Francis emphasized diverse initiatives. After 1945, while the spirit of service and innovation unquestionably continued, the hospital increasingly stressed particular niches, including some new departments in which its strengths could be effectively utilized.

As the new century began, the general hospital was well equipped to serve patients suffering from an array of disorders, and the sisters, in an attempt to fulfill their mission, continued to provide patients with the most up-to-date equipment and care. Although the hospital continued to suffer from a lack of funds, it was the sisters' "intention to persevere in this policy of extending to the poor every aid that medical science offers, trusting in the help of an All-Kind Providence to reward as He has promised even a drink of water given in His Name." Not only did they intend to provide for the sick and indigent, but they were to offer the most modern and up-to-date services.[1] Characteristic of the prewar period is the sisters' attempt to adopt and implement new diagnostic services, and to increase areas of specialization.

[1] *Report of the St. Francis Hospital*, June 1, 1921–May 31, 1923, p. 6.

91

Reflecting the trends of medical practice at that time, doctors began to choose particular specialties, responding to the ever increasing knowledge in medical science, reforms in medical education and the development of sophisticated technological equipment which demanded specialized expertise.

In the twentieth century, the sisters at St. Francis demonstrated a tendency to be both innovative and opportunistic, while broadening their scope of services. There is no doubt that the tradition of innovation was grounded in spiritual concerns, but in light of the new dependence upon modern science, it must have been evident to the sisters that modern technology would serve to attract that absolute necessary entity, the paying patient. As noted earlier, without the reliance on fees from patients, the sisters would have been unable to serve the destitute. The sisters' attempts to modernize and change their facility reflects not only their insight into community attitudes, but also their foresight in anticipating the efficacy of the programs and policies which they implemented. The end product, of course, is one of the largest health care systems in Western Pennsylvania, but this did not develop without some problems for the institution itself. The sisters attempted to offer services in all areas of medicine, desiring to be a general hospital in the fullest sense. Not until after the second world war would they begin to define their areas of expertise.

As the sisters strove to keep their facilities current in the early twentieth century, they obtained and utilized the latest inventions and discoveries in the growing field of medical technology, which played an increasingly important role in the practice of medicine during the years prior to the Great Depression. New technology exemplified by diagnostic equipment, laboratory procedures and new anesthesiology techniques all enabled physicians to make objective measurements and diagnoses. As Americans discovered the role science played in improving their lives, and as they became more respectful of, and confident in, scientific technology, they naturally became more reliant on scientific health care. St. Francis Hospital, like so many other institutions of the era, improved its facilities by adding technological innovations, but always with the goal of improving patient services.[2]

In a way, the development of technology and expansion of research could not have been achieved, nor would it have been very effective, without the specialization of physicians that occurred simultaneously. The medical staff had grown during the first part of the twentieth century and, reflecting the

[2]Joel D. Howell, "Machines and Medicine: Technology Transforms the American Hospital," in *The American General Hospital, Communities and Social Contexts*, (Ithaca: Cornell University Press, 1989), p. 110.

trend of the period, new specialists were added to the staff. By 1911, there were physicians associated with the hospital in the fields of medicine, surgery, psychiatry, gynecology, genito-urology, rhino-laryngology, pediatrics, ophthalmology, otology, and dermatology. In addition, a radiologist and pathologist were available to perform diagnostic studies. Historian Charles Rosenberg has noted that not only were specialists becoming more and more accepted in the early twentieth century in the United States, but general hospitals gradually began to assign beds to specialty wards.[3] By 1911, St. Francis Hospital had designated beds for particular specialties. The children's department, psychiatry department and the ward for skin diseases kept patients separate from people admitted to other departments.[4] As of 1921, a department of obstetrics had been added, reflecting the beginning of the trend towards hospitalized childbirth. Departments in dentistry and proctology had also been established. Throughout the period from 1909 to 1923, the three largest departments, in terms of inpatient admissions, were medicine, surgery, and psychiatry. From June 1, 1910, to May 31, 1911, the department of medicine admitted 580 patients, the general surgery department admitted 578 individuals and psychiatry/neurology admitted 526 people. From June 1, 1922, to May 31, 1923 those numbers increased to 1,320, 1,291 and 1,158, respectively. Total in-patient admissions grew from 2,847 in 1909 to 7,421 by 1923.[5] Some of the new departments mirrored trends occurring nationally, but in others, St. Francis was much more progressive and innovative.

1900 to World War II—Cardiology

St. Francis Hospital played a pioneering role in the development of electrocardiography. Although it was not the first hospital in the nation to utilize such technology, it was quite possibly the first in Western Pennsylvania, and one of the first in the United States to do so. In 1914, Dr. James Delavan Heard, Professor of Medicine at the University of Pittsburgh and senior staff member at St. Francis Hospital, persuaded Richard Beatty Mellon that electrocardiography (EKG) had diagnostic value. Mellon subsequently agreed to

[3]Charles E. Rosenberg, *The Care of Strangers; The Rise of America's Hospital System*, (New York: Basic Books, Inc., 1987), pp. 172–173.

[4]*Report of the St. Francis Hospital*, June 1, 1921–May 31, 1923, pp. 6–7.

[5]*Report of the St. Francis Hospital*, June 1, 1921–May 31, 1923, p. 46.

purchase the apparatus, and established the first fellowship in medicine at the University.[6] In June 1914, Dr. Heard and Dr. Andrew P. D'Zmura, who had done his internship at St. Francis in 1912, and was then a medical resident, went to the laboratory of Thomas Lewis (later Sir Thomas Lewis) at University College Hospital Medical School in London to learn the procedure and interpretation of the electrocardiograph machine.[7] Sir Thomas Lewis published approximately one hundred papers and three books between 1909 and 1920, and is given credit for establishing the electrocardiogram as a necessary part of the examination of the heart. As early as 1912, he unequivocally introduced the electrocardiogram into clinical medicine, stating "if the routine examination of patients who present rapid heart action by modern methods, and especially by electrocardiographic means is not undertaken the condition will often escape detection."[8]

St. Francis Hospital, eager to cooperate in the venture, furnished space for the cumbersome new machine and provided room and board for D'Zmura, the first Mellon fellow. With his salary provided by Richard B. Mellon, D'Zmura, as a post-graduate, was free to do research in the field of cardiology. The new machine arrived in many packing cases from England in 1914. One of D'Zmura's most difficult tasks was in encouraging someone to volunteer to be the first subject. "They thought I was crazy when I suggested we actually use the thing." Dr. Harold B. Gardner, an intern, agreed to be the first subject. Bystanders feared he would be electrocuted, or at the very least, a little singed, but all applauded when the first graph appeared. D'Zmura subsequently collaborated with engineers from Westinghouse from 1926 until 1931, and helped to develop one of the first self-contained portable electrocardiographs, which had been clinically tested at St. Francis. Fifty units were produced, and in 1956, the Smithsonian institution sought one of the original EKG machines for their collection. This exemplifies what Sister Adele referred to as a "tradition of innovations."[9]

Not only did the Sisters of St. Francis Hospital possess a willingness to explore new technology, but they also exhibited their propensity for sharing

[6] A fellowship refers to a specialized course of study following the residency.

[7] Andrew P. D'Zmura, "Forty Years of EKG at St. Francis General Hospital," 1955 ScientificDay Presentation; Robert W. Nickeson, "Looking Back: James Delavan Heard, 1870–1967," *Alumni News* (Fall 1991): 16.

[8] George E. Burch and Nicholas P. DePasquale, *A History of Electrocardiography*, (Chicago: Year Book Medical Publishers, Inc. 1964), p. 162.

[9] Interview with Sister M. Adele Meiser, 1993; Andrew P. D'Zmura, "Forty Years of EKG at St. Francis General Hospital," 1955 Scientific Day Presentation; *St. Francis*, Spring 1950; Unpublished manuscript, 1979, St. Francis Hospital Archives; Pat McCormack, "Museum Seeking Heart Machine," *Sun-Telegraph* 8 January 1956.

their services in the interest of the community's health. Evidence abounds which proves the willingness of the hospital physicians and administration to promote the general welfare of the community at large. The hospital may have been the first institution in the area to own an electrocardiograph machine and they willingly shared it. The machine was available to any reputable member of the medical profession without charge if the patient was without means. Interestingly, and a source of frustration for Dr. D'Zmura, apart from members of the St. Francis staff, few physicians referred patients for study within the first six years. The one exception was the Magee Hospital and Dispensary, which referred patients with heart disease to the St.Francis Hospital Cardiac Dispensary. This possibly reflects a reluctance on the part of some physicians to utilize and place faith in new diagnostic equipment.[10] It has been noted that, in general, hospitals were somewhat reluctant to rush right out and purchase the electrocardiograph machine, unlike the X-ray, which became instantly popular. Clearly, St. Francis was cognizant of its value from the earliest days of its discovery.[11]

D'Zmura actively sought participation of the community in the formation of a 'Pittsburgh Association for the Prevention and Relief of Heart Disease.' His desire was that physicians, the general public, convalescent homes, trade schools and social workers would join together to study the disease and strive to prevent it. He noted that "a nucleus for the work in Pittsburgh already exists at St. Francis Hospital, where the medical school has a cardiographic laboratory." He added that, "with the cooperation of the hospital management, a cardiac dispensary has been organized." D'Zmura assured private practitioners that this type of Association would not impinge upon their private practice but would, in fact, require their referrals for private patients' acceptance into any of the agencies of the association.[12]

By the 1920s, St. Francis was one of only four institutions in the country approved by the American Medical Association for a residency in cardiovascular disease, exemplifying once again the value which the sisters placed on education in their institution. The cardiac dispensary was the first in Pittsburgh to be approved by the American Heart Association in accordance with the standards set up by Dr. Alfred Cohn of the Rockefeller Institute.[13] In the

[10] A. P. D'Zmura, M.D. "The Organized Care of Cardiac Patients," *Pittsburgh Medical Journal* (December 31, 1921): 15–17.

[11] Joel D. Howell, "Machines and Medicine: Technology Transforms the American Hospital," in *The American General Hospital, Communities and Social Contexts*, (Ithaca: Cornell University Press, 1989), pp. 118–119.

[12] A. P. D'Zmura, M.D. "The Organized Care of Cardiac Patients," *Pittsburgh Medical Journal* (December 31, 1921): 16–17.

thirties, St. Francis Hospital offered intensive post-graduate courses on the interpretation of electrocardiograms.[14]

By the end of the second world war, St. Francis remained only one of seven hospitals nationally which continued to offer a residency program in cardiovascular disease, approved by the American Medical Association. They were in the company of Massachusetts General Hospital and Pennsylvania Hospital. By 1947, two more hospitals offered cardiology residency programs, and a year later eighteen hospitals had established residencies in the field. Clearly, St. Francis was a pioneer in this area.[15]

1900 to World War II—Pathology Laboratory

Mirroring nationwide trends to establish more sophisticated diagnostic techniques, St. Francis' laboratories were equipped with all of the necessary "apparatus and instruments." Until September 1910, the pathological laboratory was housed in a small room in the basement of the old hospital, but later that year the labs were moved to the first floor of the new building. Six years later, the pathology laboratory was moved to a separate building across Forty-fifth Street from the hospital and connected to the hospital by an underground tunnel.[16] By 1921, the laboratories had been enlarged considerably and had been divided into several distinctive departments. One of the few problems with which the hospital administration had to be concerned was that few medical graduates were interested in devoting their careers to work in the laboratories. Rarely discouraged, however, the sisters resolved the problem by training sisters as technicians because they were the least likely to leave following training. Medical residents were also hired. The medical school attempted to deal with the issue by incorporating related subjects, such as neuropathology, into the medical school curriculum at the University of Pittsburgh. The pathology laboratory was responsible for conducting autopsies, which served to furnish "many interesting clinicopathological lessons and discussions." In order to inform interested physicians that an autopsy was ready to commence,

---

[13] Andrew P. D'Zmura, "Forty Years of EKG at St. Francis General Hospital," 1955 Scientific Day Presentation.

[14] Andrew P. D'Zmura, "Forty Years of EKG at St. Francis General Hospital," 1955 Scientific Day Presentation.

[15] *Journal of the American Medical Association* 131 (1946) and 134 (1947).

[16] Sister M. Clarissa Popp, *History of the Sisters of St. Francis of the Diocese of Pittsburgh 1868–1938*, (Millvale: Sisters of St. Francis, 1939), p. 123; "St. Francis Hospital," manuscript c. 1940, St. Francis Hospital Archives, p. 10; *Report of the St. Francis Hospital*, 1910–1911, pp. 45–46.

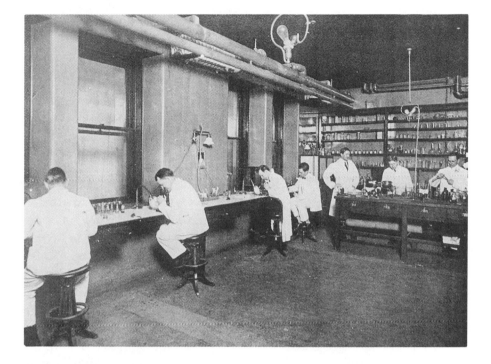

Pathological Laboratory, 1913

a megaphone was used to announce the autopsy throughout the hospital.[17] New technological advances established at the hospital were always implemented with the objective of providing educational experience to students and physicians alike.

Physicians also utilized the laboratory for research projects, reporting on pellagra, tuberculosis, pancreatitis, coronary stenosis, carcinoma and anthrax, to name a few. The hospital boasted that the laboratories were manned by scientists, but it was not unusual for researchers to have their findings corroborated by scientists in the government laboratories.[18] In 1924, a tumor clinic was established along with a frozen sections laboratory and Dr. Nealon, staff obstetrician, received a grant to study cervical carcinoma in women.[19] It is imperative to note that although research and education were not the

[17] *Report of the St. Francis Hospital,* June 1, 1921–May 31, 1923, pp. 27–30; *Weighing the Evidence,* 1927 campaign brochure.

[18] *Report of the St. Francis Hospital,* June 1, 1921–May 31, 1923, pp. 27–30; *Weighing the Evidence,* 1927 campaign brochure.

[19] "A Great Medical Center," unpublished manuscript, n.d., St. Francis Hospital Archives.

sisters' primary goals, they were cognizant of their importance, and strove to initiate such services whenever possible, but never at the expense of patient care.

1900 to World War II—Dispensary

The hospital dispensary, which first began operation sometime in the latter part of the nineteenth century, was not widely used until the twentieth century. In the late 1890s, less than a dozen patients were seen within an entire year, according to the records of the Board of Public Charities. In 1896, a large dispensary was added to the first floor, but apparently was not widely utilized at first.[20] In 1900, only 37 outpatients were treated; by 1901, that had risen to 97. By 1906 and 1907, approximately 150 patients were treated in a given year, but after the new dispensary opened in 1908, the dispensary physicians saw over 750 patients in one year.[21] In 1910, the dispensary moved into the new building. Housed on the ground floor, it consisted of a waiting room, pharmacy and five examining and treatment rooms, all of which had "hot and cold running sterile water." The dispensary work was divided into eight different services: general medicine, general surgery, gynecology, genitourinary surgery, pediatrics, diseases of the eye, diseases of the skin and diseases of the ear, nose and throat. Each department was supervised by a medical staff member. Daily consultations were offered in the major branches, and the specialties had office hours several times weekly. The only patients admitted to the dispensary were those who were unable to pay a private physician.[22] Within a short time, the work of the dispensary multiplied dramatically. In 1912, the dispensary physicians treated 3,117 patients, and for the next few years, the number of patients treated annually stabilized around 2,500.[23]

Dispensaries, first established in America in the late eighteenth century, were designed to provide an alternative to hospital care for the urban poor, but their primary role was that of dispensing prescriptions. They also offered clinical experience for young medical students and for newly trained physicians desirous of more experience while they built their private practices. By

[20]St. Francis Day Address, April 11, 1953, W. S. McEllroy, M.D.

[21]*Annual Report of the Board of Commissioners of Public Charities of the Commonwealth of Pennsylvania,* for years 1897, 1898, 1900, 1901, 1902, 1903, 1904, 1906, 1907, 1908, 1909.

[22]*Report of the St. Francis Hospital,* 1911, pp. 7, 8.

[23]*Annual Report of the Board of Commissioners of Public Charities of the Commonwealth of Pennsylvania,* for years 1909, 1912, 1913, 1914, 1916.

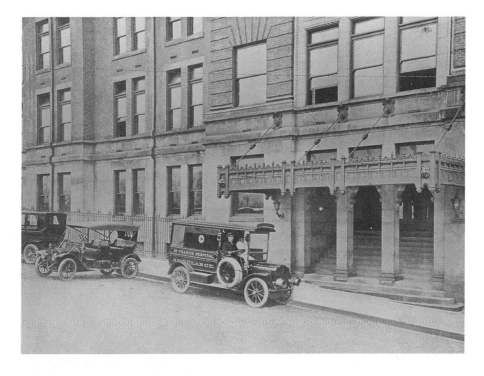

Main Entrance, Forty-fifth Street, 1913

the 1920s, most independent dispensaries had disappeared as hospital out-patient departments, capable of offering additional diagnostic and laboratory facilities, generally replaced the outdated clinics. St. Francis Hospital pre-sumably altered their methods of practice to conform with changing medical technology and capabilities, and merely changed the name of their facility for the ambulatory poor to reflect current trends.[24]

Within ten years, the out-patient department grew markedly. In the year from June 1922 to May 1923, the hospital recorded 9,882 return visits and 5,741 new patients for a total of 15,623 patient visits in one year. The follow-ing departments were represented in the dispensary: medicine, surgery, dental, eye, ear, nose and throat, pediatrics, dermatology, genito-urinary, neurology, gynecology, obstetrics, proctology and cardiology. True to the hospital's mis-sion to provide care for the community, the dispensary physicians also offered the cardiac clinic in the evening for workmen, "so that they may be examined

[24]Charles E. Rosenberg, "Social Class and Medical Care in the 19th-Century America: The Rise and Fall of the Dispensary," in *Sickness and Health in America, Readings in the History of Medicine and Public Health,* Judith Walzer Leavitt and Ronald L. Numbers, eds. (Madison: University of Wisconsin Press, 1985), pp. 273–283.

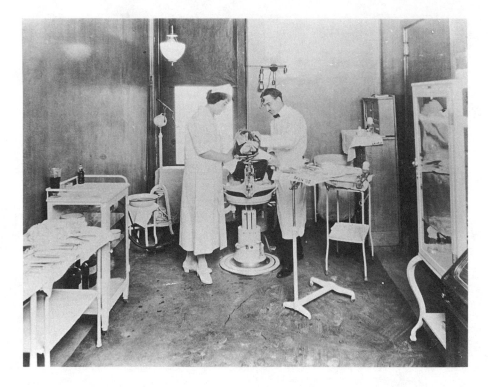

Dental Clinic Room, 1923

and advised as to proper employment without loss of time from their present occupation." The dispensary continued to treat patients who were unable to afford a private physician. A social service worker determined patient need which was based on the patient's income, size, character and responsibilities of the family, in conjunction with a reasonable standard of living, and also the character and probable cost of adequate medical treatment. When a patient could afford it, he paid ten cents per visit or per prescription, but "the lack of a dime is no barrier to those who need treatment." X-rays and additional therapeutic treatments were also given without additional charge. The out-patient clinic cooperated with the various charitable agencies of the city, including the school and city welfare nurses, offering care to patients referred by those agencies.[25]

The out-patient department, established to serve the urban poor directly,

[25] *Uniting the Armies of Health and Industry,* published for Industrial Pittsburgh by St. Francis Hospital, c. 1927, St. Francis Hospital Archives; *Report of the St. Francis Hospital,* June 1, 1921–May 31, 1923, pp. 22–24; *Weighing the Evidence,* 1927 campaign brochure.

also provided diagnostic services to middle income families unable to afford consultation or laboratory fees who were referred by private outside doctors. The dispensary physicians recommended the treatment of choice to the re-ferring physicians. Apparently, this service offered by St. Francis was fairly unusual in Pittsburgh. Philip Klein noted in his monumental study of the thirties that there were no diagnostic services available on an out-patient basis for private patients of moderate income. St. Francis, however, had been fulfilling that very need.[26]

The dispensary, not surprisingly, also had an educational function. Pa-tients served as clinical subjects for physicians, interns, fourth year medical students, social workers and student nurses. This was not unusual, as the pa-tient receiving gratuitous care often did so in exchange for agreeing to allow students to observe and examine them as part of an educational program. Dr. F. B. Utley, director of the dispensary, recommended to the board that the dispensary physicians be permitted to follow their patients if they were admitted to the hospital wards. He felt that it would be beneficial to the students if they could study their patients in the hospital under the helpful guidance of the attending staff. In addition, the medical staff, more aware of dispensary physicians' abilities, could then promote them to a higher level on the medical staff.[27] The dispensary, or out-patient clinic, exemplifies the sisters' policies quite clearly. The clinic grew enormously to serve the local indigent population, but always with community service in mind; the hospital administration offered the hospital services to other physicians and middle income families, while also providing for educational experiences for students in the various divisions of medicine.

1900 to World War II—Industrial Medicine/Surgery

Industrial medicine has always played a major role in the St. Francis Hospital history, reflecting a national interest in the field during the second decade of the century.[28] In the latter half of the nineteenth century, large compa-

---

[26] *Report of the St. Francis Hospital*, June 1, 1921–May 31, 1923, pp. 22–24; Philip Klein, *A Social Study of Pittsburgh: Community Problems and Social Services of Allegheny County*, (New York: Columbia University Press, 1938), p. 763.

[27] *Report of the St. Francis Hospital*, June 1, 1921–May 31, 1923, p. 22.

[28] Rosemary Stevens, *In Sickness and In Wealth, American Hospitals in the Twentieth Century*, (New York: Basic Books, Inc., 1989), p. 83.

nies appointed company doctors whose primary responsibilities were largely confined to the surgical repair of industrial accident victims. By the early twentieth century, however, physicians became more involved in conducting periodic and preemployment examinations and health supervision of workers. Following the adoption of workmen's compensation laws around 1910, industrial medicine included preventive medical engineering of the workplace as part of its focus. By the 1920s, organized medical departments with full-time physicians within the larger companies were common. By this time, too, it was not unusual for companies to make arrangements with area hospitals to treat their employees.[29]

Many of Pittsburgh's wage earning men were employed in jobs that imposed great physical risk. In 1916, for example, of the 250,000 wage earners in the city, 70,000 were employed in the steel mills, 20,000 worked in the mines, and 50,000 were employed by the railroad. A study of injuries in a three month period in the spring of 1907 showed that the hospitals in the county treated and admitted over 509 men. This does not include those that were treated and released the same day, or those injured outside of Allegheny County. In the entire year, 526 men were killed in industrial accidents. Clearly, there was a need not only for improved industrial conditions, but for adequate emergency care as well.[30]

At the turn of the century, in fact, Pittsburgh had an excessive number of deaths when compared to other cities, especially among certain age groups of males. In 1900, Pittsburgh ranked eighth among large cities in general mortality levels, sixth in overall male mortality, but third for men between the ages of fifteen and fifty-four. The death rate for men between the ages of twenty-five to thirty-four was one-third higher than the death rate for other large cities. Industrial accidents were one of the leading causes of those deaths. Interestingly, three-fifths of all fatal industrial accidents among adult men happened to unskilled and semiskilled workers.[31]

In the second decade of the twentieth century, Pittsburgh's numerous hospitals and dispensaries, most of them adequately equipped and progressively managed, lacked any system of coordination between them. Many of the hospitals had an overabundance of unoccupied beds, but refused admission to the sick poor and those with communicable diseases in spite of their

[29] Paul Starr, The Social Transformation of American Medicine: The Rise of a Sovereign Profession and the Making of a Vast Industry, (New York: Basic Books, Inc., 1982), pp. 200–202.

[30] Paul Underwood Kellogg, ed. The Pittsburgh Survey, vol. by Crystal Eastman, Work-Accidents and the Law, (New York: Russell Sage Foundation, 1916) pp. 7, 11.

[31] S. J. Kleinberg, The Shadow of the Mills, Working-Class Families in Pittsburgh, 1870–1907, (Pittsburgh: University of Pittsburgh Press, 1989), p. 28.

subsidies. There was no organized method of ambulance service. The injured and sick were often transported long unnecessary distances at great risk to the patient. Frequently, a police patrol wagon would pick up an accident victim without the aid of a medical attendant. Visiting nurses were unorganized as well. Probably due to this lack of systematization, the Carnegie Steel Co., in 1909, instituted an elaborate, effective, and organized method to deal with their accident victims, and St. Francis Hospital played a major role.[32]

The Carnegie Steel Company program involved appointing a chief surgeon in the town where the works were located. He was paid a yearly salary commensurate with services rendered. In works employing over twelve hundred men, the surgeon had an assistant. These doctors were to be available at all times, constantly within telephone communication. Their duties included the provision of medical care and educational services. They were responsible for giving first aid lectures and instructions, making home visits to the injured and rendering whatever surgical attention was necessary.

Plants which employed over eighteen hundred men had their own Standard Emergency Hospital, which included a waiting room, redressing room, operating room, ward room, bathroom, nurses' room, laboratory and X-ray room. When a patient was first injured, if it was minor, he was seen in the redressing room. Otherwise, he was observed in the ward room, in cases of shock, for example. Patients had surgery in the operating room. Workers who had been injured previously also visited the hospital to have their dressings changed at an appointed time. Graduate nurses were in attendance constantly.[33]

The medical practitioners were also responsible for informing employees of the services available to them and their own responsibilities in heeding the advice given. A circular was sent to the men to remind them to seek help from the company surgeon, even for minor injuries, and not to treat themselves. For example, there was a strict rule prohibiting employees from removing foreign bodies from the eyes of other employees. Workers were essentially forced to follow these directives because the foreman was not permitted to allow an employee to return to work after an injury until he received the signature of the company surgeon. If an employee had not followed the surgeon's advice and, therefore, was not recovering appropriately, he would be delayed in returning

[32] Paul Underwood Kellogg, ed. *The Pittsburgh Survey*, vol. *Wage-Earning Pittsburgh*, (New York: Russell Sage Foundation, 1914) pp. 11, 12.

[33] William O'Neill Sherman, M.D., Appendix XV, "Surgical Organization of the Carnegie Steel Co." in Paul Underwood Kellogg, ed., *The Pittsburgh Survey*, vol. *Wage-Earning Pittsburgh*, (New York: Russell Sage Foundation, 1914) pp. 455–460.

to work. This strict adherence to policy was intended to promote more rapid return of the injured to the work force.[34]

The steel mills provided first aid education as part of their program. First aid squads composed of workers were organized throughout the works. Each class utilized the American Red Cross textbook and attended twelve lectures and demonstrations. Competitions were held and prizes given to the winning crews in order to stimulate and maintain interest in first aid. Squad members were given examinations to test efficiency. They were responsible for administering on-site treatment for minor injuries or transporting accident victims via stretcher to the Emergency Hospital on the premises. After the patient was treated, he was either sent home or to the hospital via ambulance. Home bound patients had the benefit of a visiting nurse who not only provided care, but also gave advice on nursing, child care, sanitation and housekeeping.[35]

The works often maintained their own wards in the local hospitals. The Carnegie Steel's first ward was at West Penn, but St. Francis subsequently provided a ward for the company under Dr. William O'Neill Sherman's direction. Employees were admitted regardless of whether or not they had been injured on the job. If they required hospitalization for other reasons, they were still cared for on the industrial ward. The sisters took special care of their patients on the industrial wards, often providing flowers and even a canary. Dr. Sherman was considered to be a Pittsburgh pioneer in the field of industrial medicine, having done research in the treatment of fractures by the open reduction method with self tapping stainless steel screws. Early rehabilitation work within St. Francis received great impetus through him.[36]

Apparently, Carnegie Steel's educational and treatment program was very effective. Infection rates were reduced to a fraction of 1 percent, and the periods of convalescence were markedly reduced. The company's goal was to provide prompt medical care in order to reduce the convalescent period, thereby reducing the charge on the relief fund. Proper care also guarded against relapse due to premature reemployment.[37]

---

[34] William O'Neill Sherman, M.D., Appendix XV, "Surgical Organization of the Carnegie Steel Co." in Paul Underwood Kellogg, ed., *The Pittsburgh Survey*, vol. *Wage-Earning Pittsburgh*, (New York: Russell Sage Foundation, 1914) pp. 455–460.

[35] William O'Neill Sherman, M.D., Appendix XV, "Surgical Organization of the Carnegie Steel Co." in Paul Underwood Kellogg, ed., *The Pittsburgh Survey*, vol. *Wage-Earning Pittsburgh*, (New York: Russell Sage Foundation, 1914) pp. 455–460.

[36] William O'Neill Sherman, M.D., Appendix XV, "Surgical Organization of the Carnegie Steel Co." in Paul Underwood Kellogg, ed., *The Pittsburgh Survey*, vol. *Wage-Earning Pittsburgh*, (New York: Russell Sage Foundation, 1914) pp. 455–460; Interview with Dr. George Wright Jr., 10/25/93; "St. Francis Launches Biggest Expansion," May 1955, source of publication unknown, copy in St. Francis Hospital Archives; Interview with Sister M. Adele Meiser, 1993.

[37] Paul Underwood Kellogg, ed., *The Pittsburgh Survey*, vol. *Wage-Earning Pittsburgh*, (New York: Russell Sage Foundation, 1914) pp. 12 and 247.

The physicians of the industrial medicine department, which was a part of the department of surgery, utilized progressive new techniques in the treatment and rehabilitation of industrial injuries. During the period 1921–1923, approximately half of the surgery department's two thousand cases belonged in this category. The surgeons were especially advanced in the implementation of orthopedic and burn therapy. Doctors were insistent that their patients ambulate as soon as possible, an unusual idea for the period. One of the more advanced therapies of the time was that of blood transfusions, which were given to patients in shock. Interestingly, donors were readily secured at any time from patients on the ward service, "because of the high morale and existing esprit de corps." Other forms of therapy which aided rehabilitation were also employed, such as hydrotherapy, light and heat treatments, occupational therapy and machines designed for scientific exercise of limbs. The hospital took pride in the fact that "an industrial community finds added value in the various phases of therapy treatments for through them can be rectified many of the disabilities that attend workmen." The hospital noted that in the occupational therapy department "muscles that have fallen into disuse through long sickness, are given occupation at the dictation of doctors who diagnose the need and prescribe the type of work with the same precision that a course of medical treatment would be ordered." In the late twenties, two "trained" occupational therapists were in charge.[38]

It is interesting to note that St. Francis Hospital may have been unique in its establishment of an industrial ward which provided acute care as well as rehabilitative services. Historian Rosemary Stevens notes that, even as late as the 1920s, "there were few adequate facilities for industrial accident cases in hospitals anywhere in the United States. The average hospital organization, geared to undertake 'careful and daring surgery,' was just not attuned to effective reconstruction work, including the 'unremitting aftercare' of massage, exercises, electrical treatment, education and appliances ... the continuous care of an injured worker, both as inpatient and as long-term outpatient was generally unavailable."[39]

The hospital viewed itself as providing a service to the industrial community and, as a result, solicited funds from local employers, appealing to their desire to maximize employee productivity. "Every employer fully realizes the direct benefit that accrues from the general hospital that serves the community of his plant. He appreciates the out-patient and bed-patient service of the

[38] *Report of the St. Francis Hospital*, June 1, 1921–May 31, 1923, p. 39; *Uniting the Armies of Health and Industry*, published for Industrial Pittsburgh by St. Francis Hospital, c. 1927, St. Francis Hospital Archives; *Weighing the Evidence*, 1927 campaign brochure.

[39] Rosemary Stevens, *In Sickness and In Wealth, American Hospitals in the Twentieth Century*, (New York: Basic Books, Inc., 1989), p. 88.

general hospital ... where his employees receive the care that returns them to productivity in a minimum length of time ... brings peace of mind and full efficiency." It is important to note that although U.S. Steel, which had absorbed Carnegie Steel, was the only industry which had their own specified ward, other companies, such as Crucible Steel, also brought their injured employees to St. Francis.[40] The industrial wards were present for many years, and by 1950, thirty-nine patients were accommodated on one ward, and fifty outpatients were seen every other day. Dr. J. H. Wagner, the chief surgeon for the Carnegie Illinois works, directed the work on the ward at that time.[41]

In the early years of the industrial wards, St. Francis Hospital, with only one ambulance, transported injured workers to the hospital. Sister Adele recalled how she worried that the ambulance would be in use in one place when it was needed in another. Her worries were well founded because the hospital ambulance was the only vehicle which the sisters owned, so it doubled as a taxi for the sisters, who at that time did not drive.[42]

The industrial medicine department played a role in education and research in the community. In 1929, Edward Bindley of the Pittsburgh Steel Company left $100,000.00 to the School of Medicine of the University of Pittsburgh for an education program in industrial medicine. As a result, the school enhanced the curriculum by adding lectures on industrial medicine as part of a preventive medicine program. In 1936, the medical school of the University of Pittsburgh established the Department of Industrial Hygiene in response to a survey conducted in the early thirties, which revealed that nearly eighty percent of its recent graduates had some contact with organizations involved in the treatment of injured workers. Wanting to train their students adequately, the new department required senior students to take fourteen hours of industrial medicine. A Westinghouse Electric grant, as well as funds from other corporations and foundations, enabled the department to begin to undertake serious research in 1937. In time, the school offered an intensive course of graduate study, and by 1944, a graduate fellowship was established. This research oriented fellowship featured a rotating internship at the Industrial Hygiene Foundation of Mellon Institute, the Pennsylvania Department of Health, the TB League and Western State Psychiatric Hospital, followed by a six-month residency in traumatic surgery and rehabilitation at St. Francis Hospital.[43] Before the war, the industrial hygiene department

[40]*Uniting the Armies of Health and Industry*, published for Industrial Pittsburgh by St. Francis Hospital, c. 1927, St. Francis Hospital Archives; Interview with Sister M. Adele Meiser, 1993.

[41]*St. Francis*, (Fall 1950).

[42]Interview with Sister M. Adele Meiser, 1993.

[43]Barbara I. Paull, *A Century of Medical Excellence, The History of the University of Pittsburgh School of Medicine*, (Pittsburgh: University of Pittsburgh Medical Alumni Association, 1986), pp. 147–148.

at the University of Pittsburgh, directed by Dr. T. Lyle Hazlett, also organized a study of fever therapy in which St. Francis Hospital participated. The aim of the study was to determine the uses to which fever therapy could be used, and to correlate the results obtained in the various affiliated hospitals. Although fever therapy was very popular at the time, there had been no documented studies organized in Pittsburgh. The work was pioneered in Pittsburgh at St. Francis with the development of a fever machine by Mr. Houghten and Dr. Ferderber, who also carried out experimental and clinical studies.[44]

The industrial medicine department illustrates the hospital administration's willingness to be innovative in order to serve the community. Not only was industrial medicine a distinctive hospital service for the time, but its aspect of rehabilitative care was even more so and set the foundation for a major rehabilitation center developed several decades later.

1900 to World War II—Pediatrics

The first doctors interested in child health were generally obstetricians, but by the 1880s, pediatrics had developed into a field in its own right. The American Medical Association devoted a special section to pediatrics in 1880, and in the subsequent decade, several scientific journals focusing entirely on pediatric medicine had developed. By this time, too, numerous clinics and specialty hospitals had been established to cater to the needs of children. The emergence of pediatrics as a medical specialty reflects the late nineteenth century trend towards specialization in medicine and the move towards professionalization; but it also was part of a general reorientation of attitudes towards children whereby childhood had come to be seen as developmentally unique.[45]

St. Francis, with a history of being as progressive as any institution of its time, established the children's department in May 1910. The entire wing of one floor was divided into small wards accommodating approximately seven

[44]Letter from T. Lyle Hazlett, M.D., director of the Department of Industrial Hygiene, University of Pittsburgh to Sister M. Thomasine, 10/20/37, St. Francis Hospital Archives; Fever therapy, also known as pyrotherapy or thermotherapy, was popularized before the advent of antibiotics. High fever, 105 to 106 degrees was produced by the inoculation of the organisms of malaria, rat-bite fever, typhoid or with the use of specially designed 'fever boxes.' The rationale was that high fever was considered to be germicidal or bactericidal and would therefore be effective in the treatment of resistant forms of syphilis, gonorrhea and other infections; W. Wayne Babcock, *A Textbook of Surgery, for Students and Physicians*, (Philadelphia: W. B. Saunders Co., 1935), p. 480.

[45]Richard A. Meckel, *Save the Babies; American Public Health Reform and the Prevention of Infant Mortality, 1850–1929*, (Baltimore: Johns Hopkins University Press, 1990), pp. 45–47.

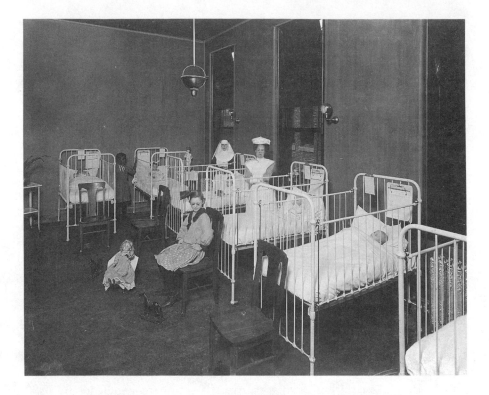

Children's Ward, 1913

children. These small wards allowed for the isolation of patients with contagious diseases. The children's dispensary made it possible for the children
to receive the necessary follow up care during their convalescence at home.
The department was generally filled to capacity by the nineteen twenties.
In addition to patients referred by the dispensary or other private patients,
the hospital also cared for sick children from St. Rita's Home for Children.
Physicians studying pediatrics were "given the privilege" of seeing the newborn babies in the obstetrics department so that they could study pediatrics
of the newborn. The establishment and resultant growth of the pediatrics
department reflects the interest in child health of health care professionals
at the time. Infant mortality was recognized as a major health care concern,
and in fact, Dr. J. Everhart, director, felt the work in the department might
help to combat the problem. Many children were treated through cooperation with the Rotary and Kiwanis clubs of many surrounding communities.
At the end of 1927, the hospital had given 1,217 days of care to thirty-one
crippled children for the Rotary clubs of Dubois, Franklin, Oil City, Butler,

Clairton, Meadville, Blairsville and McKeesport, and the Kiwanis club of Reynoldsville.[46]

1900 to World War II—Genito-urinary Department/ Venereal Disease

As early as 1911, there was a genito-urinary specialist on the medical staff, and by 1921, there was a separate department for that particular surgical specialty. Although operative cases made up a substantial portion of the work of the department, the dispensary cases were much larger in number. During the period June 1, 1921–May 31, 1923, the department physicians saw 687 new patients and 3,440 return patients. Out of that total number, 1,701 patients received Salvarsan treatments. The fact that 41 percent of the patients treated had syphilis emphasizes the flexibility of the hospital's admission policies even further. Even more so, it points out how important those policies were in terms of maintaining the health of the community. Further, specialists from the hospital, recommended by the Allegheny County Medical Society, would lecture to groups of men or women regarding the prevention of "social diseases."[47] In the mid-thirties, the hospital continued to provide Salvarsan treatments for those suffering from syphilis, but by 1935, the numbers had declined somewhat, perhaps proving the efficacy of educational programs. In that year, 541 patients with syphilis were seen in the dispensary.[48]

At the turn of the century, patients with venereal disease, regarded with much social stigma, were often denied admission to hospitals and clinics on the grounds that they were not worthy of assistance. Even after diagnostic tests and effective treatments had been developed, hospitals and clinics had difficulty establishing facilities for patients with venereal disease.[49] The existence of this particular service exemplifies the administration's priority of serving the community regardless of the policies of other facilities.

In the first few years of the twentieth century, many strides had been

---

[46]*Report of the St. Francis Hospital,* June 1, 1921–May 31, 1923, pp. 35–37; *Report of the St. Francis Hospital,* 1911, p. 43; *The Weekly News of St. Francis Hospital,* published weekly for the Friends of the Hospital, 1 (13 May 1927).

[47]*Report of the St. Francis Hospital,* June 1, 1921–May 31, 1923, p. 40; *Uniting the Armies of Health and Industry,* published for Industrial Pittsburgh by St. Francis Hospital, c. 1927, St. Francis Hospital Archives.

[48]Letter from William D. Cutter, American Medical Association to Sister M. Thomasine, January 6, 1936, St. Francis Hospital Archives.

[49]Allan M. Brandt, *No Magic Bullet, A Social History of Venereal Disease in the United States Since 1880,* (New York: Oxford University Press, 1987), pp. 40, 44.

made in an effort to combat syphilis. In 1906, August Wassermann, Albert Neisser and Carl Bruck published an account of their successful efforts in developing a diagnostic test for syphilis. Historians have noted, however, that as late as 1912, few physicians had the necessary technical and laboratory facilities to conduct these tests. As early as 1909, St. Francis Hospital laboratories were conducting Wasserman reactions, and by the early twenties, the hospital performed 8,205 blood Wassermann tests and an additional 1,539 spinal fluid Wassermann tests within a two year period.[50] Shortly thereafter, the first effective treatment for syphilis was discovered by Nobel laureate immunologist Paul Ehrlich. Salvarsan, an arsenical compound, was given with some risk, and the course of injections was often lengthy and unpleasant, but most patients could be rendered non-infectious and avoid the miserable consequences of late and tertiary syphilis.[51]

1900 to World War II—Obstetrics

By 1923, the hospital had a thriving obstetrical department which had increased the number of deliveries by 20 percent from 1921–1923, reflecting the increased use of hospitals for deliveries in the twentieth century. Although indigent and single women frequently turned to institutions for care during childbirth in the nineteenth century, it was not until the twentieth century that middle and upper class women chose to have their babies in hospitals, reflecting their belief in the promise and hope that scientific medicine would prevent the maternal and infant mortality and morbidity so common in the nineteenth century. By 1933, 35 percent of all births in the nation occurred in hospitals.[52]

The obstetrics department at St. Francis was one of the busiest in the city. From 1921–1923, the hospital recorded 510 spontaneous deliveries, 35 forceps deliveries, 49 breech deliveries by manual extraction and 10 Caesarean sections. St. Francis recorded 437 deliveries in 1926, and 699 in 1930. By 1926, there were at least eighteen institutions in the city of Pittsburgh

[50]*Report of the St. Francis Hospital*, June 1, 1921–May 31, 1923, p. 30; *Report of the St. Francis Hospital*, 1911, p. 44; Allan M. Brandt, *No Magic Bullet, A Social History of Venereal Disease in the United States Since 1880*, (New York: Oxford University Press, 1987), pp. 40, 44.

[51]Allan M. Brandt, *No Magic Bullet, A Social History of Venereal Disease in the United States Since 1880*, (New York: Oxford University Press, 1987), p. 130.

[52]Judith Walzer Leavitt, *Brought to Bed, Childbearing in America, 1750–1950* (New York: Oxford University Press, 1986), pp. 73, 173, 188.

which provided obstetrical services, but only three other hospitals recorded more deliveries than St. Francis; and in 1930, only West Penn and Magee Hospital served more parturient women.[53] The facility was also offered to outside physicians who were permitted to utilize St. Francis for deliveries as long as they "faithfully carried out the routine of the Obstetrical Department and have shown every desire to cooperate with the management, the Sister in charge, and the chief of the department." Clearly, the administration was interested in elevating the department to a very high standard, but the sisters also wanted to open their doors to outside physicians in their desire to serve the community. The obstetrics chief, Dr. W. A. Nealon, noted that in the endeavor of improving the department, the management of the hospital was very cooperative. The hospital at that time also had established a prenatal clinic, which serves to emphasize the hospital's focus on preventive care.[54]

1900 to World War II—Social Service Department

During the first decades of the twentieth century, social service departments began to be established in hospitals. The tasks of social workers included providing medical advice to discharged patients and monitoring patients' compliance with instructions as well as evaluating the patient's social and economic status, cooperating with other private and public welfare agencies whenever necessary.[55] The St. Francis Hospital's social service department, established in January 1918, was instrumental in implementing the policies established by the sisters early in the hospital's history. The social service workers visited patients in their homes regularly to determine a patient's financial status so that no patient would be charged who was unable to pay. However, because of the hospital's unstable financial situation, it was imperative that those who could afford to pay did so, since the sisters relied upon patient receipts in order to remain financially solvent.[56]

Workers visited patient homes for other reasons. The social service workers attempted to assess and, whenever possible, correct the social and living

[53]"Reported Births in Institutions, 1926–1935," Department of Health, City of Pittsburgh, Allegheny County Health Department Archives.

[54]*Report of the St. Francis Hospital*, June 1, 1921–May 31, 1923, p. 26.

[55]Charles E. Rosenberg, *The Care of Strangers, The Rise of America's Hospital System*, (New York: Basic Books, Inc., 1987), p. 314.

[56]*Report of the St. Francis Hospital*, June 1, 1921–May 31, 1923, pp. 19, 22.

conditions of the patients. They found ways to provide material relief, legal aid and temporary or permanent adjustments of their home environment through relatives, friends, employers, private and public agencies. Workers also assisted in the placement of infants in temporary homes or day nurseries during the confinement of the mother. They arranged baptisms when necessary, and dealt with problems of illegitimacy. The social workers' tasks, then, to be sure, were widely varied.[57]

In some ways, the social workers acted more like a visiting nurse staff. For example, they visited patients in order to assess the progress of dispensary patients. This determination of the results of any treatments the patients received was then added to their permanent medical record. These medical histories were invaluable to physicians as they evaluated the care which they provided. Social service personnel visited obstetrical patients in their homes following their discharge from the hospital, advising them in their care.[58]

Interestingly, St. Francis stands out as an exception through its establishment of a social service department. Again, tradition and the desire to be distinctive among Catholic hospitals produced an innovative approach. In 1930, Dr. John O'Grady urged Catholic hospitals to establish such departments so that workers may "reach out into the homes of its ward and clinic patients in order that they may be relieved of the worries and anxieties that play such an important part in ill-health and recovery, ... set the mind of the sick mother at rest in regard to the care of her children." Medical social service workers were needed to understand home condition and patients' habits, such as diet, so the hospital would be in a better position to diagnose and treat illness. The only way a doctor could be assured that his advice would be followed was through the social service department. Dr. O'Grady's description mirrors the department already established by that time at St. Francis. By 1929, only seventeen of the 641 Catholic hospitals had a medical social service department. This was attributed to a lack of funds.[59] St.Francis, too, had to close their department for several years during the Depression for that very reason, but they reestablished the department as soon as possible. During this interim, the tasks previously performed by the social workers were not ignored, but were allocated to the sisters.[60]

[57] *Report of the St. Francis Hospital*, June 1, 1921–May 31, 1923, pp. 21, 48.

[58] *Report of the St. Francis Hospital*, June 1, 1921–May 31, 1923, pp. 19, 26.

[59] John O'Grady Ph.D., U.D., *Catholic Charities in the United States: History and Problems*, (Washington, D.C.: National Conference of Catholic Charities, 1930).

[60] Interview with Sister M. Adele Meiser, 1993.

1900 to World War II—Medical Staff Organization

As many of the hospital's departments became more systematized and specialized, and as the patient load increased dramatically in the early twentieth century, it was imperative that the medical staff organize. This occurred on a wider scale nationally as hospitals complied with the standardization requirements of the American College of Surgeons during the second decade of the twentieth century. By the 1920s, the medical staff at St. Francis Hospital was organized into two distinctive hierarchies of dispensary physicians and hospital staff. Assistant staff physicians were at the lowest level, but could rise to the level of associate before proceeding to the highest level, that of staff physician. The separate dispensary staff included in each department someone from the regular hospital staff, but positions were also held by doctors not appointed to the regular hospital staff. Apparently, the title of associate in one hierarchy did not ensure the same title in the other. In addition, the hospital had a large house staff of residents and interns which was responsible for the direct care of ward patients under the direction of staff members. The physicians not only cared for patients, but also were responsible for clinical teaching of medical students from the University of Pittsburgh School of Medicine.[61]

1900 to World War II—Conclusion

During the first half of the twentieth century, the sisters had established a firm foundation for the development of services, as well as for a philosophy of care which remains today. Not only would they focus on providing for those already injured or ill, but they also endeavored to prevent the need for such services. Public policy by this time had begun to emphasize prevention as a way to improve the health condition of the American population. Discoveries in bacteriology, with the resultant developments of preventive immunological techniques, popularized medicine's ability to eradicate disease. A diphtheria antitoxin was developed in the 1890s. Vaccines against typhoid and tetanus were introduced at the turn of the century. In addition, improvement in

---

[61] *Report of the St. Francis Hospital*, June 1, 1921–May 31, 1923, pp. 3–5, 16; Rosemary Stevens, *In Sickness and in Wealth, American Hospitals in the Twentieth Century*, (New York: Basic Books, Inc., 1989) p. 78.

public hygiene by filtering the water supply and regulating milk supplies, for example, also lent credibility to medical science's ability to prevent disease.[62] Preventive medicine, however, by the time of the first world war, was still not a major focus of America's hospitals. Hospitals were generally seen as short-term repair shops rather than centers for preventive medicine or long term care.[63]

St. Francis Hospital had already implemented such preventive care policies by 1921, however. The sisters felt the hospital was designed to provide the most efficient medical and surgical care available, but also to aid in the prevention of disease. In the dispensary, patients were not only treated for their chief complaint "but his daily regime with reference to diet, exercise, rest, tobacco, alcohol, recreation, and ventilation is outlined. . . . In this way preventive medicine is practiced in its best sense." Social service workers handed out medical blanks which were to be filled out by healthy patients' private physicians. This was to encourage preventive examinations, and thereby ensure good health. Preventive care was marketed to industrial employers "that there may be the least amount of shut down of human machinery."[64] The sisters' progressive attitude at such an early time period was unique.

The sisters' primary concern was always caring for the sick and injured, especially those without adequate financial resources, but they did not achieve this without some strains amongst personnel within the institution. New growth, organization and specialization introduced new tensions. The physicians had other concerns which historians have claimed directed American hospital development. Charles Rosenberg has noted that the "decisions that shaped the modern hospital have been consistently guided by the world of medical ideas and values . . . the attitudes and aspirations that gave the profession its peculiar identity."[65] The decisions of the Sisters of St. Francis were guided by spiritual and religious beliefs and aspirations. The staff of St. Francis, although their interests reflected those of physicians elsewhere, were never able to gain enough control within the institution to implement all of the changes which they advocated. In the early 1920s, for example, the doctors

[62] Paul Starr, The Social Transformation of American Medicine, The Rise of a Sovereign Profession and the Making of a Vast Industry, (New York: Basic Books, Inc., 1982), p. 135.

[63] Rosemary Stevens, In Sickness and in Wealth, American Hospital in the Twentieth Century, (New York: Basic Books, Inc., 1989), pp. 81, 90.

[64] Report of the St. Francis Hospital, June 1, 1921–May 31, 1923, pp. 8, 21, 48; Uniting the Armies of Health and Industry, published for Industrial Pittsburgh by St. Francis Hospital, c. 1927, St. Francis Hospital Archives.

[65] Charles E. Rosenberg, The Care of Strangers; The Rise of America's Hospital System, (New York: Basic Books, Inc., 1987), p. 7.

were very concerned that a hospital the caliber of St. Francis should be far more involved in "scientific investigation and contribution to the knowledge of disease." One of their proposed solutions was to enlarge the junior and assistant staffs in order that senior staff members be relieved of some of the burdensome routine work, and therefore have time to pursue research activities. In addition, the doctors perceived that an assembly room, seating one hundred or more people, would allow the hospital to hold important meetings, previously held at other local hospitals and, therefore, add to the hospital's prestige.[66] The sisters' goal was always to serve the community, and however their funds were spent, it was always with that in mind. Research was important, and to be sure, valuable contributions were made, but it never took precedence over patient care. Since the hospital suffered from a perpetual limitation in funds, the doctors' goals were never fully realized.

During the first forty years of the new century, the sisters' funds were limited, and they were unable to build a new facility. Undaunted in their mission to serve the sick, however, they found other ways to promote the development of their hospital. Attention was paid to the development of a specialized and educated medical staff and the acquisition of new diagnostic equipment. New departments were formed in order to serve the community. By the end of the second world war, the sisters were able to foresee the time when financial difficulties would be alleviated somewhat so that they could expand their facility, develop services even further and become much more involved with the community.

World War II to 1979

Following the second world war, the previously established hospital departments were expanded, and new services and programs implemented in order to reach out and serve more people in an attempt to care for those whose needs were not being met in the community. Because the sisters had been able to enlarge the physical plant, their goals were easier to attain. In addition, several research projects were developed and educational opportunities were established. Characteristic of this period, too, was a growing partnership between the Sisters of St. Francis and other agencies as they endeavored to

[66] *Report of the St. Francis Hospital,* June 1, 1921–May 31, 1923, p. 16.

aid the community more efficiently. To be sure, they never lost sight of their mission to provide holistic care for all in need.

The sisters built on the foundation established in the period prior to the second world war by expanding services and developing new ones in order to be competitive in the changing medical environment. St. Francis has a history of being innovative and progressive, having often been the first hospital in the Pittsburgh area to utilize new equipment or techniques. In 1945, Sister Thomasine encouraged Dr. S. S. Allen to go to Ann Arbor to study under one of the nation's leading neurosurgeons. St. Francis Hospital, as a result, may have been the first hospital in Pittsburgh to have a surgeon trained in neurosurgery.[67] The hospital was probably the first hospital in Pittsburgh to use radioactive elements in the form of the Cobalt 60 machine which was installed in 1953.[68] With the opening of the new addition in 1960, the hospital was able to develop many more new educational and patient care services. The inhalation therapy department was established in 1960.[69] In 1967, the coronary care unit, radiation therapy department and nuclear medicine center were all developed to meet changing patient needs.[70] In 1973, the hospital established the city's first cardiac electrophysiology laboratory, and in 1975, they brought the first CAT scanner to the area.[71] Clearly, the hospital continued the pattern of remaining up-to-date medically.

Cardiovascular surgery was developed early in the hospital, not surprising considering the hospital's history in cardiology. Dr. James W. Giacobine performed open heart surgery at St. Francis Hospital in 1959.[72] Two years later, he organized and headed the first open heart team. The heart-lung machine, necessary to the surgery, had first been used at the University of Cincinnati, where Giacobine had done his residency. In addition, Dr. Giacobine developed a homemade heart-lung machine which he tested on dogs for six months before performing the procedure on people.[73]

Although the hospital sisters were proud of this first accomplishment, patient care remained foremost in their minds. The administration's response to this new technology is reminiscent of their attitudes following the development of electrocardiography in the second decade of the century. Sister

[67]"Hospital in Modern America," unpublished manuscript, n.d., c. 1960s, St. Francis Hospital Archives.

[68]"29th Annual Personnel Picnic," program, 1990, St. Francis Hospital Archives.

[69]Sister M. Adele Meiser, points for 'On Location' TV interview, manuscript, n.d. but c. 1986, St. Francis Hospital Archives.

[70]"Partners in Progress," c. 1967, St. Francis Hospital Archives.

[71]"29th Annual Personnel Picnic," program, 1990, St. Francis Hospital Archives.

[72]Manuscript, 1979, St. Francis Hospital Archives; there is some discrepancy regarding this date. Some sources suggest that the surgery was performed in 1958.

[73]Probe—On Call 11 (February 1966).

Adele recalled the positive relationship she had with the administration at West Penn Hospital in that time period. Although St. Francis had pioneered in providing cardiovascular surgery, Sister Adele encouraged the administrator at West Penn to do the same, in order that they continue to provide modern up-to-date care, reflecting, perhaps, her belief that care of the patient was more important than hospital competition.[74]

World War II to 1979—Rehabilitation Department

The rehabilitation department of St. Francis, which had its roots in the industrial medicine and physical medicine departments, was the first of its kind in Western Pennsylvania. Other facilities providing rehabilitation services existed, but St. Francis was the first general hospital to incorporate those services within the hospital setting.[75] Although the idea to establish such a facility in the area was first proposed as being affiliated with the University of Pittsburgh, St. Francis Hospital was first to accomplish the task in 1960.[76]

Before the second world war, work in physical rehabilitation was directed mainly towards crippled children, with funds provided largely from the state or voluntary organizations. Title V of the Social Security Act of 1935, as a response to the U.S. Children's Bureau, provided for case finding of children with handicaps. The use of teams of professionals became widespread. Orthopedic surgeons, neurosurgeons, plastic surgeons, physical therapists, speech therapists and occupational therapists, as well as public health nurses and medical social workers, worked together with a focus on rehabilitation. Before the war, there were few services for adults. Only several adult out-patient rehabilitation centers existed in New York City and Cleveland. For over twenty years, state governments had taken advantage of matching federal funds for vocational rehabilitation, but funds for physical restoration were not part of state programs until 1944. The rehabilitation of World War II veterans provided incentive to care for civilians, whose numbers were much greater that the veterans.[77]

The interest in a rehabilitation center in Pittsburgh was first recognized

[74]Interview with Sister M. Adele Meiser, 1993.
[75]Interview with Sister M. Adele Meiser, 1993.
[76]"Hospital in Modern America," manuscript, n.d., c. 1960s, St. Francis Hospital Archives.
[77]"A Plan for Community Rehabilitation Center of Pittsburgh," manuscript, March 1952, St. Francis Hospital Archives.

in 1947, following the report made by Dr. Claude W. Munger and Mary Jarrett for the Health Division of the Health and Welfare Federation. In that same year, the Chamber of Commerce of Pittsburgh brought Dr. Howard A. Rusk to speak at an open meeting about work in New York. A year later, the Council of Medical Social Service Board brought Rusk to speak at a large meeting which included industrialists, personnel department heads, doctors, lay board members and health care workers. A steering committee was organized in July 1950 to develop plans for a community rehabilitation center in Pittsburgh. The committee was composed of representatives from the Allegheny Conference on Community Development, the Health and Welfare Federation of Allegheny County, the Hospital Council of Western Pennsylvania and the State of Pennsylvania Bureau of Rehabilitation. In addition, there were representatives from the University of Pittsburgh's graduate school of Public Health and the School of Medicine. Other representatives from the United Vocational and Employment Service, and the Welfare and Retirement Fund of the United Mine Workers also participated. Dr. Howard Rusk served as a consultant to the committee. The plans discussed called for affiliation with the University of Pittsburgh, with the ultimate goal of eventually building a new facility within the University of Pittsburgh Medical Center.[78] It simply is not clear why the goals of this committee, to establish a rehabilitation center within the university, were never realized. Although a community rehabilitation center was eventually established, it was situated within the St. Francis hospital.

St. Francis Hospital had an interest in establishing a rehabilitation facility as early as 1953. Clearly, because of its industrial medicine department, it had many of the elements of a rehabilitation institution already in place. Sister Adele, frequently the pioneering leader whenever change occurred, recalled that there was a woman involved in the Catholic Hospital Association who was very involved in rehabilitation medicine. Sister knew her from meetings and followed her work in publications, so she was aware of new trends in the delivery of those types of services. When the new building was being planned, Sister Adele had also been advised to incorporate something new and different into the facility in order to capture the interest of the community, which would aid in raising funds.[79] Plans were underway when Drs. Griffith,

---

[78]"A Plan for Community Rehabilitation Center of Pittsburgh," manuscript, March 1952, St. Francis Hospital Archives; Claude W. Munger, M.D., and Mary C. Jarrett,"Report of a Survey of the Care of Chronic Disease in Pittsburgh and Allegheny County," (Pittsburgh: Health and Welfare Federation, 1947), AIS, 68: 14.

[79]Interview with Sister M. Adele Meiser, 1993.

Wagner and Thomas, along with board member Mr. Carl Kirschler, went to New York to visit a rehabilitation center in order to make recommendations to the St. Francis board, staff and administration.[80] Sister Adele had sought the advice of the medical staff, who recommended Dr. Thomas C. Hohmann as one of the best choices to head the new department. He declined at first, but later accepted.[81] Dr. Hohmann did his internship and residency at St. Francis, followed by training at the Warm Springs Georgia Foundation and at the Institute for Physical Medicine and Rehabilitation in New York. The St. Francis administrators engaged Dr. Howard T. Rusk as a consultant to aid in the planning of the new department. In addition, in preparation for the new rehabilitation department, the hospital administrators sent a physical therapist to the Rusk Institute in New York in 1956, and Sister M. Ricarda Pahler OSF studied rehabilitation nursing.[82]

In 1960, the new rehabilitation center was established by combining the old department of physical medicine, which included physical therapy, the occupational therapy department, a new brace and orthotic center, vocational counseling, social service and an activities of daily living, or self help, section. The unit which included forty in-patient beds, occupied two stories in the new nine story wing. The department also had a cafeteria dining room, lounge, library and sun deck. The occupational therapy department provided looms, a printing press, electronics such as radios and oscilloscopes and a kitchen for developing skills. The purpose was to make it possible for patients to resume daily living activities as normally as possible. Out-patient services were also offered. The philosophy behind the department was that in order to achieve maximum success, the rehabilitation must commence with the onset of the disability. It claimed to be the first department of rehabilitation medicine in a general hospital in Western Pennsylvania, providing "all the facilities of medical, surgical, psychiatric and training skills pooled to offer the most complete service possible to every patient."[83] The center was not designed to serve any particular type of disability. During the department's first five years,

[80]Minutes, Board of Managers, 9/28/53.

[81]Interview with Sister M. Adele Meiser, 1993.

[82]Sister M. Adele Meiser, "Intermediate Rehabilitation Care," *Hospital Progress*, September 1968; "Faces the Facts," advertisements which ran in the *Pittsburgh Press*, 1983, 1984; Dorothy Naumann, ed, *Equitable News* 13 (May, 1962); *St. Francis Forward*, (Spring 1958, Winter 1959); Minutes, Board of Managers, 5/28/56.

[83]Sister M. Adele Meiser, "Intermediate Rehabilitation Care," *Hospital Progress*, September 1968; "Faces the Facts," advertisements which ran in the *Pittsburgh Press*, 1983, 1984; Dorothy Naumann, ed., *Equitable News* 13 (May, 1962); *St. Francis Forward*, (Spring 1958, Winter 1959); Minutes, Board of Managers, 5/28/56.

1,863 individuals were admitted; thirty percent of those patients had suffered cerebral vascular disorders.[84]

The hospital's rehabilitation department not only served the patients of the community, but provided educational opportunities for myriad health professionals. The American Medical Association approved a residency program in physical medicine and rehabilitation. Affiliated with the University of Pittsburgh, orthopedic residents also rotated through the program. Drs. Joseph Novak and Thomas C. Hohmann, both diplomats of the American Board of Physical Medicine and Rehabilitation, were in charge of the training. Physical therapy students from the University of Pittsburgh and Indiana University of Pennsylvania, as well as occupational therapy students from eight different university programs, benefited from the training offered at St. Francis. Social service students from the University of Pittsburgh also enjoyed the educational services provided.[85]

St. Francis Hospital proved to be the exception rather than the rule by their willingness to establish a rehabilitation facility. Partially as a result of new federal legislation, such as the Hill-Burton act, hospitals expanded and increased their numbers markedly in the period between 1946 and 1960. The new hospitals, like those before them, however, concentrated on providing short-term cures with no major shift to long-term treatment of rehabilitation. There were approximately five thousand short-term general hospitals compared to three hundred hospitals for long-term care. Short-term hospitals which did attempt to change their function were heralded as major experiments. Although St. Francis Hospital does not appear in the literature as such an experiment, that may reflect the sisters' long standing history of maintaining a low profile publicly. Their establishment of rehabilitation services, in fact, demonstrates their exceptional flexibility in expanding and redefining hospital functions.[86]

As the center proved successful, it became apparent over the years that the number of individuals on the waiting list increased, and therefore, patients were not treated immediately. St. Francis devised a priority system whereby those who were thought to be the best candidates for treatment were admitted immediately. An intermediate care unit was established to meet the needs of the still untreated group who were not in the top priority for immediate reha-

---

[84]"St. Francis General Hospital's Facilities and Plans for the Future," manuscript, 1966, St. Francis Hospital Archives.

[85]"St. Francis General Hospital's Facilities and Plans for the Future," manuscript, February 1966, St. Francis Hospital Archives.

[86]Rosemary Stevens, *In Sickness and in Wealth, American Hospital in the Twentieth Century*, (New York: Basic Books, Inc., 1989), pp. 229–230.

bilitation. The patients who were admitted to this unit were not terminally or acutely ill, but were those who it was deemed would not benefit from full-scale rehabilitation, possibly because of a chronic disability, but would still need help with activities of daily living. This prevented patients discharged from the hospital from being dependent on others for their daily personal care. The intermediate unit was also used for patients in the intensive rehabilitation program who had to halt the program due to development of other medical problems. The fourteen bed unit was established in October 1966. The average length of confinement to the unit was 23.4 days, and 70.6 percent of the patients were discharged to their homes. Although the intermediate care unit was not an official part of the rehabilitation department, since patients were under the direct care of their attending physicians, patients still had access to social workers and occupational and physical therapists.[87]

World War II to 1979—Out-patient Department

Out-patient care continued to be provided by the hospital, but immediately following the war, the numbers of patients in most of the departments declined. Falk Clinic opened during this period, and many other out-patient clinics were also established resulting in fewer cases cared for at St. Francis. In the year 1938–1939, 20,070 patients were seen, compared to 11,229 individuals seen in the year ending May 31, 1947. The number of people seen in the neurosurgery dispensary increased, however, probably due to the development of neurosurgical techniques.[88] In 1948, it was noted that there was also an increase in the number of allergy patients, but a decrease in the number of medical cases. This was probably due to the patients' increasing ability to meet the expenses of medical care either themselves or with third party payment systems; they no longer needed free care at the clinic. The medical clinic, however, remained the largest department serving 1,013 patients in a given year. The second largest department, the allergy clinic, served 877 patients. The out-patient clinic physicians at that time also continued to see private patients who had been referred by their own physicians to the various specialty clinics, primarily surgical, obstetric, gynecologic and dental.[89]

---

[87]Sister M. Adele Meiser, "Intermediate Rehabilitation Care," *Hospital Progress*, September 1968; Minutes, Medical Staff, 3/1/66, St. Francis Hospital Archives.

[88]Minutes, Board of Managers, 6/9/47

[89]Minutes, Board of Managers, 6/14/48, Dispensary annual report.

World War II to 1979—Obstetrics

Clearly, when departments expanded or changed, they did so on an already established foundation. And once that foundation was in place it was not easily removed. In 1976, the Health Systems Agency (HSA), a regional health planning board comprised of sixty-one members, recommended the closing of maternity wards in thirteen district hospitals in an attempt to eliminate duplication of facilities and minimize escalating hospital costs. The HSA estimated that four million dollars would be saved annually by eliminating underused maternity beds in Southwestern Pennsylvania. In Allegheny County alone, the estimated savings would be approximately 1.2 million dollars annually. The HSA expected that the anticipated savings would reduce the number of Blue Cross premiums and tax increases used to pay patients' bills, including Medicaid. The HSA used eleven hundred births annually as the criteria to determine which hospitals should close their maternity units. Understanding that St. Francis Hospital had about five hundred births annually, the HSA proposed that they be one of the hospitals to close their maternity unit.[90]

The hospital board and administration were adamantly opposed to the closing of the obstetrical unit, fearing the hospital would lose gynecologists and pediatricians who were "highly valued staff members." The hospital executives felt the entire 757 bed hospital, the largest in the city, would suffer if they were forced to close their twenty-five bed unit, as physicians who delivered and cared for babies were attracted to the hospital because it provided them with an opportunity to treat other patients, primarily women and children. The sisters, board and medical staff were concerned that in order for the hospital to benefit the people of the area, they could not be deprived of the services provided by gynecologists, obstetricians and pediatricians. There is also some evidence to suggest that they had financial concerns, not surprising considering the hospital's history of monetary difficulties. Dr. Robert E. Davis, medical director of the hospital, also claimed that the hospital's birth statistics were grossly inaccurate as understood by the HSA. In July 1976, Sister Adele and Dr. H. R. Dailey, chairman of obstetrics and gynecology, each notified the HSA by letter that they were opposed to the recommendation; they also

[90]Dolores Frederick, "St. Francis, Attorney Labor Over Obstetrics Cut Letters," *Pittsburgh Press*, 18 March 1977; Dolores Frederick, "Hospital Battles Ward Closing Plan," *Pittsburgh Press*, 19 March 1977; Henry W. Pierce, "St. Francis Hospital Fights Maternity Unit Shutdown," *Pittsburgh Post-Gazette*, 18 March 1977.

requested that they have the opportunity to take part in the development of the HSA's plan, but their requests were ignored. No one from the HSA contacted anyone at the hospital. The following March, hospital officials publicly accused officials of the HSA of ignoring them while proposing to eliminate the hospital's maternity ward. It is difficult to determine how the issue was finally resolved, though the end result was clear. Sister Adele telephoned someone from HSA at one point to voice her unwillingness to comply with the proposed plan. The gentleman with whom she spoke suggested to her that she was not looking at both sides of the situation but only saw things one way. She agreed that he was absolutely correct, stating, "one way, my way!" In August 1977, the Health Systems Agency announced a revision in their original plan which had called for only Shadyside hospital to provide obstetrical services to eastern Allegheny county. The obstetrics department at St. Francis Hospital was never closed and continues to thrive, serving parturient women of the community.[91]

World War II to 1979—Outside Agencies

Following the second world war, as the sisters continued in their mission to provide necessary services, they began to associate with other agencies in order to deliver care more efficiently. The administration was obviously always cognizant of prevailing trends in hospital services and intent on remaining current. In the early forties, Pennsylvania hospitals were criticized for not having blood and plasma banks in hospitals with bed capacities exceeding two hundred beds. St. Francis Hospital, at that time, got their supply from Magee Hospital, but soon began to plan for their own service.[92] Physicians on staff recommended the hospital start with fifteen to twenty pints of blood, and also advised that all employees be typed and classified.[93] The Blood Bank was officially opened on February 1, 1948. During the first four months, 706 pints of whole blood had been taken and 457 pints were transfused. Thirty pints

[91]Dolores Frederick, "St. Francis, Attorney Labor Over Obstetrics Cut Letters," *Pittsburgh Press*, 18 March 1977; Dolores Frederick, "Hospital Battles Ward Closing Plan," *Pittsburgh Press*, 19 March 1977; Henry W. Pierce, "St. Francis Hospital Fights Maternity Unit Shutdown," *Pittsburgh Post-Gazette*, 18 March 1977; Interview with Sister M. Adele Meiser, 1993; Henry W. Pierce, "St. Francis Wins Reprieve In Maternity Unit Battle," *Pittsburgh Post-Gazette*, 16 August 1977.

[92]Minutes, Board of Managers, 6/8/42.

[93]Minutes, Medical Staff, 6/3/46.

were given to other hospitals, twenty-four of those to the Veterans Administration, reflective of the sisters' willingness to share their services.[94] In 1959, however, St. Francis Hospital joined the Central Blood Bank, a service which provided blood to many area hospitals. By then, the hospital required four thousand pints, annually, partially due to the new open heart surgery program. It was anticipated that the requirements would exceed four thousand pints so a recruitment program was begun among the one thousand employees.[95] Clearly, as one phase of the hospital's services grew, such as the neurosurgery and cardiovascular surgery departments, demands were placed on other services, providing incentive for growth. It is imperative to remember, however, that behind the expansion were sisters with foresight and a strong desire to provide for those God had placed in their care.

In 1959, St. Francis entered into an agreement with the Pennsylvania State Bureau of Vocational Rehabilitation (BVR), exemplifying again the new trend to establish relationships with outside agencies. The main goal of the BVR was to provide service to qualified individuals with physical disabilities that incapacitated them from formal occupations. They provided rehabilitation of the physically disabled where there was work potential, striving to make producers out of tax consumers. The bureau did not perform clinical services, but assisted in providing state or federal funds by which the patient received the necessary training or equipment to make him a tax-paying citizen. The Sisters of St. Francis, believing that rehabilitation was a significant part of comprehensive medical care and that the hospital through its own resources or other community resources should offer this service to its patients, consequently considered it appropriate to cooperate with BVR.[96] The hospital agreed to accept patients under the Bureau of Rehabilitation program, and to render services to them as authorized by BVR. In return, BVR would pay at rates not to exceed those charged the general public.[97]

The program commenced in September 1961. An official relationship was established whereby the hospital provided 250 square feet for a counselor and two secretaries appointed by BVR. Hospital staff was informed of the availability of the new service. All referrals to the bureau were made by staff physicians, but actual case findings could have been done by any member of

[94] Minutes, Board of Managers, 6/7/48.
[95] *Pittsburgh Press*, 17 November 1959.
[96] Sister M. Adele Meiser and Thomas C. Hohmann, M.D., "Hospital and State Merge in Rehabilitation Program," *Journal of the American Hospital Association* 39 (8/1/65), reprint.
[97] Minutes, Board of Managers, 12/14/59.

the staff or the bureau counselor. It was deemed advisable to commence voca-tional counseling early in the patient's rehabilitation process. BVR members collaborated with physicians, nurses, members of the admissions department, the public health nurse, social workers and those on the psychology ser-vice. Periodic group discussions of counselors, staff psychologists and BVR counselors avoided an overlap of services. The specialized BVR counselors, aware of the patient's ability to perform and function, and also familiar with the employment possibilities within the areas in which the patient lived, made judgments concerning vocational rehabilitation.[98] By 1967, BVR had a backlog of five to six thousand individuals in need of evaluation. The hos-pital, then, opened an Evaluation Center, also financed by the state BVR, which was to be supervised by Dr. Hohmann, although other staff were to be consulted.[99]

The hospital administration not only cooperated with other agencies in the direct provision of care, but also in the financing of specific projects. The Variety Club of Pittsburgh has a long history of providing funding for programs in the rehabilitation department. The Variety Club, which was first founded in Pittsburgh, grew into an international organization, composed of men in show business, which has raised millions of dollars to help needy and handicapped children in the world. In 1968, Variety's Mother Tent #1 helped to establish the Variety's Center for Handicapped Children at St. Francis, a pilot program for psychiatric and physical rehabilitation for children. The unit consisted of an eight bed physical rehabilitation unit and an eight bed psychiatric rehabilitation unit. They also established a Brace Shop in 1961 and Speech Clinic in 1964 at St. Francis, and gave grants for other related projects.[100] In November 1965, Sir Billy Butlin of London, came to Pittsburgh to receive the International Variety Personality of the Year award, presented by Variety Club, Tent #1. He was the largest individual benefactor to Variety clubs, donating five thousand dollars to St. Francis Hospital.[101] Over the years, they continued to support rehabilitation at St. Francis. In 1979, for

[98]Sister M. Adele Meiser and Dr. Thomas C. Hohmann, "Hospital and State Merge in Rehabilitation Program," *Hospitals, J.A.H.A.* 39 (August 1, 1965); "Partners in Progress," c. 1967, St. Francis Hospital Archives; Sister M. Adele Meiser, "Rehabilitation Counselors Meet," *The Bulletin—Hospital Association of Pennsylvania,* (November, 1963): 4; Sister M. Adele Meiser and Dr. Thomas C. Hohmann, "A State Rehabilitation Program in the General Hospital," pp. 2–3, manuscript, n.d., St. Francis Hospital Archives.

[99]Executive Director's Report to the Board of Managers, 10/23/67.

[100]"A Working Partnership," manuscript in St. Francis Hospital Archives; article in St. Francis Hospital archives, n.d.; *Signs of Life* 6 (Spring/summer 1969), 5 (Summer/Fall 1968).

[101]"Gift Check from Sir Billy," article, n.d., c. 1966, St. Francis Hospital Archives.

example, the Variety Club International donated a van, the Sunshine Coach, to the hospital to be used to transport handicapped children to clinics and recreational events.[102]

World War II to 1979—Research

Research continued to be one of the hospital's interests although, as Sister Adele noted, it never took precedence over providing care and services to patients. Noting the lack of adequate funds or academicians, Sister Adele took great pride in the hospital's focus. Nevertheless, the hospital was able to contribute to the myriad studies performed in medical academia. For example, in 1967, the hospital conducted a pilot study for the United States Public Health Service, the purpose of which was to determine if early intensive medical and nursing care of victims of cerebral thrombosis or cerebral hemorrhage improved recovery rate.[103] The hospital was also involved in participating on a safety panel board which was organized at St. Francis to research safety practices within operating rooms. The board worked in conjunction with researchers at the United States Bureau of Mines, the Mellon Institute and the University of Pittsburgh.[104] Sister Adele always noted the tremendous value of research, but felt that other institutions were better equipped for large scale studies.

St. Francis directly influenced medical research by training a physician who later received international recognition. Dr. Philip S. Hench was given credit for working to develop cortisone. He began his research to explore drugs to combat rheumatic heart disease while he interned at St. Francis Hospital. In 1950, he was granted a five thousand dollar Passano Foundation award for pioneering in the treatment of rheumatic diseases. He directed the department involved with rheumatic diseases at Mayo clinic, and later won the Nobel prize in medicine for "discoveries regarding the hormones of the adrenal cortex."[105] Although the hospital's research endeavors may have been minimal, they were not without merit.

[102] "St. Francis Gift," *Pittsburgh Catholic*, 23 November 1979.

[103] "Partners in Progress," c. 1967, St. Francis Hospital Archives.

[104] "St. Francis Launches Biggest Expansion," May 1955, source of publication unknown, copy in St. Francis Hospital Archives.

[105] "St. Francis Launches Biggest Expansion," May 1955, source of publication unknown, copy in St. Francis Hospital Archives; *St. Francis*, (Spring 1950, Winter 1950–1951).

World War II to 1979—Pastoral Care

It had always been the sisters' mission to aid in healing by providing spiritual care, and in the late seventies an organized department was developed to meet those needs. In keeping with the hospital's policy of providing spiritual and ecumenical care, Sister Adele established the pastoral care department in 1979. Since the hospital's founding, spiritual care was always offered to patients, whether by the sisters or clergy from other faiths, who were encouraged to administer to non-Catholic patients. Since 1874, the Capuchin fathers from St. Augustine's church have held the chaplaincy at the hospital. The concept of holistic care, caring for spiritual needs as well as physical and mental, was established in the first days of the hospital's history and continues to the present day.[106] The idea of 'holistic care' although not unique to St. Francis, quite likely had greater emphasis in Catholic hospitals.[107]

Beginning in the mid-sixties, many Catholic institutions established pastoral care departments either in response to the decline in numbers of sisters who were entering the Order, or due to an increase in the numbers who left religious life in this period. As nursing sisters became less numerous, there was an increasing concern regarding how to provide spiritual care. New pastoral care departments were developed to provide a coherent plan of addressing the spiritual aspect of health service. In many hospitals, lay individuals were also active members of the department.[108]

The pastoral care department, officially organized as a department in 1979, was in keeping with the sisters' philosophy. The nine members of the pastoral care department, directed by Sister Adele until just several years ago, minister to the physical and spiritual person. The first members of the department represented the Lutheran and United Presbyterian denominations as well as Roman Catholic. The purpose was not to lead people to any particular practice, but to God. Not only do the pastoral care department members counsel or pray with people, but they also work to notify home churches

---

[106]Written history, "St. Francis Hospital," manuscript, n.d. but c. 1940, St. Francis Hospital Archives.

[107]See also Mary Louise Sullivan M.S.C., "Mother Cabrini: Missionary to Italian Immigrants," *U.S. Catholic Historian*, 6 (1987), p. 270; Susan Carol Peterson and Courtney Ann Vaughn-Roberson, *Women With Vision: The Presentation Sisters of South Dakota, 1880–1985*, (Urbana: University of Illinois, 1988), p. 189.

[108]Mary Carol Conroy, "The Transition Years," in *Pioneer Healers: The History of Women Religious in American Health Care* eds., Ursula Stepsis, CSA, and Dolores Liptak, RSM, (New York: Crossroad Publ. Co., 1989), p. 156.

and to call requested clergy, exemplifying the sisters' belief in providing ecumenical care.[109]

Conclusion

By the late seventies, the hospital had clearly developed into one of the largest general hospitals in Western Pennsylvania and, to its credit, had provided more care for the indigent than any other institution in the region. Because of the sisters' insistence on maintaining their mission to serve the poor, other goals were not completely met, however. Neglecting to raise or direct funds into research, as well as the institution's organizational structure, has limited the number of American physicians interested in seeking medical staff privileges there. As an institution endeavoring to offer all basic medical services to the community at large, it has excelled, but as a research or teaching institution, it has fallen slightly short of its goal.

Clearly, the hospital sisters established a tradition of innovation that has continued into the latter half of the twentieth century. Competition from the medical school at the University of Pittsburgh and other facilities, some quite well endowed, have made it difficult for St. Francis Hospital to remain as competitive in all areas as it was in the first part of the century. As the hospital sisters reevaluated their services in the latter half of the twentieth century and determined that the hospital would develop expertise in specific areas, they wisely chose to focus on departments in which they could compete. As a result, they have established a rehabilitation department and furthered a psychiatric department that remain highly competitive within the region. The administration's foresight proved to be beneficial not only to the development of the institution, but to the community as well.

To be sure, the Sisters of St. Francis of Millvale established a hospital which is in line with their own philosophy. Believing that "as human beings we are composed of body and soul with an eternal destiny," they developed an institution which serves to heal the body, mind and spirit. "Everyone who approaches us for care, regardless of race, creed, nationality, age, sex, handicap, or economic status, is entitled to share in the fruits of our ministry. . . . We are committed to protecting, nurturing and enhancing life . . . as members of a major medical teaching Health Center, we uphold Judeo-Christian principles and values in the moral and professional education of our men and women."

[109]"Bottom Line," *Probe*, (May 1982).

The sisters, by maintaining absolute authority within the institution, have been able to proceed as they desired in fulfilling the four components of their mission, which includes not only providing for patient care, but also offering educational activities and encouraging research as well as participating in any activity intended to promote individual and community health.[110]

[110]The "Logo" and "Mission" of the St. Francis Hospital.

Chapter Four

Healing the Mind—Psychiatry

Probably more than any other department, the psychiatric division exemplifies how the sisters struggled to uphold their spiritual principles in the context of change in the field of medicine. New theories and treatment modalities in psychiatry challenged the sisters to make decisions which occasionally resulted in tension with the hospital physicians, other hospitals and the community at large. In some ways, too, however, the sisters' mission to provide holistic care to every individual directly caused the establishment of new and innovative programs in the hospital. Characteristic of the period following the second world war is the wider focus on provision of community service. The importance of the psychiatric department to the development of the hospital cannot be overemphasized. Providing care for the mentally ill set St. Francis Hospital apart from the other private general hospitals in the region. As the sisters maintained their authority within the institution, they laid the foundation for what became one of the leading psychiatric facilities in Western Pennsylvania.

The historiography of mental illness has largely neglected the role played by religious orders in the twentieth century, and further, has focused generally on the periods prior to World War II. Studies have analyzed mental illness in the context of Progressive reform, or the professionalization of physicians. Other social historians have argued, somewhat controversially, that confinement in an asylum served as a method of social control; the bourgeoisie over the lower classes. More recent studies have explored the impact of changing mental health policies and practices on society and the victims of mental illness in America. The history of St. Francis Hospital demonstrates the tension inherent in the struggle to maintain a traditional mental health facility which

131

provided care during a period of recurrent upheaval in mental health theory, practice and policy. The sisters also dealt with the conflicts within themselves as they recognized the unmet needs of so many psychiatric patients while they desired to establish what was perceived to be modern mental health care services, and comply with government mandates.[1]

The study of mental health care in America can easily be divided into two separate and distinct parts. The period prior to World War II is characterized by institutionalized care and largely empirical treatment methods. The impact of World War II, however, affected trends in psychiatric care, changing dramatically the mental health practices and policies in the following decades. Psychiatrists introduced numerous new theories regarding the etiology of mental illness as well as innovative treatment modalities. The end result, of course, was the implementation of new mental health policies altering the provision of care for the mentally ill.

1900 to World War II

In the early 1900s, the hospital continued what was established in the latter part of the nineteenth century and maintained two distinctly different divisions of the hospital, the general hospital and the "nervous side," or psychiatric division. The psychiatric department stood out as the epitome of what innovative psychiatrists recommended as an up-to-date modern facility for the treatment of mental disorders. Early in the twentieth century, there was a new effort to establish psychiatric wards in general hospitals. According to psychiatrists at that time, there were numerous benefits, including the possibility for an increasing number of patient referrals. Psychiatrists hoped that new clientele, such as children, might be attracted, and that other physicians of other specialties might become sensitized to the psychological and emotional needs of patients. By 1930, however, of the 421 general hospitals approved by the AMA for intern training that responded to the survey, only 56 hospitals had wards for psychiatric patients. By 1938, only 153 hospitals of the approximately 5,000 general hospitals in the country accepted mental patients. Approximately 2.5 percent of general hospitals in the United States in 1939 had provisions for even the mildest psychiatric cases. In 1937, St. Fran-

---

[1]Constance M. McGovern, "Mental Illness," in *Encyclopedia of Social History*, ed. Peter N. Stearns, (New York: Garland Publishing, Inc., 1994), p. 466; Gerald N. Grob, *From Asylum to Community: Mental Health Policy in Modern America*, (Princeton: Princeton University Press, 1991).

cis Hospital was the only privately owned general hospital in Pennsylvania that maintained a department for neuro-psychiatric patients.[2]

St. Francis Hospital argued the advantages of having a psychiatric department as part of a general hospital. The psychiatrists felt it was necessary to have ready access to medical and surgical services, such as a laboratory, X-ray department or operating room, which only a general hospital could provide. Many of their patients suffered from other ailments of a non-psychiatric nature, and there was a connection between some medical/surgical disorders and psychiatric abnormalities.[3] It was widely known that numerous patients who exhibited symptoms of mental disease had a disorder of somatic origin, such as a brain tumor, for example. Not only did the psychiatrists support the view that a psychiatric department was necessary to the general hospital and vice versa, but the sister administrators openly advocated the policy and encouraged other hospitals to follow. Sister Adele was adamant that in order to provide comprehensive care for patients in the general hospital who might suffer from temporary psychotic episodes, or for those in the psychiatric unit who might have medical or surgical problems, a psychiatric unit had to be an essential component of any general hospital.[4]

Reflecting conditions noted in other institutions in the early twentieth century, many of the patients hospitalized in the St. Francis psychiatric department did, in fact, suffer from somatic disorders. Between 1922 and 1940, historians have suggested that in other institutions the percentage of patients whose behavior was due to somatic etiology rose from 33 percent to 44 percent.[5] In the period 1921–1923, St. Francis physicians identified fifty-two cases of "psychoses with other brain and nervous disease." Patients were diagnosed as having psychoses and other related disorders such as brain abscess, cerebral embolism, cerebral hemorrhage, encephalitis, meningitis and chorea. In addition, the hospital cared for 137 cases of "psychoses with other somatic diseases," which included anemia, asthma, burns, carcinoma, diabetes, cholecystitis, infectious diseases, pregnancy, puerperal sepsis, otitis media, phlebitis

[2]Gerald N. Grob, *From Asylum to Community: Mental Health Policy in Modern America*, (Princeton: Princeton University Press, 1991), pp. 165–166; Gerald N. Grob, *Mental Illness and American Society, 1875–1940*, (Princeton: Princeton University Press, 1983), p. 241; C. C. Wholey, "Psychiatric Facilities in Pittsburgh," *American Journal of Psychiatry*, 93 (March 1937), p. 1188.

[3]C. C. Wholey, "Psychiatric Facilities in Pittsburgh," *American Journal of Psychiatry*, 93 (March 1937), p. 1188.

[4]Sister M. Adele Meiser, OSF, "Psychiatric Unit: Pro and Con," *Modern Hospital*, 53 (December 1939). Interviews with Sister M. Adele Meiser, 1993.

[5]Gerald N. Grob, "The Chronic Mentally Ill in America: The Historical Context," *Mental Health Services in the United States and England: Struggling for Change; collected papers prepared for the Joint United States/England Conference on Mental Health Services*, (Princeton: Robert Wood Johnson Foundation, 1991), p. 10.

and tuberculosis.[6] These admissions serve to emphasize the psychiatrists' belief that psychiatric disorders and somatic diseases were often closely related. Although in many areas the hospital pioneered new trends, in terms of those accepted for admission, they mirrored other facilities of the time. The diagnoses of the patients admitted to St. Francis resembled those of other institutions, while supporting the new belief at that time that general hospitals and psychiatric departments should be closely linked.

Innovative psychiatrists went further, however, and not only advocated the establishment of a psychiatric department within the general hospital, but adhered to the idea that those departments should develop 'psychopathic' wards. The concept of a "psychopathic" hospital was first developed at the turn of the twentieth century. Reflecting current trends, the Pennsylvania Committee on Lunacy also advocated the establishment of psychopathic wards in general hospitals. The purpose of such a ward was to provide a place for the acute and recent insane to be sent for ten to sixty days for diagnostic purposes, study and observation. It was to be equipped with a laboratory and, ideally, was to be under the supervision of a medical school, whereby students could furnish labor while preparing to work in state institutions. They could also assist the state and municipalities in sharing the costs. Presumably, this would allow some patients to avoid being hastily pronounced insane. Only St. Francis initiated such a project which the Committee on Lunacy felt promised "to be a valuable adjunct to the hospital." In 1912, the same year that new sun porches were added to the nervous side, plans to establish a "psychopathical ward" were delayed because the hospital was unable to appropriate any funds for maintenance. By 1913, however, the psychopathic ward was open and "doing good work." Evidence suggests that the ward did not remain open. The hospital may have been unable to properly fund the psychopathic ward because the 1916 report of the Committee on Lunacy continued to recommend the establishment of such wards in the vicinity of Philadelphia and Pittsburgh, as the "city of Pittsburgh has no such hospital."[7]

By 1923, however, the entire Neuropsychiatric Department, and not just a separate ward, was referred to as the Psychopathic Department. It functioned as it was described ten years earlier, providing for those thought to be curable. It is not clear if the ward actually had closed after its opening, or whether the records ignoring its existence were merely inaccurate. At any rate, the

[6]*Report of the St. Francis Hospital*, June 1, 1921–May 31, 1923, pp. 33, 82, 83. Note that these refer to numbers of cases and not individual patients.

[7]*Annual Report of the Board of Commissioners of Public Charities of the Commonwealth of Pennsylvania*, the report of the Committee on Lunacy for year 1908, p. 8; 1912, p. 390, Report of the assistant general agent, p. 81; 1913, p. 69; 1916, p. 297.

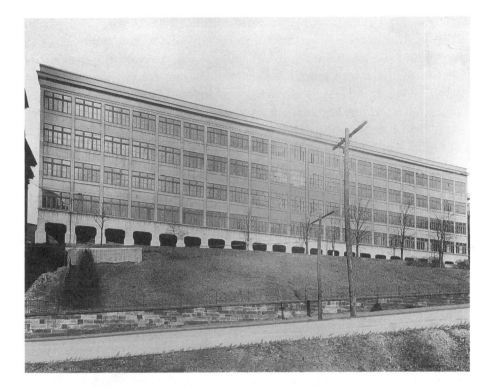

Psychopathic Department Sun Porches, 1923

policy had been implemented whereby all patients were admitted for study and diagnosis, and only those patients whose recovery seemed possible were treated over extended periods of time. The administration claimed that during the hospital's first fifty years, they had "turned thousands back into productive life, and made them fully independent producers, rather than to allow them to become inmates of public asylums for the remainder of their lives, there to be a constant drain upon taxpayers. Last year alone (1926), 465 were cured of mental illness and again made assets instead of liabilities to the community."[8] In the psychiatric ward could be found "men, women, even children, being brought out of the darkness into light. They were learning again to keep step with the stride of doers, again to take their places in life-production, economic assets, rather than possible inmates of some asylum for the remainder of their lives."[9] Those patients who were deemed incurable were transferred

[8]*Uniting the Armies of Health and Industry,* published for Industrial Pittsburgh by St. Francis Hospital, 1927; *Weighing the Evidence,* campaign brochure, 1927.

[9]*For All of Us,* building campaign brochure, c. 1927, St. Francis Hospital Archives.

to the appropriate public or private institution. By 1920, then, the hospital functioned entirely according to the philosophy of a "psychopathic" institution, acting also as a clearing-house, caring for acute cases and transferring others to mental institutions in Western Pennsylvania, as well as parts of Ohio and West Virginia. This practice continued for many years. The Sisters of St. Francis felt they were developing the "idea of a mental hospital in its strictest sense," and believed they were the only institution of this type in Western Pennsylvania. State and other public institutions were viewed as facilities for long-term or chronic care patients. The psychiatric department, which had two hundred beds by the early twenties, was generally filled to capacity. Over one thousand patients from West Virginia, Ohio and Pennsylvania were admitted annually.[10]

Historian Gerald N. Grob has noted that by 1920, only four institutions were clearly identified as psychopathic institutions, they included Pavilion F of the Albany Hospital, the Boston Psychopathic Hospital, the Michigan Psychopathic Hospital and the Henry Phipps Psychiatric Clinic at Johns Hopkins. The Boston Psychopathic Hospital, one of the most influential, did not provide long-term custodial care, and did not confine patients for extended periods. It acted as a clearing-house for Boston's mentally ill, providing intensive treatment for acute patients who were returned to homes or admitted later to state hospitals for more extended treatment. It was also intended as a center for research. It is apparent, however, that St. Francis also had begun to develop a 'psychopathic' facility around the same time period. Clearly, over time, the idea of treating the acutely ill became the hospital's philosophy for all of the psychiatric patients admitted. Theory and practice, however, did not necessarily exist together in reality.[11] The sisters' intent to serve all patients sometimes conflicted with this policy, especially in the years following World War II.

1900 to World War II—Treatment Methods

The psychiatric department of St. Francis Hospital established the foundations for comprehensive and up-to-date treatment of numerous psychiatric disorders very early in its history. Its early philosophy regarding the care of the

---

[10] *Report of the St. Francis Hospital*, June 1, 1921–May 31, 1923, pp. 34–35; *Worker's confidential Handbook*, *St. Francis Hospital Campaign*, 1927; C. C. Wholey, "Psychiatric Facilities in Pittsburgh," *American Journal of Psychiatry*, 93 (March 1937), p. 1189.

[11] Gerald N. Grob, *Mental Illness and American Society, 1875–1940*, (Princeton: Princeton University Press, 1983), pp. 126–139.

acutely ill mental patient reflected the ideology of contemporary innovative psychiatrists. As the hospital expanded over the years, these foundations were built upon, resulting in a treatment center which provided care and treatment for myriad psychiatric maladies.

In the early twentieth century, therapies to treat psychiatric disorders were generally non-specific and empirical, although occasionally supported by rationale. For example, it was commonly believed that chronic or masked focal infections, in the tonsils or mouth, played an important role in the etiology of psychoses. Many accepted the theory, but surgery to remove the infection was not widespread. Two of the most common therapies were hydrotherapy and elimination drugs. Therapeutic innovation, not nihilism, characterized this period.[12]

Treatment methods for St. Francis' psychiatric patients included hydrotherapy, occupational therapy and physiotherapy, as well as psychotherapy.

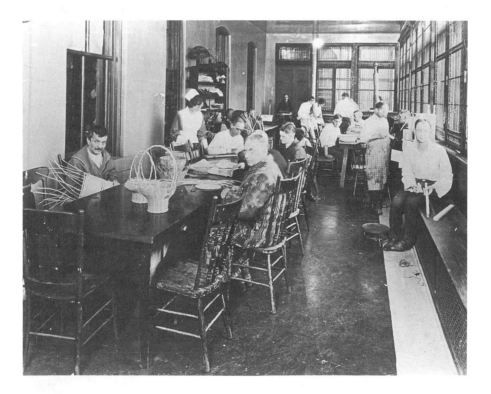

Occupational Therapy Workroom, 1923

[12]Gerald N. Grob, *Mental Illness and American Society, 1875–1940*, (Princeton: Princeton University Press, 1983), pp. 121–122.

Occupational therapy, first implemented in the hospital in 1917, allowed patients to use creative and motor skills to create baskets and other items, which were occasionally exhibited for hospital personnel and visitors. When prescribed by the physician, men generally became involved in carpentry, painting or weaving, and women were engaged in sewing, embroidery, weaving rugs or basket making. Hydrotherapy included various forms of water treatments. The department of physical medicine, which housed the hydrotherapy unit, had opened in 1910. The physiotherapy department provided an assortment of treatments for the general hospital as well as the psychiatric department. These treatments included electric cabinet baths, rubs with alcohol or salt, massages, bakings, medical gymnastics, high frequency vacuum treatments and treatments with electricity (galvanic, faradic, ionization, diathermy). Psychiatrists also employed other analytic methods in treating their patients. Most simply, it was understood that allowing the patient to talk was beneficial. "A valuable start in freeing the patient from his symptoms is made when he is allowed to tell his story, with the consequent release of his pent-up feelings.

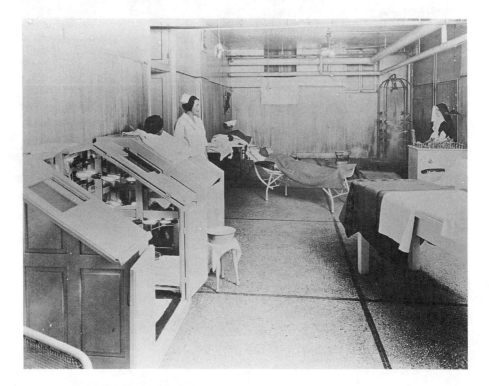

Electric Cabinet and Hydriatic Room, 1923

The therapeutic value of a sympathetic attitude toward the patient's story can hardly be overemphasized."[13]

The psychiatric department also utilized the newest diagnostic methods. The electroencephalogram (EEG) was first used as a diagnostic tool at St. Francis in 1915. Evidence suggests that St. Francis, false to their tradition of innovations, may have been the first hospital in Pittsburgh to do so.[14]

Innovations in treatment continued at St. Francis into the next decades. The psychiatric department during this period was very active, admitting fifteen hundred to eighteen hundred patients per year.[15] Electric Shock Therapy (EST), first utilized nationally in the 1930s, was introduced at St. Francis in 1936.[16] By the early forties, insulin and metrazol therapies were also widely used, typical of other psychiatric facilities as well, but by 1940, electroshock therapy began to replace metrazol as the treatment of choice.[17] When the census of the hospital was approximately 260 per day, the hospital recorded performing electroshock therapy on fifty to sixty-five patients daily. Seclusion and restraint were other treatment modalities, but were not used "excessively."[18]

Although these treatments of the twenties, thirties and forties sound barbaric, they were, by contemporary standards, the epitome of excellent psychiatric treatment methods. The therapeutic claims may not have been based on conclusive data, but they reflected the confident outlook of psychiatrists who believed in the efficacy of treatments.[19] "Mild and convalescent psychotic patients" were materially helped toward recovery.[20]

St. Francis also had a long history of treating patients with venereal diseases, willingly admitting patients diagnosed with syphilis to the psychiatric department. In the early twentieth century, the Committee on Lunacy listed syphilis as one of the myriad causes of insanity. Notably, the St. Francis Hos-

[13] *Report of the St. Francis Hospital*, June 1, 1921–May 31, 1923, pp. 25, 33–34; C. C. Wholey, "Mental Symptoms in Relation to General Medicine," *Journal of the American Medical Association* 89, (December 3, 1927), p. 1948.

[14] *Report of the St. Francis Hospital*, June 1, 1921–May 31, 1923; "History of Services," *Community Mental Health / Mental Retardation Center Bulletin* 1 (September 1971); Written history, "St. Francis Hospital," manuscript, n.d. but c. 1940, St. Francis Hospital Archives.

[15] C. C. Wholey, "Psychiatric Facilities in Pittsburgh," *American Journal of Psychiatry*, 93 (March 1937), p. 1189.

[16] *Sun-Telegraph*, 8 January 56

[17] Gerald N. Grob, *Mental Illness and American Society, 1875–1940*, (Princeton: Princeton University Press, 1983), pp. 295–304.

[18] Minutes, Board of Managers, 12/14/42, includes report of Dr. Eugene L. Sielke, inspector for the Bureau of Mental Health, St. Francis Hospital Archives.

[19] Gerald N. Grob, *Mental Illness and American Society, 1875–1940*, (Princeton: Princeton University Press, 1983), p. 308.

[20] *Report of the St. Francis Hospital*, June 1, 1921–May 31, 1923; "History of Services," *Community Mental Health / Mental Retardation Center Bulletin* 1 (September 1971); "St. Francis Hospital," manuscript, n.d. but c. 1940, St. Francis Hospital Archives.

pital attributed their patients' mental disorders to this disease more frequently than any other state or private psychiatric facility in the state at that time. By 1912, syphilis was no longer listed as either a diagnostic category or as a cause of disease, reflecting changes in determining the etiology of psychiatric diseases. Clearly, however, at the turn of the century, St. Francis cared for a group of patients perhaps not readily accepted in other institutions.

Number of Patients Admitted Whose Insanity Was Deemed Caused by Syphilis, by Year, and Percentage of that Total Admitted to St. Francis.[21]

Year	St. Francis	Private	State	Total	% at St. Francis
1900	11	3	14	28	39
1905	20	4	9	33	61
1906	13	2	13	28	46
1907	13	2	12	27	48
1908	9	4	20	33	27
1909	15	4	37	56	27

Within the next two decades, with the discovery of new diagnostic and treatment methods for syphilis, the genito-urinary department cared for many patients diagnosed with the disease. Those in the tertiary stages of syphilis, those with marked neurological symptoms, continued to be cared for in the psychiatric division.

1900 to World War II—Substance Abuse

Toward the end of the nineteenth century, St. Francis Hospital began to develop the foundation for their alcohol and chemical dependency programs, solidifying their reputation in the region as one of the institutions of choice to deal with such problems. In 1892, for example, the hospital treated seven patients, four males and three females, whose insanity was allegedly caused by alcoholism. None of the other licensed private psychiatric hospitals in the state had such patients, and only one state hospital had a patient whose insanity was due to alcoholism.[22] This may suggest that St. Francis, unlike

---

[21] *Annual Report of the Board of Commissioners of Public Charities of the Commonwealth of Pennsylvania,* the report of the Committee on Lunacy for years: 1900, 1905, 1906, 1907, 1908, 1909; Note: Before 1907, there were seven state and six private institutions. After 1907, there were six state hospitals listed.

other hospitals of the period, freely admitted alcoholics. By 1898, alcoholism was still viewed as a cause of insanity and not a disease in its own right. In addition, it was perceived to be a moral problem, not physical. Ten men and one woman were insane because of 'intemperance.' Interestingly, just as six years earlier, state institutions did not seem to readily admit alcoholic patients since none of them had patients whose insanity was attributed to alcoholism. Two alcoholic patients, however, were housed at the Asylum for the Chronic Insane at Wernersville. By this time, however, other private facilities, such as the Friends Asylum and Pennsylvania Hospital, were accepting alcoholic patients.[23] Clearly, St. Francis played a pioneering role in the acceptance of alcoholics into their psychiatric facility.

By 1900, the St. Francis Hospital continued to be a leader in the care of alcoholics within its psychiatric department. Of seven state and six private institutions throughout the state, St. Francis housed 56 percent of all patients whose insanity was deemed due to alcoholism. Within the first decade of the twentieth century, however, more and more of the patients in state and private institutions were considered to be insane because of alcoholism, so by 1909, St. Francis housed only 10 percent of the state's patients listed under that category.[24] This suggests that St. Francis was either more willing to accept alcoholics than other institutions, or that the hospital's physicians were more willing to attribute insanity to the alcoholic condition, but in either case, the hospital was a forerunner in the care of alcoholics.

Within the next ten years, attitudes toward alcoholism began to change in the United States. It was no longer believed to be a cause of insanity, reflecting the change from the nineteenth century custom of defining the etiology of psychiatric disorders in terms of external predisposing causes such as drugs, domestic difficulties, uterine dysfunction, inherited predisposition or alcohol.[25] The beliefs of the physicians at St. Francis mirrored national trends. Alcoholism was seen as an expression of a definite neurosis or psychoneurosis, more as the result or symptom of insanity or of other underlying nervous, mental or organic diseases. Physicians at St. Francis further believed that alcoholism was often caused by "faulty habits of living." Alcoholism was also viewed as a state innocently acquired by the victim who

[22] *Annual Report of the Board of Commissioners of Public Charities of the Commonwealth of Pennsylvania,* the report of the Committee on Lunacy for year 1892.

[23] *Annual Report of the Board of Commissioners of Public Charities of the Commonwealth of Pennsylvania,* the report of the Committee on Lunacy for year 1898.

[24] *Annual Report of the Board of Commissioners of Public Charities of the Commonwealth of Pennsylvania,* the report of the Committee on Lunacy for years 1900, 1905, 1906, 1907, 1908, 1909.

[25] Gerald N. Grob, *Mental Illness and American Society, 1875–1940,* (Princeton: Princeton University Press, 1983), p. 37.

attempted to find relief from various mental and physical ailments, such as migraines, neuralgia, dysmenorrhea or indigestion, for example. It was believed that if the causes could be determined and eradicated, then the alcoholism could be abated. Further, it was thought that if those cases were properly treated "in the incipient stage the prognosis is very favorable for a permanent cure."[26]

By 1911, St. Francis had a separate department for the treatment of inebriety and other drug addictions, under the direction of Dr. Cornelius C. Wholey. Regular staff members made a specialty of the "diseases of inebriety and drug addiction." Upon admission, patients addicted to alcohol or narcotics were interrogated by the staff physician and the resident. Attempts were made to ascertain the various reasons which led to the habit, and then a plan of treatment was decided upon whereby the "unnatural craving" would be destroyed. Patients who "either culpably or blamelessly allowed themselves to become the victims of this obnoxious passion, and who are desirous of subduing it," were admitted to private rooms, cared for by nurses, and endured an assortment of diagnostic tests. The staff's goal was to clean up the patient and quiet his/her craving. It was clearly understood that permanent abstinence in the case of the alcoholic would be achieved only when "an enduring incentive has been established which is a stronger urge than the intoxication impulse." Hospitalization protected the patient for a period of time from conditions which created what seemed to him a necessity for that first drink. A rigid scientific treatment was enforced which was "based on the personal character and habits of the particular patient under observation." Drug therapy involved a "judicious application, widely varying with individuals, of a sedative, eliminating, and supporting therapy." Psychotherapy was employed as a method of treatment for those felt to be suffering from a form of neurosis or psycho-neurosis. Implicit in this description of care during the period just prior to World War I is the notion that there was hope in 'scientific' treatment, reflective of the times. Implicit, too, is the suggestion that patients could be cured and returned to the community as productive members of society, mirroring fairly early the philosophy of leading psychiatrists of the period who advocated the implementation of 'psychopathic' wards.[27]

[26]*Report of the St. Francis Hospital,* 1911, p. 37; C. C. Wholey, "Dangers and Inconsistencies in Some Notable Short-Time Treatments for Drug Addictions," *Journal of the American Medical Association* 64 (April 24, 1915), pp. 1390–1392.

[27]*Report of the St. Francis Hospital,* 1911, pp. 36, 37; C. C. Wholey, "Dangers and Inconsistencies in Some Notable Short-Time Treatments for Drug Addictions," *Journal of the American Medical Association* 64 (April 24, 1915), pp. 1390–1392.

Evidence suggests also that the St. Francis physicians were beginning to perceive alcoholism as a separate disease entity. The hospital staff, seemingly, had not lost sight of a concept which had begun to be developed and disseminated many years before, but which was widely ignored by most medical institutions by the turn of the century. In fact, a view of chronic drunkenness as a disease had "became rather generally diffused in the medical community in the decades before the Civil War." Dr. Joseph Turner of Bath, Maine led a crusade calling for medical treatment of alcoholics, and he urged the construction of inebriate asylums for that purpose. In 1864, after a twenty year campaign, Turner opened the New York State Inebriate Asylum in Binghamton, New York, for the study and treatment of alcoholics. He believed that studying a patient population would lead to breakthroughs in the medical battle against alcoholism. By 1900, there were over fifty public or private facilities established for the purpose of treating alcoholics. Other members of the medical establishment also actively sought methods of dealing with alcoholics. In 1870, Drs. Joseph W. Parrish and Willard Parker founded the American Association for the Cure of Inebriates (renamed Association for the Study of Inebriety). The purpose of the organization was to research treatment for addiction to narcotics and alcohol.[28]

There is some evidence to suggest that, in fact, staff physicians at St. Francis were not only beginning to consider alcoholism as a separate disease, but also that they were separating it from the other psychiatric disorders. In 1911, twenty-nine patients were admitted to the neurological (psychiatric) service with the diagnosis of alcoholism under the category of poisonings. The following year, the hospital admitted seventeen men and four women with "alcoholic psychosis" listed as the diagnosis. This implies the consideration of alcoholism as a separate disease. Much more significant, however, is the fact that in the same year, 1,168 patients were admitted to the department of medicine with the primary diagnosis, under the category of "diseases due to chemical and physical agents," of "dipsomania," an archaic term meaning alcoholism. This provides strong evidence that alcoholism was perceived as a separate disease. The fact that the hospital admitted alcoholics to the department of medicine suggests that physicians may have been questioning whether or not alcoholics should be considered to be 'insane.'[29] It is important to note, too, that this was the single largest diagnostic group of

[28]Mark Edward Lender and James Kirby Martin, *Drinking in America, A History*, (New York: Free Press, 1982), pp. 119–120.

[29]*Annual Report of the Board of Commissioners of Public Charities of the Commonwealth of Pennsylvania*, the report of the Committee on Lunacy for years 1912, 1913.

several hundred listed. The diagnosis with the second largest number of cases was lobar pneumonia, which afflicted only 101 patients. St. Francis physicians were taking notice of the alcoholic, and were interested in studying the disorder. The patient, quite obviously, was no longer being blamed for his affliction, although clearly, he was expected to be held responsible for wanting a cure.[30] Alcoholism was no longer considered to be a cause of psychotic disorders, but, rather, a symptom of a mental affliction, or as a disease in and of itself.

As early as 1911, the recorded diagnostic categories suggest that staff physicians were cognizant of the relationship between alcoholism and other physical disorders, suggesting that various physical maladies were due to alcohol or other chemical agents. This reflected a significant change. Whereas a decade before alcoholism was deemed a cause of insanity, it was subsequently seen as a causal factor in the development of an assortment of physical ailments. Note the following table:

Diagnostic Category:
Diseases Due to Chemical and Physical Agents

Alcoholism, acute

"	rheumatism—1
"	alcoholic edema of brain—1 (died)
"	asthma—1
"	uremic poisoning—1
"	wound of foot—1
"	bronchitis—2
"	gonorrhea conjunctivitis—1

Alcoholism, chronic

"	eczema external genitalia—1
"	pleurisy—1
"	delirium tremens—3

Patients were also diagnosed with other disorders apparently linked to alcoholism, but not implicitly caused by it. Note the following table:

[30] *Report of the St. Francis Hospital,* 1911, pp. 12–16, 36, 37; C. C. Wholey, "Dangers and Inconsistencies in Some Notable Short-Time Treatments for Drug Addictions," *Journal of the American Medical Association* 64 (April 24, 1915), pp. 1390–1392; *Annual Report of the Board of Commissioners of Public Charities of the Commonwealth of Pennsylvania,* the report of the Committee on Lunacy for years 1912.

Disorders Linked to Alcoholism

	improved	died
Diagnostic Category: Acute Infectious Diseases		
pneumonia, lobar, alcoholism	6	12
Diagnostic Category: Digestive system		
gastritis, chronic, alcoholism	7	
hemetemesis, chronic alcoholism		1
cirrhosis, ascites, alcoholism	1	
Diagnostic Category: Respiratory system		
bronchitis, acute, alcoholism	1	
Diagnostic Category: Nervous system		
neurasthenia, chronic alcoholism	1	

St. Francis Hospital's recognition of the nature of alcoholism may have reflected current theory. The Committee on Lunacy stopped listing alcoholism under causes of insanity in 1912, but, interestingly, listed alcoholic psychosis as a "form of disease."[31] Legally, though, alcoholics were not considered by the state of Pennsylvania to be insane, at least by 1907, and, therefore, could not benefit by the legislation which appropriated funds for the maintenance of the indigent insane. For that reason, in 1912, the president of the Board of Public Charities recommended to the Pennsylvania state legislature that they establish a state institution for the care and proper treatment of "alcohol and drug victims." "Such persons need institutional care and a certain amount of restraint." The president also recommended adoption of legislation permitting temporary detention of inebriates and drug addicts.[32] As early as 1907, alcoholics were not considered to be insane by the state legislators and many doctors began to make the same assessment.

The exclusion of alcoholics from such legislation may explain why St. Francis, willing to accept patients regardless of their ability to pay, had such a large percentage of alcoholic patients. Though the state legislators did not categorize alcoholism with insanity, and inebriates did not come under the supervision of the Committee on Lunacy for that reason, it was widely recognized that there was a close connection which existed between "mental deficiency and the conditions of drug addiction and dependency," which helps to explain why psychiatric institutions dealt with alcoholic patients.

[31] *Annual Report of the Board of Commissioners of Public Charities of the Commonwealth of Pennsylvania,* the report of the Committee on Lunacy for years 1912, 1913.

[32] *Annual Report of the Board of Commissioners of Public Charities of the Commonwealth of Pennsylvania,* 1912, p. 14.

In 1917, the Committee on Lunacy noted that there had been an increase in the resources for the care of those "mentally inferior groups" in the state, reflecting the concern which five years earlier had already been apparent at the St. Francis Hospital.[33]

Just prior to the 1920s, many of the nation's citizens were becoming increasingly apathetic towards alcoholic rehabilitation. This was due in part to the increased hostility towards alcoholics on the part of "drys" as criticism of prohibition increased. A focus on the Depression in the thirties and war in the forties discouraged private or public sector efforts on behalf of individual alcoholism. As a result, alcoholism treatment was largely ignored through the 1940s.[34] St. Francis Hospital, however, continued to admit and treat alcoholics throughout the period. By 1923, St. Francis Hospital continued to identify more cases of alcoholism than any other psychiatric disorder. There were 126 cases of alcoholic psychoses, and 1,800 cases of alcoholism without psychosis. This suggests that the physicians had resolved that alcoholics would be cared for in the psychiatric department, whether or not they were deemed to be insane. 'Alcoholism' comprised 51 percent of the total 3,751 conditions recorded under the category of mental diseases.[35] Treating and caring for alcoholic patients was a fundamental objective of the psychiatric facility. As in so many other areas, the foundation was laid very early in the history of the institution. By the late 1920s, the treatment of alcoholics had become "more serious today than previously, because of large numbers of emergency cases created by synthetic and poisonous liquors now consumed." In this, too, St. Francis definitely stood out. In its desire to maintain its mission of accepting all in need of care, the administration continued to admit alcoholics during prohibition. Many hospitals, at that time, chose to refuse admission to those who were possibly in violation of the law.[36]

By the end of the 1930s, however, there was some renewed interest in alcoholism on the national level on the part of scientists and physicians. They began identifying the condition as some kind of psychiatric disorder that could have medical complications, although the St. Francis medical staff had obviously been cognizant of that relationship at least two decades earlier. In 1938, the Research Council on Problems of Alcohol was established by

---

[33] Annual Report of the Board of Commissioners of Public Charities of the Commonwealth of Pennsylvania, the report of the Committee on Lunacy for year 1917, p. 243.

[34] Mark Edward Lender and James Kirby Martin, Drinking in America, A History, (New York: Free Press, 1982), pp. 159–160, 181.

[35] Report of the St. Francis Hospital, June 1, 1921–May 31, 1923, pp. 82, 84.

[36] Uniting the Armies of Health and Industry, published for Industrial Pittsburgh by St. Francis Hospital, 1927; Weighing the Evidence, campaign brochure, 1927; Worker's confidential Handbook, St. Francis Hospital Campaign, 1927; Telephone interview with Dr. David Musto, New Haven Connecticut, 2/11/94.

scientists. In addition, the Yale University Center for Alcohol Studies was established, reflecting a reignited scientific and academic interest in alcohol abuse. The Yale Center subsequently began publishing the *Quarterly Journal of Studies on Alcohol*, which later became *The Journal of Studies on Alcohol*. The Center's most important contribution was the popularization of the modern disease concept. Laymen and professionals began to see the disease concept as a breakthrough in dealing with alcohol related issues, forgetting that the view had been advanced by the medical community almost a century before. It is interesting to note that the evidence suggests that St. Francis Hospital did not wait for the Yale Center or the AMA to popularize the disease notion which they had noted as early as the twenties.[37]

St. Francis Hospital has a long history of accepting and treating patients for chemical abuse. In 1911, the hospital admitted only two patients with the primary diagnosis of "morphinism," addiction to morphine, but clearly, they were interested in treating people for the disorder, laying the foundation for many of the programs established in the second half of the twentieth century. By the early twenties, the number of patients admitted for narcotics addiction had grown considerably. Within a two year period, nine individuals were admitted with the diagnosis of psychosis due to opium and derivatives. An additional seventy-nine people were admitted with the diagnosis of drug addiction without psychosis. Psychiatrists at St. Francis clearly viewed narcotics addiction as a neuropsychiatric problem. The primary etiological factor was that of inherent mental instability, since it was perceived that the majority of addicts became victims during adolescence before character could have become stabilized. Only a small few succumbed through therapeutic necessity.[38]

Physicians at St. Francis mirrored the trends in narcotic addiction therapy. Until the 1920s, physicians believed that withdrawal and a few weeks of after care would lead to the cure of addiction. Researchers nationwide sought an effective treatment plan. The first three decades of the twentieth century were characterized by a therapeutic enthusiasm which was reflected in the psychiatric department at St. Francis. By 1930, it was fairly clear that the search for an effective medical cure for addiction had failed, and in 1942, physicians' suspicions were confirmed with the United States Public Health Service study of addicts treated at Lexington Narcotic Hospi-

[37] Mark Edward Lender and James Kirby Martin, *Drinking in America, A History*, (New York: Free Press, 1982), pp. 185–190.
[38] *Report of the St. Francis Hospital*, 1911, p. 13; *Report of the St. Francis Hospital*, June 1, 1921–May 31, 1923, pp. 82, 84; C. C. Wholey, "The Mental and Nervous Side of Addiction to Narcotic Drugs, A Neuropsychiatric Problem," *Journal of the American Medical Association* 83 (August 2, 1924), p. 324.

tal, which noted that 75 percent of the patients treated for narcotics addiction relapsed.[39]

Treatment methods for narcotics addiction varied over the years. From 1909, when the Towns-Lambert method was first introduced, until the early twenties, when the efficacy of the treatment was questioned, St. Francis' Dr. C. C. Wholey utilized a variation of that method. Although he felt the treatment had to be adapted to individual idiosyncrasies, he felt it was the "best method for morphin and allied habits." Before treatment, the patient's bowels were evacuated completely and the largest tolerable dose of the addicting substance was given. Thirty minutes later, the patient received a formula made of extracts of prickly ash bark and hyoscyamus in addition to 15 percent tincture of belladonna. The formula was given at half hour intervals until the patient demonstrated signs of the atropine effect: dilation of pupils, dry throat and redness of the skin. Twenty-four hours later, after another cathartic, the addicting drug was given in one-half or one-third of the previous amount. Twelve hours later a third cathartic was given, and six to eight hours later, this was followed by a dose of one or two ounces of castor oil. Strychnine was sometimes given to combat exhaustion. Dr. Wholey, however, in the interest of safety, varied the prescribed treatment by administering the belladonna mixture and purgatives over two, three or many times the length of the period outlined in the original treatment, and they were given in correspondingly less intensive amounts. The belladonna mixture was given at hourly intervals only when the patient was awake. Sleep was provided for from the beginning through such drugs as sulphonal, trional, veronal, paraldehye and bromides. The addictive drug was administered before meals and at bedtime, and was rapidly cut down until the end of anywhere from one to three weeks. No patient ever was made to conform to a set course of treatment.[40] By the late twenties, Dr. Wholey continued to rely on cathartics, especially in confused and delirious patients whose psychosis was related to alcohol addiction.[41]

Dr. Wholey, in contrast to pioneers in the field who were advocating various specific short-term treatment methods such as the Towns-Lambert method, believed this treatment to be only a preliminary step. Addiction to morphine was "rarely finally obliterated by a short-time treatment." It got the patient off the drug, but this was just a beginning step towards a permanent

[39] David F. Musto, *The American Disease, Origins of Narcotic Control*, (New York: Oxford University Press, 1987), pp. 77–78, 85.

[40] David F. Musto, *The American Disease, Origins of Narcotic Control*, (New York: Oxford University Press, 1987), pp. 81–82; C. C. Wholey, "Dangers and Inconsistencies in Some Notable Short-Time Treatments for Drug Addictions," *Journal of the American Medical Association* 64 (April 24, 1915), pp. 1390–1392.

[41] C. C. Wholey, "Mental Symptoms in Relation to General Medicine," *Journal of the American Medical Association* 89 (December 3, 1927), p. 1945.

cure. As he believed that addiction was often due to neurosis, psychosis or a bad environment, a correction of the environment or psychotherapy was often imperative if a cure was to be expected.[42] Part of Wholey's treatment plan called for the patient to be willing to cooperate, and to understand fully that the ability to give up the habit was up to him. It would require a "fight," and from the first hour it was largely the patient's responsibility. Wholey did not drug his patients so that they were in a semi-delirious state unaware later of the struggle they went through. It was his philosophy that the "character fibers are not toughened by passing through any such twilight sleep."[43]

In the late twenties, Narcosan was another treatment method under study. Supposedly, the drug was designed to relieve patients of the craving for narcotics with minimum discomfort. By 1928, New York City was spending twenty-five thousand to fifty thousand dollars annually on Narcosan treatments. St. Francis was one of the first general hospitals to explicitly investigate the use of Narcosan, and was the first general hospital outside of New York to use the treatment. By the end of the decade, however, it was revealed, after additional clinical studies in New York, that Narcosan had no merit as a treatment for narcotic addiction.[44] St. Francis, then, willingly utilized new treatment methods advocated by researchers and scientists in their attempt to care for their patients, setting the stage for the following decades.

St. Francis Hospital served individuals of the community by providing psychiatric care and treatment for alcoholics, chemical dependents and those with venereal disease. The hospital also provided other services, showing a predilection for community involvement, which developed on a much wider scale following the second world war.

1900 to World War II—Commitment to the Community

One of the new trends in psychiatry in the 1920s was the concept that early treatment made subsequent institutionalization unnecessary. There is some

---

[42] David F. Musto, *The American Disease, Origins of Narcotic Control*, (New York: Oxford University Press, 1987), pp. 81–82; C. C. Wholey, "Dangers and Inconsistencies in Some Notable Short-Time Treatments for Drug Addictions," *Journal of the American Medical Association* 64 (April 24, 1915), pp. 1390–1392.

[43] C.C. Wholey, "Dangers and Inconsistencies in Some Notable Short-Time Treatments for Drug Addictions," *Journal of the American Medical Association* 64 (April 24, 1915), pp. 1390–1392.

[44] *Uniting the Armies of Health and Industry*, published for Industrial Pittsburgh by St. Francis Hospital, 1927; *Weighing the Evidence*, campaign brochure, 1927; *Worker's confidential Handbook, St. Francis Hospital Campaign*, 1927; David F. Musto, *The American Disease, Origins of Narcotic Control*, (New York: Oxford University Press, 1987), p. 316n46.

evidence to suggest that neuropsychiatric patients were seen in the dispensary at St. Francis in the early 1920s, a time when few outpatient facilities were available. In 1920, there were only nine outpatient clinics in the entire state. The dispensary physicians included several 'neurologists' on staff. At that time, the distinction made between neurologists and psychiatrists was not yet clear, and in fact, the St. Francis department was sometimes called the department of 'neuropsychiatry.' Diagnoses listed under "Neurology" were often not clearly different from those listed under psychiatry. Approximately two percent of the visits made to the dispensary were to the neurology department, but the early foundation for out-patient care had been established.[45]

The psychiatrists serving the hospital in the mid-thirties were active themselves throughout the community. Dr. C. C. Wholey served as the consulting psychiatrist to the Western State Penitentiary, where research and various studies were routinely carried out, often under the direction of academicians from the University of Pittsburgh. Case studies were continually tabulated. Other doctors were more directly involved at the University of Pittsburgh. St. Francis' Dr. W. K. Walker established the department of psychiatry in the medical school in 1910, and was succeeded as director of that department in 1928 by Dr. C. H. Henninger, a staff member at St. Francis.[46]

The St. Francis Hospital department of psychiatry also provided educational resources for students in local institutions. Social workers and psychology students from colleges, universities and agencies within a radius of one hundred miles utilized the facility. The St. Francis school of nursing always included psychiatry in their program and by 1937, the school offered three-month affiliation programs to students from other schools, including Mercy and St. John's in Pittsburgh, Latrobe Hospital and New Castle Hospital. The hospital had also provided clinical experience for psychiatric teaching in the department of medicine of the University of Pittsburgh since 1910. Clinical and didactic lectures were given weekly through the fourth year. In addition, two residents and twelve visiting psychiatrists benefited from the department's services.[47] As the hospital moved into the post world war period, the foundation for comprehensive psychiatric services had been established.

[45]Gerald N. Grob, *Mental Illness and American Society, 1875–1940*, (Princeton: Princeton University Press, 1983), pp. 239–240; *Report of the St. Francis Hospital*, June 1, 1921–May 31, 1923, pp. 5, 86.

[46]C. C. Wholey, "Psychiatric Facilities in Pittsburgh," *American Journal of Psychiatry*, 93 (March 1937), pp. 1189–1191.

[47]C. C. Wholey, "Psychiatric Facilities in Pittsburgh," *American Journal of Psychiatry*, 93 (March 1937), pp. 1189–1190.

World War II to 1977

The post-war period in the history of St. Francis Hospital is characterized by changing theories regarding the etiology and treatment of psychiatric illness, a much deeper involvement in the community and an intensified struggle for the sisters as they attempted to maintain their spiritual principles in the midst of policy changes in the community at large. Although new theories developed, and the government played a more active role in the care of the nation's mentally ill, St. Francis remained at the forefront of these changes as they relied more on community efforts to deal with psychiatric and related problems.

Following the Depression and the war, conditions in the nation's mental health facilities had deteriorated significantly. Buildings were in need of extensive repairs, institutions were severely overcrowded and the war caused a shortage of physicians. But the war experience itself resulted in monumental changes in the field of psychiatric medicine. The role of psychiatrists in war time created a sharp expansion of the specialty's boundaries. Psychiatrists had been assigned the duty of screening out those deemed unfit to serve because of mental disorders. They played an extensive role in rehabilitating battlefield psychological casualties, and psychiatrists also exerted some effort to maintain military and civilian morale. The physicians' experiences led to new theories regarding the definition of insanity and its etiology, resulting in new treatment modalities and a greater emphasis on the part of doctors on prevention.[48] In addition, the gradual weakening of kinship and family networks and religious institutions, which in the past had provided the major supports for individuals requiring some sort of personal assistance, fueled changes in the mental health field.[49]

Following the war, many psychiatrists began to accept new theories regarding the definition of mental health. The traditional model was based on the assumption that there was a sharp distinction made between health and disease. New concepts of psychodynamic psychiatry argued that behavior occurred along a continuum that commenced with the normal and concluded with the abnormal, blurring the traditional demarcation. This new concept of health and disease resulted in a greater emphasis on psychological therapies, leading to the development of new specialties such as clinical psychology,

---

[48]Gerald N. Grob, *From Asylum to Community: Mental Health Policy in Modern America*, (Princeton: Princeton University Press, 1991), pp. 8–10.

[49]Gerald N. Grob, *From Asylum to Community: Mental Health Policy in Modern America*, (Princeton: Princeton University Press, 1991), pp. 7, 93.

psychiatric social work and psychiatric nursing.[50] New beliefs regarding eti-ology, prevention, treatment and disease provided the basis for an expansion and elaboration of mental health services.

It is interesting to note that the traditional model of psychiatry, based on the assumption that there was a sharp distinction between health and disease, which was challenged in the post world war two period, was con-sidered to be obsolete by one of the St. Francis Hospital physicians prior to the first world war. Dr. Theodore Diller suggested that "the very existence of insanity is a matter of opinion.... There are some individuals who rep-resent so much mental disorder that everyone recognizes them as insane, and another large group of individuals who are so sound in their mental op-erations that they are called by everyone sane. Then in society we could grade down from the insane to the still less insane and so on, and from the sane to those a little less sane, until we came to middle ground in which were found a certain number of individuals whose sanity became question-able."[51]

With these new theories in mind, military physicians advocated new and different treatment methods as they began to see environmental stress as playing a role in the etiology of psychiatric disorders. The war unified beliefs that human interventions and immediate treatment, often sedation, food, rest, psychotherapy and emotional support, could alter psychological outcomes. Soldiers had been treated immediately in close proximity to their units, which enabled service men to maintain established social relationships and a sense of cohesion and integration. The low incidence of severe disorders helped to support the allegation that early treatment in a non-institutional setting represented an effective preventive strategy. The obvious implication for psychiatry was that community and private practice would become the norm instead of the exception.[52]

A renewed spirit of therapeutic optimism and activism was, thereafter, carried back to civilian life. Perceiving the hospital environment as a social organization, researchers emphasized the need to employ a holistic approach that took into account all of the relevant social and emotional factors relating to mental illness. Recognizing the significance of the environment, interper-sonal relationships and the social needs of the patients is characteristic of

[50]Gerald N. Grob, *From Asylum to Community: Mental Health Policy in Modern America*, (Princeton: Princeton University Press, 1991), pp. 7, 93.

[51]Theodore Diller, M.D., "The Problem of Insanity as it confronts Practitioners," *The Weekly Bulletin* [of the Allegheny County Medical Society], (January 8, 1916), pp. 11–12.

[52]Gerald N. Grob, *From Asylum to Community: Mental Health Policy in Modern America*, (Princeton: Princeton University Press, 1991), pp. 15–18.

the "therapeutic community" concept which is based on the proposition that patients as well as staff had to take active participatory roles in the therapeutic process. Advocates believed this approach stood in stark contrast to traditional therapies, whereby authoritative ideology fostered dependency and "actually strengthened pathological symptoms characteristic of the mental illness." Psychiatric services had to be integrated along an unbroken continuum to ease release of patients into the community, reflecting the then prevailing theory regarding the definition of insanity. The range of services was therefore to include a day hospital, or part-time care.[53] In addition, supporters of this new "milieu therapy," believing that isolation and the prison-like antitherapeutic character of traditional mental hospitals could be altered, advocated the "open-door" hospital, recommending that features such as locked doors, barred windows and fences be eliminated.[54]

These new methods of treatment, intervention and "milieu therapy" became even more salutary with the introduction of psychoactive drugs in the 1950s. Studies proved that certain drugs were beneficial in modifying behavior such as anxiety, agitation and manic states. In addition, these pharmaceutical agents enhanced patients' receptivity to other psychodynamic therapies. The drugs resulted in an entirely different atmosphere in the wards, enabling patients to participate in social events. Chlorpromazine, or Thorazine, was the first of the psychoactive drugs to be introduced, and was followed shortly thereafter with the introduction of the antidepressants iproniazid and imipramine.[55]

The renewed interest in psychiatric disease was reflected in the National Mental Health Act, passed by Congress in July 1946, which created the six member National Mental Health Advisory Council, and established the National Institute of Mental Health. In addition, three goals were recognized. The first was to support research relating to the cause, diagnosis and treatment of psychiatric disorders. The second was to train mental health personnel by providing individual and institutional grants. The third was to award grants to states to assist in establishing clinics, and to fund demonstration studies dealing with the prevention, diagnosis and treatment of neuropsychiatric disorders.[56]

---

[53]Gerald N. Grob, *From Asylum to Community: Mental Health Policy in Modern America*, (Princeton: Princeton University Press, 1991), pp. 143–145.

[54]Gerald N. Grob, *From Asylum to Community: Mental Health Policy in Modern America*, (Princeton: Princeton University Press, 1991), pp. 143–145.

[55]Gerald N. Grob, *From Asylum to Community: Mental Health Policy in Modern America*, (Princeton: Princeton University Press, 1991), p. 146.

[56]Gerald N. Grob, *From Asylum to Community: Mental Health Policy in Modern America*, (Princeton: Princeton University Press, 1991), p. 28.

World War II to 1977—The Hospital and Its Patients

By the mid-fifties, St. Francis Hospital, as one of the largest hospitals within the city, continued to offer psychiatric care on a large scale, incorporating many of the prevailing theories into the services it provided. The hospital had three major components in its psychiatric division. It offered a psychiatric emergency service to which 650 people were admitted in 1956. The second service, a short-term service for alcoholic patients generally in the acute states of intoxication, admitted 1,000, or 21 percent of the total patients admitted that year. The third and largest service offered private care for other committed or non-committed patients. Approximately half of the beds were in a ward, 39 percent were semi-private and only 12 percent of the beds were in private rooms. There were seventeen psychiatrists on staff, and the nursing service was directed by a sister who had completed post-graduate work in the specialty.[57]

There were generally two types of patients; those who were not committed were admitted to the small open ward in the general hospital, and those who were committed were admitted to the closed wards in the psychiatric wing, which had beds for 162 female patients and 126 male patients. The wards housed four to as many as thirty patients. The first floor had beds for alcoholic and aged men. Depressed, agitated and aged women were on the second floor, and acute and convalescent women were housed on the fourth floor. The third floor housed acute and convalescent men. The most disruptive and "noisiest" patients were confined to a ward which the medical residents nicknamed the "bull pen."

The psychiatric patients were expected to adhere to certain rules and regulations. The patients in the closed wards were not permitted to have visitors for the first two weeks, but following that time, they could have up to three visitors on Thursdays and Sundays from two to four in the afternoon. The family received three visiting cards upon the patient's admission, which were to be presented when visiting, allowing the family to determine who was to call. Patients were required to wear their own clothing, and were to be dressed by ten in the morning. The family was responsible for laundering clothing. Staff believed that wearing one's own clothes raised the patient's morale, and created a sense of well-being.[58] The non-committed patients in the open ward, where there were eleven beds for men and twenty-eight for

---

[57]Data needed for the classification of Private Mental Hospitals, sent to the American Psychiatric Association Central Inspection Board, November 1955, St. Francis Hospital Archives; Sister M. Adele Meiser, "Care of the Mentally Ill in the General Hospital," *Journal of the American Hospital Association* (September 1951).

women, were treated somewhat differently. By 1962, some patients, with a doctor's permission, could leave overnight or for weekends with members of their families, similar to a half-way house idea. Others in the open ward were occasionally permitted to leave the hospital unescorted.[59]

The hospital in the mid-fifties admitted patients with a wide array of psychiatric diagnoses. The largest group of admissions, under the heading of personality disorders, was diagnosed with "alcoholism (addiction)," which represented 23 percent of the patients admitted for the year. Clearly, the commitment to alcoholics continued unabated. The second largest number of patients were listed as schizophrenics, under the heading psychotic disorders. They comprised 17 percent of the total admissions for the year ending in December 1954.[60]

The hospital treated patients of all ages, but most of them were young to middle aged adults. Seventy-eight percent of the patients admitted in 1954 were between the ages of twenty and fifty-nine. Although the hospital would accept children, only 1 percent of those admitted were under sixteen, and another 3 percent fell between the ages of sixteen and nineteen. The aged, those over seventy, comprised only 6 percent of the patient admissions.[61]

By the 1950s, the sisters paid careful attention to the physical surroundings in the psychiatric department, a response to the changing post-war views regarding the etiology of mental illness, noting that the environment influenced behavior. Color was utilized in the interior decor with an attempt to create a home-like appearance. Detention screens replaced bars on the porches, and locks in the interiors of patients' rooms were removed, as were suicide hazards.[62]

[58]John R. McGibony, M.D., Mental Health: A Community Program, (Pittsburgh: Health and Welfare Association of Allegheny County, 1958), Section D, "General Hospitals," pp. 44–45; Sister M. Adele Meiser, "Care of the Mentally Ill in the General Hospital," Journal of the American Hospital Association (September 1951); "How It Began," Community Mental Health, Mental Retardation Center—Bulletin 1 (November 1971); AMA Council on Medical Education—Fellowships and Residencies in Psychiatry and Neurology, form letter, n.d. but c. 1948–1950, St. Francis Hospital Archives; Minutes, Board of Managers, "Report of St. Francis General Hospital and Rehabilitation Institution concerning the Psychiatric Survey Initiated by the Department of Welfare," 1956; Interview with Dr. George Wright, 10/25/93.

[59]Sister M. Adele Meiser, "Care of the Mentally Ill in the General Hospital," Journal of the American Hospital Association (September 1951); "How It Began," Community Mental Health, Mental Retardation Center—Bulletin 1 (November 1971); AMA Council on Medical Education—Fellowships and Residencies in Psychiatry and Neurology, form letter, n.d. but c. 1948–1950, St. Francis Hospital Archives; Minutes, Board of Managers, "Report of St. Francis General Hospital and Rehabilitation Institution concerning the Psychiatric Survey Initiated by the Department of Welfare," 1956.

[60]Report sent to the American Psychiatric Association Central Inspection Board, November 1955, St. Francis Hospital Archives.

[61]Data needed for the classification of Private Mental Hospitals, sent to the American Psychiatric Association Central Inspection Board, November 1955, St. Francis Hospital Archives.

[62]Sister M. Adele Meiser, "Care of the Mentally Ill in the General Hospital," Journal of the American Hospital Association (September 1951).

By the mid-fifties, numerous treatment modalities were offered. Somatic treatment modalities were still of an empirical nature, but even though their mode of action was unknown, various treatments did offer promising results.[63] By this time, electric, insulin and metrazol shock treatments were still prescribed frequently, an average of fifty treatments per day.[64] Treatments were given in patient rooms every day except Sunday. Hydrotherapy and occupational therapy continued to be utilized. The rationale behind the occupational therapy was the belief that mastering a skill gave patients satisfaction. Eventually, patients became self confident, and their social attitudes were strengthened. The dual purposes of the therapy were to assist patients to adjust as individuals and to associate with other people. Tranquilizers, a major breakthrough in the treatment of psychiatric illnesses, were used at St. Francis beginning in 1955.[65] They had the effect of quieting patients, which the residents of Lawrenceville will attest to since, before their widespread use, people in the community claimed they could hear the patients all the way up Butler Street.[66]

Recreational opportunities had expanded by this time, reflecting national trends toward increased use of socialization therapies. Patients often dined together or attended movies, which were shown to the patients once every week in the auditorium. Playing cards, checkers, pool, ping-pong, radio, TV, magazines and books were available. Staff members directed sing-a-longs, parties, dancing, games and competitive amusements. Badminton, shuffle board and horse shoes could be played outdoors. The objective of recreational therapy was to aid in restoring the patients to a normal social life. Barber shops and beauty parlors encouraged interest in personal appearance. Evidence suggests that socialization therapies became more common after results from studies of the 1950s were known. St. Francis' history, however, demonstrates that it had been cognizant of the benefits of some of these therapies since the late nineteenth century.[67]

Socialization therapies continued to expand at St. Francis in the sixties. In 1962, the hospital combined the occupational and recreational therapy departments into an expanded Diversional Therapy department which func-

---

[63]Gerald N. Grob, *From Asylum to Community: Mental Health Policy in Modern America*, (Princeton: Princeton University Press, 1991), p. 127.

[64]Sister M. Adele Meiser, "Care of the Mentally Ill in the General Hospital," *Journal of the American Hospital Association* (September 1951).

[65]"Adult Out-Patient Services," *Community Mental Health, Mental Retardation Center—Bulletin* 1 (November 1971).

[66]Caren Marcus, "St. Francis Wing, Image to Fall," *Pittsburgh Press*, 8 August 1975.

[67]Sister M. Adele Meiser, "Care of the Mentally Ill in the General Hospital," *Journal of the American Hospital Association* (September 1951); Gerald N. Grob, *From Asylum to Community: Mental Health Policy in Modern America*, (Princeton: Princeton University Press, 1991), p. 143.

tioned sixteen hours per day, six days per week, in and out of the hospital. In 1964, the Patient Activity Council (PAC) was formed to provide patients with the opportunity to share in planning and presentation of recreational activities. PAC activities included two discussion groups, "New Horizons," and "Dynamic Speaking," as well as the "Pak-Yaks," a debate team and the *Paczette*, a weekly newsheet generated by the patients.[68]

St. Francis Hospital never changed its view that having the psychiatric department within the general hospital benefited patients throughout the entire institution. It was not unusual for patients in the general hospital to become delirious or psychotic as a result of toxic, infectious, exhaustive or traumatic causes. In addition, interdepartmental consultations were readily available. Psychiatric patients also were more willing to be admitted to St. Francis because they felt there was less stigma attached to admission in a general hospital.[69] With the advent of the Hill-Burton Act, which provided funds for expansion of psychiatric divisions (as well as other construction), more hospitals were willing and able to provide some psychiatric services. In addition, in 1955, Congress passed the Mental Health Study Act, which authorized the National Institute of Mental Health, with the aid of the National Mental Health Advisory Council, to select an investigatory organization to analyze the human and economic problems of mental illness. The investigatory body, The Joint Commission on Mental Illness and Health Study group, was organized in 1955 by the American Medical Association and the American Psychiatric Association. One of their key recommendations was the establishment of psychiatric units or, at least, psychiatric beds in general hospitals of one hundred or more beds. These high quality facilities could offer immediate care at the onset of acute illness, and also keep the patient near home. By 1963, apparently, hospitals were beginning to respond to the recommendation. Four hundred sixty-seven of 5,291 (8.8 percent) general hospitals had separate in-patient units. An additional 578 hospitals admitted psychiatric patients, but not in separate wards, and 2,137 hospitals accepted psychiatric cases for diagnosis and treatment pending transfer to other institutions.[70] Clearly, St. Francis Hospital, in maintaining their full psychiatric department, stands out as an ongoing exception.

---

[68]Malcolm Frank Berman, "A Comprehensive community Mental Health Center Directed from a General Hospital Base," (M.S. Theses, University of Pittsburgh, 1966).

[69]Sister M. Adele Meiser, "Care of the Mentally Ill in the General Hospital," *Journal of the American Hospital Association* (September 1951).

[70]Gerald N. Grob, *From Asylum to Community: Mental Health Policy in Modern America*, (Princeton: Princeton University Press, 1991), pp. 165–166; Joint Commission on Mental Illness and Health, *Action for Mental Health, Final Report of the Joint commission on Mental Illness and Health*, (New York: Basic Books, 1961), pp. xxvii–xxviii, 265.

Of the twenty-seven general hospitals in Allegheny County, only six hospitals had wards for psychiatric patients. Suburban General Hospital opened a psychiatric unit in 1950 which had nineteen beds in an unlocked unit. It accepted only voluntary admissions, emergencies being sent to St. Francis. Suburban General provided electric shock therapy three times per week. Gratuitous care was given only occasionally, and no occupational therapy, physical therapy or social services were offered. Shadyside Hospital opened their psychiatric department, only for women, in 1944. It also accepted only voluntary admissions, and nearly all of the patients were private patients of staff psychiatrists. Shadyside, too, offered shock therapy. St. Margaret's Hospital established a seven bed research ward for the study and treatment of alcoholism or problems related to drinking. Although it was supported by the State Department of Health, as well as by patient fees, it too, had admission restrictions. Patients in the acute phase of intoxication were not admitted. The ward was administered by the faculty of the University of Pittsburgh Graduate School of Public Health. In addition, the Veterans Administration managed two facilities, in Oakland and in Aspinwall. Although the V. A. cared for patients with long-term chronic psychoses or brain damage, it was unable to handle severely disturbed psychotic patients, and only admitted veterans. Of the remaining twenty-one hospitals, twelve hospitals had no psychiatric ward, but did have an organized psychiatric service of the medical staff. The remaining nine facilities had neither a ward nor a psychiatric service.[71] By 1966, several other general hospitals also offered psychiatric services. Sewickley Valley hospital had three beds for emergency use, and St. John's General Hospital added twenty-eight psychiatric beds. Homestead Hospital had sixteen beds, and Columbia had fifteen beds.[72] St. Francis Hospital clearly filled in the gaps, serving the city's mentally ill by accepting any patient for admission, regardless of ability to pay or psychiatric condition.

World War II to 1977—Admission Policy Controversies

Not only did the hospital agree to admit any psychiatric patient, but it also assisted the city police by accepting disorderly and unmanageable psychiatric patients that under normal circumstances would have been sent to the city jail,

---

[71] John R. McGibony, M.D., *Mental Health: A Community Program*, (Pittsburgh: Health and Welfare Association of Allegheny County, 1958), Section D, "General Hospitals."

[72] Malcolm Frank Berman, "A Comprehensive Community Mental Health Center Directed from a General Hospital Base," (M.S. Theses, University of Pittsburgh, 1966), appendix.

thereby alleviating a major problem of overcrowding in the police stations. Evidence suggests, in fact, that St. Francis, as far back as the 1920s, had agreed to accept all psychiatric cases that the police picked up on weekends or holidays when Mayview was unable to commit patients. Prior to the second world war, however, all police cases sent to St. Francis for temporary care could subsequently be sent to Mayview on a temporary commitment which only required one physician seeing the patient and no affidavit. Cases moved within forty-eight to seventy-two hours. In 1941, however, Mayview was formally taken over by the state and was under state jurisdiction. This meant that all people admitted would have to have a two-man commitment form. Under the new system, it was expected to take a week or more before patients could be transferred from St. Francis to Mayview, but the hospital policy remained unchanged. By 1942, the hospital board of managers noted that St. Francis "apparently takes practically all the acute cases from the City of Pittsburgh."[73]

However, in the same year, St. Francis' open door policy was still too inadequate to serve the entire city. The Health and Welfare Federation of Allegheny county noted that the jail continued to be the primary resource for detention of mentally ill patients. Approximately five hundred individuals per year were detained there. In 1945, the Department of Welfare of the Commonwealth of Pennsylvania authorized the creation of an emergency evaluation unit at Mayview to receive persons under arrest. Ten male and ten female beds were available for patients, whose stay was not to exceed ten days, with "abnormal mental conditions other than drunkenness." The procedure, instituted to obviate the admission of mental patients through the county jail, resulted in a marked increase in the number of patients. During the biennium 1950–52, over 50 percent of new admissions had come to Mayview for observation by way of the Allegheny County Jail. Of a total of 492 male admissions, 305, or 62 percent, had come from the county jail. Of 415 female patients, 40 percent came from the that site. Included were nonresidents of Pittsburgh and Pennsylvania, as well as many patients who should have gone to Woodville.[74] At that time, Mayview officials noted that the "long-term and ideal solution would be the setting up of a processing, diagnostic, or even a complete short-term observation facility in the City of Pittsburgh." Located fifteen miles south of the city, the distance of Mayview from Pittsburgh was inconvenient for everyday use. Mayview certainly had

[73]Minutes, Board of Managers, 9/8/41 and 12/14/42, includes report of Dr. Eugene L. Sielke, inspector for the Bureau of Mental Health, St. Francis Hospital Archives.

[74]Mayview admitted city residents and Woodville admitted county patients who were not city residents.

cause for legitimate concern as the department of welfare's estimate of comfortable capacity was 2,256, whereas the institution at that time housed 3,140 patients.[75]

The policies established at Mayview and St. Francis did not completely alleviate the problem for the police, and by the early fifties the entire community was aware that the issue had become a major crisis. Hundreds of mentally ill, aged, infirm, indigent and physically unfit continued to be dumped in jail to bypass long waiting lists at state and county institutions. Drunkenness led the list of offenses. In 1952, 2,150 intoxicated people were admitted to the jail. One thousand seven hundred nineteen were admitted as vagrants, the second largest offense. Of the fifteen thousand persons admitted to jail, six hundred ended up in mental hospitals.[76] In 1953, citizens, outraged by the practice, conducted a citizens' protest over the practice of taking the mentally ill to jail.[77] In January 1953, David M. Janavitz, chairman of the Mental Health Committee of the Health Division of the Health and Welfare Federation of Allegheny County, began to work on the problem. Representatives from the Allegheny County Bar Association, Allegheny County Medical Society, Pittsburgh Neuropsychiatric Society and the Council of Churches were invited the following fall to join in the study. By October, the County Prison Board ordered all magistrates to stop admitting mental patients to the county jail. The following month, St. Francis, unwilling to let the emotionally unstable, mentally ill, vagrant or alcoholic individuals suffer neglect, agreed to set aside ten beds for emergency detention care, to last twenty-four to forty-eight hours. An agreement was formulated between St. Francis Hospital, the Allegheny County Institution District, Pittsburgh Bureau of Police, Mayview and Woodville, whereby St. Francis Hospital would supply temporary emergency care for those disturbed persons who might otherwise have been lodged in the county jail pending admission to the appropriate state institution. This agreement merely formalized what the hospital had been doing for many years.

There was controversy, however, regarding who was liable for the cost of caring for mental health patients. Early in 1955, St. Francis board members met with the county commissioners in an effort to have the county pay the hospital for the care of the city's mentally ill patients who were admitted to St. Francis. The state argued that it was only responsible for the patient after

---

[75] Annual Report, Mayview State Hospital, Fifth Biennial Report 6/1/50–5/31/52, Mayview Hospital Archives.

[76] *Post-Gazette*, 7 January 1953; *Pittsburgh Press*, 11 January 1953.

[77] Letter from Abraham Twerski, M.D., to Desmond McClarien, 5/8/70, St. Francis Hospital Archives.

admission to a state facility, but the city and county maintained that the state was responsible for the care of the indigent insane regardless of where they were treated. Under a 1951 state act, the 'applicant' was liable for the cost of temporary or emergency care, and in the case of prisoners, the director of the county institution district was the applicant. By spring of 1955, the reimbursement question was settled. The Allegheny Institution District paid for the cost of emergency care at St. Francis and transportation to the state mental hospital.[78]

St. Francis Hospital established guidelines in an attempt to control the number of emergency admissions. This emergency service was primarily meant for residents or non-residents who needed hospitalized care to protect themselves or others. Only those cases so severe as to require the police to handle and transport the patient were covered by this agreement. It was not a service that was to be requested by other institutions, such as area general hospitals, who could arrange for regular admission, under Section 311 of the Mental Health Act, to appropriate state or private mental hospitals. The service was also not to be used by patients on leave from state hospitals in Allegheny County. The rules, however, were never enforced, for they violated the sisters' long standing policy of refusing to deny care.[79]

The Social Service department workers at Mayview, on December 1, 1953, began daily duties at St. Francis, performing tasks similar to those done at the county jail. Their purpose was to clarify the city or county residence of the patient, to interview families for social histories and to make arrangement for disposition of the patient, which was usually arranged within forty-eight hours via private ambulance to the state hospital. Of 397 male admissions to Mayview, 118, or 30 percent, of the patients had been transferred from St. Francis. Of the 392 females admitted, 91, or 23 percent, were from St. Francis.[80] Throughout the next decade, St. Francis played an even larger role in the admissions to not only Mayview, but to Woodville as well.

[78]John R. McGibony, M.D., *Mental Health: A Community Program*, (Pittsburgh: Health and Welfare Association of Allegheny County, 1958), Section D, "General Hospitals," pp. 44–45; Minutes, Board of Managers, 1/6/55, St. Francis Hospital Archives; *Yesterday and Tomorrow*, (Allegheny County: Health and Welfare Federation of Allegheny County, October 1955); Report of Social Service Department, Mayview Annual Report, 6/1/52–5/31/54, Mayview Hospital Archives; *Pittsburgh Press*, 14 October 1953, 13 May 1953; *Post-Gazette*, 7 January 1953.

[79]"Psychiatric Emergency Service and Procedures, as agreed upon by representatives of St. Francis, Mayview, Woodville, the Allegheny County Institution District and Pittsburgh Bureau of Police," Revised May 1956.

[80]Report of Social Service Department, Mayview Annual Report, 6/1/52–5/31/54, Mayview Hospital Archives.

Total Yearly Admissions of Psychiatric Patients to Mayview, 6/1/55–5/30/65[81]

Year	Total	From St. Francis	Percentage from St. Francis
1955–56	726	322	46
1956–57	797	477	60
1957–58	867	514	59
1958–59	905	550	69
1959–60	785	499	60
1960–61	878	534	62
1961–62[82]	905	624	69
1962–63	787	517	64
1963–64	814	371	45
1964–65	887	445	50

For a number of years, however, the sisters and medical staff of St. Francis recognized that the agreement had been totally misused. The attitude of the public, other hospitals, the city, county and state, was that St. Francis was the receiving center and clearing house for state hospitals, but this was never the intention. Mayview only accepted patients between eight and two on weekdays, and accepted only complete commitments, requiring notarization of applicant's signature and two committing physicians. It was, therefore, impossible for Mayview to have emergency admissions. The agreement's intent was to accept patients who otherwise would have gone to jail, and subsequently transfer those emergency patients within forty-eight hours to state facilities. Other general hospitals, reluctant to accept certain types of patients and wanting to bypass problems, would not admit emergency patients, but sent them directly to St. Francis. For example, the Western Psychiatric Institute and Clinic (WPIC) in Oakland, whose primary focus was education, research and service, preferred not to deal with the usual emergency admissions, walk-ins, medico-legal problems, most alcoholic problems and, in general, any unarranged admissions. Patients had been brought to St. Francis from the lobby of WPIC. There were other general hospitals in the area that also readily sent patients to St. Francis, in lieu of a psychiatric consult or transfer to a state hospital. Outside social agencies saw St. Francis as a place to dispose of their most distressing problems, feeling that it was St. Francis' duty to accept any patient or circumstance. As a result, the hospital had patients waiting as long as four years before being transferred, partly because Mayview

---

[81] Malcolm Frank Berman, "A Comprehensive Community Mental Health Center Directed from a General Hospital Base," (M.S. Thesis, University of Pittsburgh, 1966).

limited the number of admissions of patients over sixty-five years of age. In 1955, 13.4 percent of all patients admitted to St. Francis for the year were public emergency cases.[83]

St. Francis' policy of accepting all patients, and Mayview's policy of offering care to only a limited number of elderly patients, was one of the causes of dissension within St. Francis Hospital. Although on the surface it appears that Mayview was discriminatory in its policies, it merely was setting, and enforcing, policies designed to alleviate its own situation of overcrowding. Individuals within St. Francis felt that the sisters were at fault for accepting an unlimited number of geriatric patients and then attempting to force them on Mayview.[84] It is worth noting that John Kane Hospital, a county facility primarily for geriatric cases, also had a waiting list and could not accommodate any more elderly patients.[85] In January 1959, St. Francis formalized an agreement to keep the elderly longer than stated in the original agreement (ten to fifteen days) in order to try to help the patient's family make other appropriate placement, and to try to see the elderly on an out-patient basis. This was done in spite of limited staff, including social service workers. Clearly, however, the hospital had already been accepting patients for an indefinite period of time. A year later, in 1960, when the hospital had a waiting list of ninety-seven in the general hospital and thirty-nine in the psychiatric department, the medical staff requested that the hospital limit admission of older patients and establish a maximum number of thirty beds for them. The board was willing to approve the staff's request, but added that emergency patients would be admitted at all times regardless of bed allotment. The administration of St. Francis was criticized by the medical staff for not defining their policies more clearly.[86] Even when policies were well defined, by allotting a certain number of beds for example, they were not enforced because the administration refused to deny admission to any individual.

The problem of the elderly reflected a national trend toward an increasing number of patients sixty-five or older being admitted to mental institutions. As early as 1945, the elderly constituted a disproportionately large percentage of institutionalized patients. In 1940, they represented 19 percent of all first

[83]"How It Began," *Community Mental Health, Mental Retardation Center—Bulletin* 1 (November 1971); Executive director's report, February 27, 1967; Minutes, Board of Managers, "Report of St. Francis General Hospital and Rehabilitation Institution Concerning the Psychiatric Survey Initiated by the Department of Welfare," 1956; "Psychiatry Status Report," November 15, 1963, prepared for St. Francis General Hospital, St. Francis Hospital Archives.

[84]"Psychiatry Status Report," November 15, 1963, prepared for St. Francis General Hospital, St. Francis Hospital Archives.

[85]This was the county hospital established primarily for the elderly.

[86]"Psychiatry Status Report," November 15, 1963, prepared for St. Francis General Hospital, St. Francis Hospital Archives, Exhibit B—History; Minutes, Board of Managers, 2/22/60, Motherhouse Archives.

admissions to psychiatric facilities. By 1950, that percentage had risen to 25 percent, and by 1958, nearly one-third of all state mental hospital patients were sixty-five or older. By the mid-twentieth century, the mental hospital was serving an additional role as a home for the aged. Between 1933 and 1956/58, the rate of first admissions of patients sixty-five or older increased from 156.6 to 232.7 per 100,000.[87]

Not only was St. Francis Hospital doing its share to serve the elderly population who were largely neglected by other agencies, but St. Francis was, in some ways, functioning as a municipal hospital and was perceived as such. Because of the way the state of Pennsylvania, through its agent hospitals, determined what patients would be admitted, great voids in public care existed. The County of Allegheny was "considerably derelict" in accepting any financial responsibility for their part in the care of the mentally ill, "defectives," adolescents, children and the aged. St. Francis Hospital served this purpose, as the state and county did not. In addition, the hospital did not receive adequate financial assistance for the services which it did provide. Psychiatrists within the hospital felt that outside agencies viewed the hospital with little respect and continued to "use" the hospital. There were those in the institution who felt that the policies resulted in poorer patient care, poorer public relations, a poorer image and lower personnel morale. Outside physicians, as well as the general public, perceived that the hospital was a public institution. The administration, however, was partially to blame for not adequately defining or enforcing policy.[88] Although tension existed within the institution because of the sisters' admission policies, the hospital provided a service to those whose needs were not being met elsewhere.

This entire policy debate reflects the sisters' ongoing belief about open admission and demonstrates the conflict which the sisters faced. Sister Adele, the chief executive officer, was described as one who had "the conviction that Providence has placed her in charge of a large hospital in order to make sure that people in need of help receive it, with no ands, ifs, or buts. Regulations of whatever nature from whatever government sources that restricted provision of services had no meaning for her ... it is fortunate for the people of Pittsburgh that Sister never took them (legal technicalities) seriously for so many years, and went on doing what had to be done." For example, Sister Adele

[87] Gerald N. Grob, *From Asylum to Community: Mental Health Policy in Modern America*, (Princeton: Princeton University Press, 1991), p. 159.

[88] "Psychiatry Status Report," November 15, 1963, prepared for St. Francis General Hospital, St. Francis Hospital Archives; "How It Began," *Community Mental Health, Mental Retardation Center—Bulletin* 1 (November 1971); Executive director's report, February 27, 1967; Minutes, Board of Managers, "Report of St. Francis General Hospital and Rehabilitation Institution concerning the Psychiatric Survey Initiated by the Department of Welfare," 1956.

believed that being a vagrant constituted a type of emotional illness sufficient to warrant psychiatric hospitalization, and that this was not misutilization of a hospital. Vagrants were commonly admitted until social service could find adequate shelter for them. Hospital policy, instituted by Sister Adele, did not discourage this practice, but in fact, encouraged it. The authority to admit a patient could be given by a physician over the telephone, but the decision to deny admission had to be made in person. In the middle of the night, it was often easier for the doctor to do the former.[89]

Not only did Sister Adele encourage admission of those in need, but she was concerned about those who were discharged as well. She recalled following a newly discharged psychiatric patient out of the hospital, suspicious that he had nowhere to go. She followed him out the door and up to Penn Avenue, where she caught up with him and asked him where he was going. When he responded that he had no home, Sister Adele marched him right back to the hospital where he remained until adequate housing was found for him.[90]

By 1962, aged patients continued to wait an extended period of time before transfer, and private psychiatric patients remained on a waiting list. Dr. Hugh Chavern, Clinical Director of the Psychiatric Department, requested of the board that he be given authority to make final decisions on admission of all emergency psychiatric patients. The board, reflecting the sisters' authority and committed to the same ideals, noted, "but, we knowing that these emergency patients are generally indigent, having many social problems and sometimes no home, want to make certain that no one who requires care in a home and does not have a home is turned away. It was the consensus that we should take into consideration all aspects of a person's admission including the human and social needs. The decision was left to the administration."[91]

The problem of overcrowding due to all emergency psychiatric admissions, not just the elderly, had become a full-fledged crisis by 1963. Although the Health and Welfare Federation of Pittsburgh had made some attempt to develop an overall community plan in order to take some of the responsibility and burden off of the shoulders of St. Francis, they were not successful, so the problem lurched totally out of hand. By 1963, numerous conflicts had arisen within the psychiatric department because of these policies. Many of the community psychiatrists were unable or unwilling to send their private patients to

[89] Abraham J. Twerski, Article V, manuscript, St. Francis Hospital archives; Abraham J. Twerski, "Government Health," *Pittsburgh Press*, 7 April 1976; Interview with Sister M. Adele Meiser, 1993.

[90] Interview with Sister M. Adele Meiser, 1993.

[91] Minutes, Board of Managers, 2/26/62, Motherhouse Archives.

St. Francis because of the poor condition of the physical plant. The facilities were antiquated, with poor lighting, minimal privacy for patients and poor heating. The Joint Commission for the Accreditation of Hospitals warned St. Francis that they needed a new building. Private patients resented being crowded and forced to associate with other patients. It was felt by some that the situation inhibited recovery. In addition, there was insufficient room to allow for proper stratification of recovering patients. Community physicians frequently sent their private patients to other facilities out of town. Many psychiatrists refused to consider applying for staff privileges for the same reason. There was also concern that the workload and deplorable conditions would drive away nurses and non-professional personnel who would seek more satisfying opportunities elsewhere in more organized and less traumatic surroundings.[92]

Simultaneously, increasing competition from other institutions made serious inroads into the supply of private patients, in spite of population growth. During the same period, for example, Western Psychiatric Institute and Clinic opened a thirty-five bed private unit. As private patients went elsewhere, there was concern that St. Francis would increasingly be forced to deal with "patients and family situations who are much less organized and consequently more troublesome than most private patients." The hospital would be coerced into doing more public work in order to justify its existence. The perceived loss of private patients, who were necessary to augment the hospital's meager income, was a major concern.[93]

Although the sisters' willingness to admit the emotionally unbalanced indigent is not to be undervalued, the care of patients in the institution may have suffered. The hospital's social service department, for example, was inadequate for the number of patients that were admitted. They were forced to spend so much time arranging admissions and transfers that they had no time left to do real social work.[94] One of the more dramatic outcomes of those policies occurred in 1962, when St. Francis lost the last of its three approved residency training programs. The reasons cited included the lack of adequate teaching time, the increased case load per resident, the insufficient library and the lack of basic science teaching. It is important to point out, however, that the revocation of previously approved non-university psychi-

[92]"Psychiatry Status Report," November 15, 1963, prepared for St. Francis General Hospital, St. Francis Hospital Archives.
[93]"Psychiatry Status Report," November 15, 1963, prepared for St. Francis General Hospital, St. Francis Hospital Archives.
[94]"Psychiatry Status Report," November 15, 1963, prepared for St. Francis General Hospital, St. Francis Hospital Archives.

atric residencies had increased nationwide. St. Francis, therefore, was not an exception.[95]

The problem continued unabated, and in 1965, there were eighty beds occupied by patients admitted as emergencies under the misconstrued 1953 agreement, which was to provide ten beds. Dr. Abraham Twerski met with the police and the state hospital superintendent in an attempt to work out alternative methods. St. Francis was advised to give agencies sixty days notice that the 1953 agreement would be terminated. Dr. Twerski and Dr. Harry Feather, medical director, notified the Allegheny County Board of Mental Health in February 1967 that, as of April 15, the 1953 agreement would be terminated. They suggested a prompt meeting with representative community agencies to work out alternative plans. As of May 31, 1967, other area hospitals were to participate in the caring for psychiatric emergency patients. Allegheny General, Columbia, Homestead, McKeesport, Presbyterian-University, Sewickley Valley, South Side, Suburban General, West Penn and Western Psychiatric Institute and Clinic (WPIC) were all to help to alleviate the burden which St. Francis had to bear for so many years.[96]

It is interesting to note that although the number of admissions to the emergency room did decline by one hundred patients per month, the medical staff continued to perceive that there was a monumental problem, especially in the emergency room itself. Prior to the termination of the 1953 agreement, approximately twenty-five hundred to three thousand patients were admitted annually through the emergency room to the psychiatric department. A decline by one hundred patients per month still left 100 to 150 patients per month coming through the emergency department. Staff members complained that the disruption caused by such a large number of noisy and unruly psychiatric patients in the emergency room was deterring other types of patients from seeking proper care. There were still three admission candidates for each empty bed. Some of the physicians were anxious because the psychiatric patients brought in by the police, "make for a poor image for the hospital."[97] It is difficult to determine exactly how and when the problem was completely resolved, but in time, the longstanding reputation of being

[95]"Psychiatry Status Report," November 15, 1963, prepared for St. Francis General Hospital, St. Francis Hospital Archives.

[96]Minutes, Board of Managers, June 8, 1967; Letter from Abraham Twerski and Harry Feather to David Janavitz, chrmn., Allegheny County Board of Mental Health, February 7, 1967, St. Francis Hospital Archives.

[97]Minutes, Board of Managers, October 23, 1967; Minutes, Executive Committee, Medical Staff, February 28, 1967, and April 18, 1967; Minutes, Medical Staff, December 6, 1966, and September 5, 1967; Ed Wintermantel, "Emergency Mental Care 'Pipeline' Clogs," Pittsburgh Press, 19 March 1967.

the city's clearing house for psychiatric patients began to diminish. Other hospitals began to take on greater responsibilities, especially with the implementation of government mandates in the late 1960s, lessening the burden on St. Francis Hospital. In addition, with the advent of community mental health centers, many patients were cared for on an out-patient basis, lessening the pressure to admit an unmanageable number.

World War II to 1977—Community Mental Health Centers

Following World War II and the changes in the theories regarding psychiatric illness and treatment, out-patient services increased nationally, and St. Francis was no exception. The passage of the National Mental Health Act in 1946 provided grants to states to support existing out-patient facilities, or to establish new ones. Before 1948, more than one-half of all fifty states had no clinics at all. In 1949, all but five states had at least one clinic. By 1955, there were 1,234 out-patient psychiatric clinics.[98] The Pennsylvania Department of Welfare conducted studies in August 1955, recognizing the need for services in the community to supplement institutional programs. It was noted that community mental health programs should include not only services for the mentally ill, but programs for healthy people at home, in school and in communities, as well as services for healthy people in trouble. It was also suggested that the role of the psychiatrist be expanded to include consultation and education of service personnel (social workers, nurses, ministers).[99] The Joint Commission on Mental Illness and Mental Health, established in 1955 when Congress passed the Mental Health Study Act, issued their report in 1961, which advocated the development of community based facilities, stating that "community mental health clinics serving both children and adults, operated as outpatient departments of general or mental hospitals. . . . should be regarded as a main line of defense in reducing the need of many persons with major mental illness for prolonged or repeated hospitalization. Therefore, a national mental health program should set as an objective one

[98] Gerald N. Grob, From Asylum to Community: Mental Health Policy in Modern America, (Princeton: Princeton University Press, 1991), pp. 167–168.
[99] John R. McGibony, M.D., *Mental Health: A Community Program*, (Pittsburgh: Health and Welfare Association of Allegheny County, 1958), p. 1.

fully staffed, full-time mental health clinic available to each fifty thousand of population."[100]

Subsequently, the recommendations that resulted from the various studies prompted legislation on the national and state levels, mandating community services. In 1963, President John F. Kennedy asked Congress for federal support in the development of community programs. Congress responded by passing the Mental Health Centers Act (Public Law 88-164) of 1963, which authorized the appropriation of $150 million to finance up to two-thirds of the cost of construction of community mental health centers (CMHC). Authorization of funds for staffing two years later also had a dramatic impact on the development of these centers. Legislation mandated that five essential services be offered in all CMHC's, including in-patient and out-patient services as well, as a twenty-four hour emergency department and a partial hospitalization program. The fifth primary service was that of consultation and education services, which were to be available to community agencies and mental health professionals located within the area, or serving the catchment population. St. Francis Hospital was the first hospital in Western Pennsylvania to receive a Community Mental Health Center Federal Staffing Grant. In 1966, the Pennsylvania Mental Health Mental Retardation Act mandated that four other services be available. The hospital serving the catchment area was to provide aftercare, rehabilitation and training, programs and services for the mentally retarded and unified procedures for intake and referral. Community mental health centers were not designed to focus on the chronically or severely mentally ill. The goals of the mental health policies of the 1960s were to expand community mental health services and, through preventive treatment, diminish sole reliance upon mental hospitals.[101]

It has been argued that the new mental health policies of the post-war era, in their attempt to provide a wide range of therapeutic services to a rather ill-defined population, generally on an out-patient basis, led to the neglect of those chronically and severely mentally ill who were often "cast adrift in communities without access to support services of the basic necessities of life. For such persons the transition from an institutional to a community based system proved devastating. By the 1980s the presence of homeless mentally

[100]Joint Commission on Mental Illness and Health, *Action for Mental Health, Final Report of the Joint commission on Mental Illness and Health,* (New York: Basic Books, 1961), pp. 262–263.

[101]Gerald N. Grob, *From Asylum to Community: Mental Health Policy in Modern America,* (Princeton: Princeton University Press, 1991), pp. 233, 239; "St. Francis Medical Center Department of Psychiatry Position Paper," manuscript, 6/25/87, St. Francis Hospital Archives; *Concept and Challenge, The Comprehensive Community Mental Health Center,* (Washington, D.C.: U.S. Government Printing Office, 1964), p. 4.

ill persons in many communities served as a stark reminder that the new mental health policies had negative as well as positive consequences." The policies of the period were not defined so that they integrated decent and humane care for the severely and chronically ill, but in fact strengthened the distinction between care and treatment.[102] With the main focus of post-war policy on treatment, those in need of 'care,' were neglected by many institutions. Although the sisters participated in the new community oriented psychiatric programs, their adherence to traditional 'care' policies proved to be the exception.

Characteristic of this period in the hospital's history was a greater focus on community involvement: St. Francis Hospital did not wait until the government recommended or mandated services, as the needs of the community were recognized by the board as early as the fifties. It was noted that since emotional illness comprised over 50 percent of the patients' problems for which they consulted physicians, therapeutic facilities in the community were deemed necessary.[103] Sister Adele deserves much of the credit for the establishment of the mental health centers designed to serve the community. She perceived a need, explored the possibilities and then solicited the aid of Dr. George Wright in order to carry out her plan. Sister Adele, knowing she was in need of physician support if she was to be successful, asked Dr. Wright to accompany her and another sister to San Francisco to study community mental health centers there. Although he was very skeptical of the idea, he promised her that he would not actively oppose the implementation of such centers, and agreed to travel with her to California. When the group from St. Francis was through with their task, Dr. Wright suggested that the two sisters enjoy some sightseeing before returning to Pittsburgh. Sister Adele, anxious to start on her written report, was reluctant to take the time to tour the city. At that point, Dr. Wright, reminding her that he was the acting director of the psychiatric department, told her that he felt it was his responsibility to write the report in support of the establishment of community mental health centers. He had been persuaded and was Sister Adele's best ally. Sister Adele felt they never would have established the centers had it not been for Dr. Wright's support and willingness to convince other physicians of their value.[104]

[102]Gerald N. Grob, *From Asylum to Community: Mental Health Policy in Modern America*, (Princeton: Princeton University Press, 1991), pp. 303–304; Gerald N. Grob, "The Chronic Mentally Ill in America: The Historical Context," *Mental Health Services in the United States and England: Struggling for Change; Collected Papers Prepared for the Joint United States/England Conference on Mental Health Services* (Princeton: Robert Wood Johnson Foundation, 1991), p. 14.

[103]Minutes, Board of Managers, "Report of St. Francis General Hospital and Rehabilitation Institution concerning the Psychiatric Survey Initiated by the Department of Welfare," 1956.

[104]Interview with Sister M. Adele Meiser, 1993.

In November 1962, St. Francis, with the help of the Bureau of Community Mental Health, Department of Public Welfare, Commonwealth of Pennsylvania, initiated a study to define its existing practices and services, and to canvas community social welfare and health agencies regarding unmet needs for psychiatric patients, with a particular emphasis on the provision of out-patient care. The recommendations which arose from the study included the development of several service areas, including a full-time out-patient facility, emergency evaluation coordinated with partial hospitalization services, after care and follow-up services, residential treatment for children, out-patient and day care services for geriatric patients and an alcoholic out-patient treatment facility. In compliance with those recommendations, plans were developed for services at the hospital to include in-patient, out-patient, emergency and partial hospital care. In addition, consultation, rehabilitation and educational programs and services were to be developed. The hospital administration responded quickly to the recommendations. By 1964, plans to remodel the nurses' home to convert it into the new psychiatric facility, which called for the development of an all-inclusive community mental health center, were already underway. Dr. George J. Wright, Jr., was chairman of the department of psychiatry and neurology, and was temporary director. Sister M. Lucene Fliegel, OSF, was assistant administrator in charge of psychiatry. In 1965, the hospital instituted a dramatic change in its out-patient policy, reflecting the administration's desire to respond judiciously in order to serve citizens in need of psychiatric services. The neuro-psychiatric clinic, which previously had operated only one morning per week, expanded its hours to provide services five mornings per week.[105] The hospital administration, desirous of offering comprehensive psychiatric services in order to meet the needs of the community, implemented carefully thought out plans, and was able to offer those services within a short period of time.

Sister Adele was cognizant of the pressing need to hire a full-time director of the psychiatric department. In order to apply for grant money which was necessary to establish a community mental health center, a full time director had to be appointed. She had great difficulty in the beginning, writing to the government and other institutions, and her attempts were, at first, in vain. Dr. George Wright, who was acting director at the time, wanted to be relieved of the position in order that he could attend to his private practice. Sister Adele recalled that when psychiatrists from out-of-town would come

[105]Ed Wintermantel, "St. Francis Unit A Mental Health First in State," *Pittsburgh Press* 22 March 1964. "History of Services," *Community MH/MR Center Bulletin* 1 (September 1971); "How It Began," *Community Mental Health, Mental Retardation Center—Bulletin* 1 (November 1971); "St. Francis Medical Center Department of Psychiatry Position Paper," manuscript, 6/25/87, St. Francis Hospital Archives; Interview with Dr. George Wright, 10/25/93.

to visit St. Francis, they would ask where the cows were kept, believing that all Franciscan sisters kept cows. In order to combat that image, Sister Adele requested the help of Dr. Henry W. Brosin, professor and chairman of psychiatry at the University of Pittsburgh. Sister perceived that St. Francis, which emphasized care, had many patients available for clinical research, whereas the university, which focused on teaching and research, had the academicians. Over the years, the two institutions had collaborated on joint projects, but St. Francis had to employ a full-time director of the psychiatric department in order to continue that tradition. Dr. Brosin agreed to help Sister. When he finally called her with the good news that he had found a qualified director, he warned her that upon meeting him, she would have a "social shock." Brosin warned Sister not to be alarmed because he "runs around in some kind of garb." Sister, still wearing the customary full habit, was quite amused, claiming, "Dr. I've been running around in some kind of a garb all of my life." The staff psychiatrists at that time were very supportive of the decision.[106]

In 1965, Dr. Abraham Joshua Twerski was hired as full-time clinical director of psychiatry. An ordained Jewish rabbi, Dr. Twerski had completed his residency at WPIC and been a member of the senior staff at Mayview State Hospital. He was also a clinical assistant instructor in psychiatry at the University of Pittsburgh Medical School. At the same time, Dr. George L. Alexander, Jr., was hired as director of the psychiatric out-patient clinic.[107] Dr. Twerski profoundly influenced the development of the psychiatric department, developing an institution which offered comprehensive care to a wide population area. Twerski, instrumental in obtaining a staffing grant for the community mental health centers, and in reinstituting the residency program in 1974, was also influential in consolidating and organizing the treatment programs for chemical dependency.[108] Twerski has been described as being very empathetic and understanding of his patients, whose lifestyles often contrasted dramatically with his own.[109]

The community mental health clinics did not develop without some tension, especially between the medical staff and other personnel, such as social workers and nurses. It was not unusual for new psychiatrists, who had just completed their residency programs, to work as administrators in the com-

[106]Interview with Sister M. Adele Meiser, 1993; Barbara I. Paull, *A Century of Medical Excellence, The History of the University of Pittsburgh School of Medicine*, (Pittsburgh: University of Pittsburgh Medical Alumni Association, 1986), pp. 168–170.

[107]"Rabbi, Catholic Hospital Team Up in Psychiatry," *Pittsburgh Press*, 26 September 1965.

[108]Interview with Dr. William Mooney, April 28, 1994; "County Request for 25th Anniversary Retrospective," manuscript from Adult Outpatient division, 1994, Community Mental Health.

[109]Interview with Mrs. Mary Thompson, 5/4/94.

munity mental health centers until they could establish their own private practices, at which time they would resign their positions at the community clinic.[110] Sister Adele noted that the psychiatrists were accustomed to treating patients with the expectation of curing them and helping them to return to normal living, whereas those individuals that utilized community mental health centers, although they needed assistance in functioning in life, were unlikely to change, a concept requiring adjustment on the part of staff psychiatrists.[111] More and more treatment responsibilities were given to non-physicians, sometimes even to lay people. In the beginning, the average psychiatrist looked askance at that type of treatment.[112]

Sister Adele was quite concerned about the new government mandates requiring certain hospitals to provide comprehensive psychiatric services to the community. She questioned whether they would be forced to deny care to those outside of the catchment area, but was assured that she could provide services to everyone as long as catchment area patients had priority. The hospital was unique in that it remained the only facility in the area where anyone could walk in at anytime unannounced and without an appointment, and the sisters did not want to alter that policy.[113]

The community mental health center at St. Francis was officially opened January 1, 1967, assuming the Base Service Unit responsibility for Catchment Area 9B-1 as part of the Allegheny county MH/MR program in 1969. Federal Government guidelines stated that an area could include 75,000 to 200,000 citizens. St. Francis' catchment area had a population of 190,217 within twenty-one different communities. The hospital served as a coordinating mechanism for all existing mental health resources. Federal assistance was partial, and granted only during the initial phase of the development of the program, but additional funding was subsequently provided by the Commonwealth of Pennsylvania and Allegheny County. The state paid 90 percent and the county 10 percent. Fees for service were on a sliding scale. The five basic services required by federal guidelines were offered to patients in addition to services mandated by the state.[114]

All of these services were designed to meet three goals, all emphasizing

[110]Interview with Dr. George Wright, 10/25/93.

[111]Interview with Sister M. Adele Meiser, 1993.

[112]Interview with Dr. William Mooney, April 28, 1994.

[113]Minutes of special meeting, June 1, 1966, Minutes, Board of Managers; Abraham J. Twerski, Article V, manuscript, St. Francis Hospital Archives.

[114]*Community Mental Health Center—St. Francis,* brochure, St. Francis Hospital Archives; *Community Mental Health Mental Retardation Center Bulletin* 1 (September 1971); "County Request for 25th Anniversary Retrospective," 1994, manuscript from CMHC, St. Francis Hospital Archives; Interview with Dr. William Mooney, April 28, 1994; "St. Francis Medical Center Department of Psychiatry Position Paper," manuscript, 6/25/87, St. Francis Hospital Archives.

preventive care. The primary goal was to decrease the rate of new cases of mental disorder by working to reduce harmful influences known to contribute to such disorders, and to help people at times of crises. The second goal was to decrease the prevalence of mental disability in the community through early case findings and outreach programs. The third goal was to reduce the degree of residual mental disability (sequelae) by offering aftercare programs and medications for patients returning to the community.[115]

One of the essential required services was the provision of in-patient services. Clearly, St. Francis had provided hospital care, but they specifically assigned thirty-five beds for catchment area patients. Other BSU Catchment areas, however, which did not provide comprehensive care, frequently referred patients to St. Francis to occupy beds in the Children's and Adolescents' Units, the Chemical Dependency Units and other locked Adult units. If the milieu therapy unit provided for the catchment area was filled to capacity or inappropriate for the patient's diagnosis, patients were admitted to other floors. The unit was primarily designed for patients suffering from an emotional crisis who it was deemed could be returned to the community within sixty days. Treatment consisted of individual and group therapy, chemotherapy and recreational and occupational therapy. Those in need of longer hospitalization were transferred to Woodville State Hospital. By 1974, it was clear to the hospital administration that with the drastic limitation of the patient population in state hospitals, the chronically ill who had long histories of extensive and repeated hospitalizations were also being cared for at St. Francis, but it was hoped that the expansive community services would help to alleviate the problem. In order to augment those in-patient services, the hospital established broad community networks with those not specifically in mental health areas such as the clergy, family physicians, the police and teachers, for example.[116]

Although the federal government mandated out-patient services, which the hospital already had, St. Francis committed themselves to the community at large on a much wider scale than was required. Satellite community centers developed in areas of need. Each satellite center had a life of its own, which was related to the nature of the community it was serving, in comparison to the institutional setting. The setting was often informal, allowing clients to spend the day chatting with clerical workers with whom they had established warm and friendly relationships.[117] In 1968, at the request and with the coopera-

[115]*Community MH/MR Center Bulletin* (September 1971).
[116]"The Mental Retardation Unit," *Community Mental Health, Mental Retardation Center—Bulletin* 1 (November 1971; *Community MH/MR Center Bulletin* 1 (September 1971); "St. Francis Medical Center Department of Psychiatry Position Paper," manuscript 6/25/87, St. Francis Hospital Archives.
[117]Interview with Mrs. Mary Thompson, 5/4/94.

tion of community leaders, St. Francis established a pilot outreach program, the Homewood-Brushton Trouble Center, designed to provide treatment of non-medical mental health problems in the community. Staffed by a nurse, two mental health expediters and a secretary, the two-fold functions of the center included provision of out-patient services for the mentally disabled and mentally retarded, as well as consultation and education services in order to provide a liaison between the Satellite Center and other community agencies, schools, citizens and civic groups. The center was open daily from nine until five, with evening appointments offered when necessary; in addition, the staff responded to emergencies after hours. Mrs. Mary Leach Thompson, project director, noted the benefits of the informal program, allowing individuals to comfortably remain at the center all day to socialize if they desired.[118]

In the same year, borough officials and civic leaders of Sharpsburg also requested that a satellite clinic of the Community Mental Health Program be established to serve residents of Sharpsburg, Millvale, Etna, Reserve and Shaler Townships. The purpose of the program was to prevent social and emotional strains from developing into more severe emotional illness. The program, conducted every Wednesday morning in the Sharpsburg Municipal building, also scheduled sessions on Saturday mornings and one weekday evening to accommodate day workers. Volunteers in the community arranged for secretarial and receptionist services. Although St. Francis psychiatrists, psychologists, social workers and vocational rehabilitation experts were available to provide any needed services, most of the day-to-day counseling was to be done by community clergymen, social agencies, school counselors and family doctors as this was primarily a preventive center. In the early seventies, the hospital signed contracts with the Community Action Pittsburgh, Inc., to establish outreach programs in poverty areas of the city, seemingly formalizing what had already commenced.[119]

The Garfield-Stanton Heights Satellite Center, first established as a pilot program for the treatment of children in 1970, expanded the program to provide adult services in 1972. The center offered three basic services to the community. The first, the treatment program, was designed to help people who were experiencing difficulties in their personal lives. Those struggling with marital or parent-child relationships, family or individual problems or

---

[118]Interview with Mrs. Mary Thompson, 5/4/94; "Homewood-Brushton Satellite Center," *Community MH/MR Center Bulletin* 1 (May 1972).

[119]Interview with Dr. William Mooney, April 28, 1994; *Community MH/MR Center Bulletin* 1 (September 1971); "St. Francis Medical Center Department of Psychiatry Position Paper," manuscript, 6/25/87, St. Francis Hospital Archives; "Human Relations Report," manuscript, 10/23/68, St. Francis Hospital Archives; "Hospital Going to People, Counseling Setup Planned," *Pittsburgh Press*, 3 June 1968.

other emotional crises could be treated without having to disrupt employment or family situations. Individual, group and family therapies were all provided as well as services for mentally retarded individuals. The second component of the program involved coordinating efforts between the center and other service agencies within the community. In addition, consultation and education services were offered to interested citizen's groups and other agencies. The center was open daily with evening appointments available upon request.[120]

Within a year, it became apparent that the Garfield center was unable to adequately fill requests for service, especially for residents in the East Liberty area, because of a lack of staff and a location which was difficult to reach by public transportation. Interested citizens requested that another satellite center be established in the East End. The large number of East Liberty and Highland Park residents already being seen at St. Francis attested to the need in the community, so subsequently, a new center was established in the Medical Center East Building. Children and adults received services similar to those in the preexisting satellite centers.[121]

The third essential requirement of all community mental health centers, in addition to in-patient and out-patient services, was the provision for partial hospitalization. Day Center Services, St. Francis' partial hospitalization program, was established in October 1970. The staff consisted of an interdisciplinary team whose specialties included psychiatry, rehabilitation counseling, psychiatric nursing, occupational therapy, dance therapy, casework and family therapy. Admission to the program was on a voluntary basis for adults between the ages of seventeen and sixty-five who had been referred by In-patient Services, Emergency Services, Out-patient Services and Satellites, private psychiatrists or other social agencies. The Day Center Services offered care to three types of patients. It was an alternative to in-patient hospitalization or an alternative to returning to state institutions during an acute crisis. In addition, the Center offered a phase of treatment for smoothing a patient's transition from in-patient hospitalization or state hospitalization into the community. Depending on a patient's clinical status, participation in the program extended from one to five days per week, from nine until three if necessary. Day Center Services provided milieu therapy, which included treatment as well as rehabilitation in an attempt to serve members of the community in need of psychiatric care, but who wished to maintain themselves within the community. Patients, or consumers, were encouraged to participate in the planning of their treatment. Services were also coordinated

[120] "Garfield-Stanton Heights Satellite Center," *Community Mental Health/Mental Retardation Center Bulletin* 1 (May 1972).
[121] SFGH *Community Mental Health Mental Retardation Center Newsletter* 2 (April 1974).

with a variety of community agencies, including Goodwill Industries, Vocational Rehabilitation Center, Bureau of Vocational Rehabilitation, Council House, Transitional Services and others. Obviously, the center made use of many of the services offered by St. Francis Hospital. In 1975, adult partial hospital services were established at the East Liberty Satellite, primarily for the chronically and persistently mentally ill consumers who were discharged from the state hospitals.[122]

The federal government also mandated that emergency treatment be provided. All emergency patients were evaluated and either admitted or referred to one of the many out-patient services. St. Francis expanded that service in 1970, when they hired a psychiatric nurse to provide follow-up care on all psychiatric patients presenting themselves for treatment in the emergency room. She attempted direct crisis intervention, provided preventive care and made referrals to other agencies. When the patient resided in another catchment area, the nurse corresponded with the social workers of that base service unit.[123]

The fifth essential service which the government required of Community Mental Health Centers was that of consultation and education. This element was incorporated into legislation as an attempt to fill the gap due to the limited number of psychiatric therapists. Consultation and education staff members, therefore, worked to develop the therapeutic abilities of other care-givers within the community, thereby increasing direct services to citizens in the catchment area. Another purpose of the consultation education staff was to offer information, advice and educational services to community groups or other professionals, such as teachers and doctors, who might have some influence on emotionally troubled individuals.[124]

In 1971, in order to comply with government mandates, the 9B-1 Citizens Council was established, allowing community involvement in planning community mental health programs and policy development. Community residents, hospital administrators, including Sister Adele, and CMHC staff attended regularly scheduled meetings to discuss an array of concerns. Subcommittees were formed within the council to address issues of a more specific nature, such as a children's sub-committee, consultation and education, budget and finance, mental retardation, membership and drug treatment subcommittees. Council members themselves attended seminars and lectures in

---

[122] SFGH *Community Mental Health Mental Retardation Center Newsletter* 2 (August 1974); *Community Mental Health, Mental Retardation Center—Bulletin* 1 (March 1972); "County Request for 25th Anniversary Retrospective," manuscript from CMHC, 1994, St. Francis Hospital Archives.

[123] SFGH *Community Mental Health Mental Retardation Center Newsletter* 2 (March 1974).

[124] *Community Mental Health, Mental Retardation Center—Bulletin* 1 (July 1972).

order to become more familiar with mental health issues, and they sought the views of the community in an attempt to plan and implement programs for the residents of the catchment area. Social programs were also planned for members of the council.[125]

In response to the state legislature's requirement of the community mental health mental retardation centers to provide continuous care in life management for all mentally retarded citizens who lived in the catchment area, the Mental Retardation Unit was established in July 1969. Initially, services were provided by a part-time senior psychologist, one full-time school psychologist and one half-time social worker. In-patient facilities were available primarily to determine diagnosis and outline a plan of treatment. The mental retardation unit of the community mental health center offered follow-up care and consultation to clients, families and agencies involved. Soon after, it became fairly evident that there was a need for day care and educational experiences for a population of eight to eighteen year old individuals who were not appropriate for schools or other programs because of their degree of retardation or emotional problems. Therefore, the St. Francis Growth and Development Center was established in June 1970 at the First United Methodist Church, Center and South Aiken Avenues, to provide a learning, training and socialization facility for twenty-five severely retarded children and adults who had been excluded from schools and other public services. The aim of the program was to prevent unwarranted institutionalization. The unit closed the following summer when the Right to Education Decision forced school systems to educate mentally retarded children. The same site, however, was subsequently utilized for an Adult Activities Center. Needs for services increased dramatically because of the state-wide attempt to decrease enrollments in state facilities, and eventually the site was moved to the Medical Center East Building in East Liberty. The Mental Retardation Unit provided all mandated services to mentally retarded citizens in the catchment area. By 1974, it served in excess of three hundred clients.[126]

Also in compliance with the Commonwealth of Pennsylvania's mandate, the hospital addressed the issue of aftercare. In 1973, a full-time staff member was hired to coordinate aftercare services and maintain liaison with other agencies. Planning for care following discharge was generally implemented upon the patient's admission to an in-patient institution in order to facili-

[125]SFGH Community Mental Health Mental Retardation Center Newsletter 1 (April, June 1973), 2 (June 1974).
[126]"The Mental Retardation Unit," Community Mental Health, Mental Retardation Center—Bulletin 1 (November 1971); Community MH/MR Center Bulletin 1 (September 1971); "St. Francis Medical Center Department of Psychiatry Position Paper," manuscript, 6/25/87, St. Francis Hospital Archives.

tate that patient's reorientation into the community. Eventually, liaison was established with other state institutions, county wide specialty services and other local base service units.[127]

Other programs and services were also developed during this time period, usually with a focus on the community health component. St. Francis Hospital developed new programs and services designed exclusively for children. In the spring of 1968, the hospital opened a six-bed in-patient unit for children on the second floor of the East building. The unit consisted of a nursing station, six beds, one classroom and a teacher furnished by the Allegheny Intermediate Unit. The purpose was twofold. Treatment was provided for the long term for severely disturbed children, and clinical experience was provided for the residency training program in Child Psychiatry at the University of Pittsburgh School of Medicine's WPIC. Ruth Kane, M.D., was the founder and director. In the subsequent twenty years, the children's unit treated approximately four thousand troubled children. Hundreds of students from schools of child care and child development, social work, psychology and nursing were trained. By 1972, the expanded ten-bed unit moved to the fifth floor and added two more teachers and classrooms. The unit was then restructured as a short term intervention facility, and a partial hospitalization program was initiated. In 1970, the hospital established the only short-term adolescent in-patient unit in Western Pennsylvania. The ten-bed unit was also designed as a short-term crisis intervention unit.[128]

Provisions were also made during the same time period for out-patient services for children and adolescents. In 1968, the newly established Day Hospital Program admitted patients ages two to sixteen and a half years old. Approximately 130 children were seen each week. Services included psychological testing, and group and family therapy. Several innovative programs were also initiated, such as dance therapy, music interpretation and structured art. Females participated in personal appearance classes. Other activities included swimming, track, paddleball, weight lifting, gymnastics, body-building and various field trips. The Exceptional Children's Division of the Allegheny County School System supported the Adolescent Day Care with two special education teachers, who provided formal education opportunities for all patients. In the fall of 1970, the Garfield Satellite Center Children Services was established to provide group oriented treatment and recreational services to children and their families. The Garfield center, which treated thirty chil-

---

[127] *SFGH Community Mental Health Mental Retardation Center Newsletter* 2 (March 1974).

[128] *Community MH/MR Center Bulletin* 1 (September 1971); "Children Psychiatric Inpatient Unit—Twentieth Anniversary," manuscript, n.d. but c. 1988, St. Francis Hospital Archives; "County Request for 25th Anniversary Retrospective," manuscript from CMHC, 1994, St. Francis Hospital Archives.

dren, offered various forms of therapy, including art, music, and camping. The center was run by one trained social worker and thirty volunteers. Within the next two years, children's centers were also instituted at the Sharpsburg and Homewood-Brushton centers.[129] Although St. Francis Hospital had always treated children with psychiatric disorders, this was the first attempt to establish separate programs for them, both as in-patients and out-patients. The Joint Commission, in 1961, had recommended that psychiatric clinics provide intensive psychotherapy for children, plus appropriate medical or social treatment procedures.[130]

To be sure, the advent of increased government funding and mandates resulted in an explosion of new initiatives on the part of the hospital, and eventually other agencies and hospitals followed. St. Francis stands out as an exception, however, because it was in many cases the first facility to respond to changes in mental health practice, often before funds were available or policies were changed. The sisters' commitment to the development of the psychiatric facility and the programs which they implemented set their hospital apart as a leading institution in the community.

World War II to 1977—Substance Abuse

By the time World War II had ended, the prevailing attitudes towards chemical abuse and alcoholism had begun to change. The American Hospital Association and the American Medical Association passed resolutions recognizing the disease concept in the mid-fifties. No longer perceiving addiction as a crime, the medical community at large began to offer treatment facilities to combat such problems. The Supreme Court lent credence to this view in 1962, when they officially declared addiction a disease, not a crime. In 1970, Congress passed the Comprehensive Alcohol Abuse and Alcoholism Prevention, Treatment, and Rehabilitation Act, which created the National Institute on Alcohol Abuse and Alcoholism. The objectives of the institute were research, education and public informational activities. This act gave the alcoholism constituency a voice in public health programs and research

---

[129]"The Children's Unit,"*Community Mental Health, Mental Retardation Center—Bulletin* 1 (November 1971); *Community MH/MR Center Bulletin* 1 (September 1971); "County Request for 25th Anniversary Retrospective," manuscript from CMHC, 1994, St. Francis Hospital Archives; *Community Mental Health, Mental Retardation Center—Bulletin* 1 (March 1972).

[130]*Community MH/MR Center Bulletin* 1 (September 1971); Joint Commission on Mental Illness and Health, *Action for Mental Health, Final Report of the Joint Commission on Mental Illness and Health*, (New York: Basic Books, 1961), p. 263.

planning. It was not long before states began enacting measures to substitute medical treatment for punishment of alcoholics, which also had been suggested in the first half of the nineteenth century. In 1974, President Nixon established the Special Action Office for Drug Abuse Prevention to coordinate government programs linked to the drug problem. Clearly, there was a need for substance abuse programs as substantiated by the large number of alcoholic patients admitted for treatment to the psychiatric facility at St. Francis. With the change in views regarding addiction, and the government's acceptance of that view, as well as the provision of funding, treatment programs expanded as the need to respond to an ever growing social problem was realized.[131]

St. Francis Hospital clearly had a long history of offering treatment for patients addicted to alcohol or other substances. The foundation was laid very early for the programs which continued to expand in the post-war era. More importantly, St. Francis Hospital was unique because this foundation was established at a time when other institutions neglected or ignored the widespread problem of substance abuse. Many hospitals during the 1940s had an antagonistic and negative attitude regarding these patients. When responding to a circular letter from researchers of the Committee on Hospital Treatment of Alcoholism, funded by a grant from the Research Council on Problems of Alcohol, many hospital administrators claimed to be interested in alcoholism, but were against policies to admit alcoholics because of a lack of personnel and facilities. Hospital executives felt that admitting those patients was a misuse of hospital facilities when alcoholics took up space in an already overcrowded facility, especially when they had no intention of reforming. They felt hospitals should not be used as a substitute for jail. Another administrator viewed alcoholism as a "self-induced condition." Interestingly, the same report which summarized the responses cited St. Francis as the one outstanding exception to this universal attitude. "The St. Francis Hospital in Pittsburgh has been sufficiently public spirited to fill in the void occasioned by the absence of a municipal or county general hospital in that city by providing a separate ward section for alcoholics. During 1942, 1,238 alcoholic patients were admitted to this hospital, 88 percent to the free wards and 12 percent to private rooms."[132]

By the mid-fifties, alcoholics continued to be the largest group of pa-

---

[131] David F. Musto, *The American Disease, Origins of Narcotic Control,* (New York: Oxford University Press, 1987), pp. 237, 258; Mark Edward Lender and James Kirby Martin, *Drinking in America, A History,* (New York: Free Press, 1982), pp. 185–190.

[132] Minutes, Board of Managers, 9/11/44, report for the Committee on Hospital Treatment of Alcoholism by E. H. L. Corwin and Elizabeth V. Cunningham, grant from the Research Council on Problems of Alcohol, report #7.

tients admitted, 992 of the 4,280 admissions for the year ending in December 1954. Of that group, only sixty-five were women. In addition, ninety-four patients were admitted with the diagnosis of acute brain syndrome associated with alcohol intoxication, and twenty-two patients had chronic brain syndrome associated with alcohol intoxication.[133] In the mid-sixties, alcoholics remained one of the largest groups of patients admitted to the psychiatric department, which annually received approximately nine hundred people for a week or so of 'drying out.'[134]

Following the war, and until 1965, the third floor porch area facing Mill-vale had been designated specifically for alcoholics. Treatment began with the sisters, who always cared for patients with dignity, helping patients to "walk it off." Rehabilitation during this period consisted primarily of the doctors, social workers and sister-nurses urging the patient to "quit for good." The patient was encouraged to "take the pledge," which was a solemn promise to God taken on the Bible before a clergyman, swearing total abstinence for a specified period of time. Many remained sober for a year at a time. Smoking was prohibited. In 1955, Alcoholics Anonymous meetings were introduced on the hospital's alcoholism unit.[135]

The sisters maintained their services to alcoholics in spite of the persistent animosity and controversy generated in the institution as a result of those policies. The alcoholic unit was often overcrowded, so patients were frequently admitted to other departments within the hospital. Staff physicians were annoyed because alcoholic patients were being assigned beds in the medical department, decreasing the number of beds available for the internists' patients. Some of the staff psychiatrists complained because alcoholic patients were being assigned to 9 east, a psychiatric ward, but not a ward for alcoholics. The medical staff requested that a special room be set aside for alcoholics waiting to be admitted. Staffing shortages, however, did not permit the establishment of a holding area. After May 15, 1967, under the "Psychiatric and Alcoholic Program," six area hospitals were to participate in the care and admission of alcoholics, and state hospitals, as well, were soon to be opening their doors to them.[136] The problem was eventually alleviated, but not because the sisters changed their policies.

[133] Report sent to the American Psychiatric Association Central Inspection Board, November 1955, St. Francis Hospital Archives.

[134] Abraham J. Twerski, Article VII, manuscript, St. Francis Hospital Archives; "Capital Campaign brochure for Dr. Twerski," manuscript, 5/20/83, St. Francis Hospital Archives.

[135] Report sent to the American Psychiatric Association Central Inspection Board, November 1955, St. Francis Hospital Archives; Capital Campaign brochure for Dr. Twerski, 5/20/83, manuscript, St. Francis Hospital Archives; *Welcome to the Tenth Anniversary of Gateway Rehabilitation Center*, 1/17/82, brochure, St. Francis Hospital Archives.

[136] Minutes, Executive Committee, Medical Staff, April 18, 1967, September 5, 1967.

Realizing that in-patient services were inadequate in meeting the needs of the alcoholic, the staff and administration of the hospital established, in 1958, the first outpatient alcohol program under the direction of Dr. William J. Browne. During the sessions, first offered one evening per week, Dr. Brown would meet with the patient, and a social worker would meet with the spouse. Patients sometimes were seen regularly for up to a year. Physical examinations and laboratory tests were an integral part of the patient assessment. In 1959, a grant was received from the Health Research and Services Foundation, allowing the clinic to expand its services to two evenings per week. From the very beginning of the program, staff collected data, looked at family patterns and documented findings. Family members were always involved in the program. While recognizing St. Francis' distinctive record, Dr. Browne noted that there was a long period of time when the psychiatric community did not deal with the drug and alcohol problem.[137]

Although the St. Francis Hospital's first priority was always service, it also maintained a history of involvement in medical research. As noted previously, the study of alcoholism had been given considerable attention as early as 1911. In 1954, the University of Pittsburgh requested St. Francis to cooperate in a study relating to the dietary problems in the treatment of alcoholism. The state provided funding for an additional social service worker to aid in the project.[138] In 1959, the Health Research and Services Foundation also assisted in a project entitled, "A Study for Marital Interactions of Alcoholic Patients and Their Spouses."[139]

On October 1, 1965, the first full time out-patient clinic for alcoholics in Allegheny County opened under the joint sponsorship of the county health department and St. Francis Hospital. Apparently, within the subsequent two years, funding was also provided by the state. Dr. Martin Adler, chief of the county's Bureau of Mental Health credited Sister Adele with a major role in the formation of the clinic. The clinic, held at the county's Arsenal Health Center, and directed by Dr. William J. Browne, was open five days per week, including two evenings. Services, which included casework, psychotherapy (group and individual), individual and family counseling and medication were available to anyone desiring treatment who was unable to pay for private care. The clinic provided information to employers and consultation services for attending physicians at other local area hospitals. Broad educational services included special education and therapeutic groups for adult children of al-

---

[137]"St. Francis Honors Dedicated Psychiatrist," *Pittsburgh Hospital News*, August 1989; Minutes, Board of Managers, 5/25/59.

[138]Minutes, Board of Managers, 4/26/54, 5/24/54, St. Francis Hospital Archives.

[139]Minutes, Board of Managers, 7/27/59, includes letter from Health Research and Services Foundation, 6/9/59.

coholics. It is important to note that Dr. Browne was a leader in the field, having participated in the 'People to Substance Abuse Project' in Europe and the Soviet Union.[140]

After the establishment of the community mental health centers, many of the services offered to substance abusers were encompassed within the CMHC, and therefore available to anyone regardless of their financial status. However, in the urban areas, CMHC clients tended to be younger, poorer, less well educated and disproportionately drawn from minority and nonwhite backgrounds, as compared with in-patient mental hospital populations. Many patients were referred to centers because of alcoholism and drug addiction. Congress passed a series of amendments between 1968 and 1974 expanding the therapeutic responsibilities of CMHC's to include the prevention and treatment of alcoholism and drug addiction. It is interesting to note that many other CMHC's did not provide adequate services to those seeking help for chemical abuse. Therefore, St. Francis Hospital once again picked up the slack by serving those outside their catchment area.[141]

Because the hospital had made such a commitment to the treatment of substance abuse, it was not surprising that it participated in community educational outreach programs as well. For example, in 1974, staff from the St. Francis out-patient drug program initiated a pilot project with Western Psychiatric Institute and Clinic, Peabody High School, the Board of Education and the Community MH/MR Center. The project had several components, including a creative listening seminar as an aid to education for faculty, and also a 'listening post' where students, parents or teachers could come to relate their problems and interact with their peers. Home visits were made and recommendations were made to WPIC or the St. Francis Community MH/MR Center if necessary. This mental health service was subsequently established in Schenley High School by 1977.[142] In 1974, St. Francis initiated a demonstration Alcohol/Highway Safety Program in conjunction with the Allegheny County District Attorney's office. The program, which was gradually adopted by the Allegheny County Drug and Alcohol Program, resulted

[140]"St. Francis Honors Dedicated Psychiatrist," *Pittsburgh Hospital News*, August 1989; *Regional alcoholism Treatment Center—Out-patient services*, brochure, n.d., St. Francis Hospital Archives; *Post-Gazette* 18 October 1965; Minutes, Board of Managers, Executive Director's Report, August–September 1967; The Commonwealth of Pennsylvania granted $35,919.00 to the hospital for an alcoholism outpatient center 8/29/67.

[141]Gerald N. Grob, *From Asylum to Community: Mental Health Policy in Modern America*, (Princeton: Princeton University Press, 1991), p. 255; Interview with Mary Thompson, 5/4/94.

[142]"County Request for 25th Anniversary Retrospective," manuscript, 1994, St. Francis Hospital Community MH/MR Center; *SFGH Community Mental Health Mental Retardation Center Newsletter* 2 (March 1974).

in the development of four other county alcoholism programs. The hospital subsequently hired a consultation/education coordinator to develop community/school prevention programs.[143] Clearly, the explosive growth of services that combined hospital tradition and government initiatives was applied to the services developed for chemical abuse.

In November 1971, mirroring the explosion of treatment facilities which were established nationwide, St. Francis Hospital initiated a Methadone Maintenance Drug Treatment Program located in Homewood. Geared towards persons addicted to narcotics, it was an integral part of the Community Mental Health/Mental Retardation Center, and was funded yearly by the Allegheny County Mental Health and Mental Retardation Program. Patients over 21, or those 18 to 21 with parental permission, were admitted to the program on a voluntary basis; they were to be free of addiction to alcohol and must not be involved in multiple drug abuse. Following consultation and physical examination, the patient was referred to the methadone maintenance program. Additional rehabilitation services included individual, family and group counseling as well as vocation-educational evaluations and job development. When necessary, formal psychotherapy or psychiatric treatments were provided. When the patient had reached a state of psychological and social readiness, detoxification from methadone was implemented. Although two other methadone maintenance programs were already established in the Metropolitan Pittsburgh area, St. Francis' program was unique because of its ambulatory approach. Treatment was provided entirely on an out-patient basis. It was believed that the out-patient treatment method was therapeutically beneficial in allowing the addict to continue to face his environment and the various factors which were precipitating causes of the problem. In addition, the patient's employment, schooling or family obligations would not be disrupted, and the trauma of re-entry into the community would be avoided.[144]

In August 1971, the hospital also established special out-patient services which provided treatment for abusers of other drugs who did not, for one reason or another, qualify for the methadone maintenance program. Users of amphetamines, barbiturates, hallucinogens and methaqualone, for example, had access to the program, which offered out-patient self-detoxification with supportive sessions, or in-patient detoxification when necessary. Individual,

---

[143]"St. Francis Medical Center Department of Psychiatry Position Paper," manuscript, 6/25/87, St. Francis Hospital Archives.

[144]*Community MH/MR Center Bulletin* 1 (January, 1972); David F. Musto, *The American Disease, Origins of Narcotic Control,* (New York: Oxford University Press, 1987), p. 259; *Mental Health Mental Retardation Center Newsletter* 2 (June 1974).

family and group therapy sessions, under the guidance of a registered nurse or physician, were an essential component of the program. Many of the drug addicts were 'youngsters,' as young as twelve years old. Victims of overdose were seen in the emergency room, and a nurse with special expertise was on call twenty-four hours per day for patients with drug related problems. Not only was this program available to catchment area residents, but to those from other areas as well. Clients were referred from private and CMHC psychiatrists, but could also refer themselves to the program. Other outreach consultation and educational services had been established, and were also available to schools, social agencies and interested organizations.[145]

Dr. Twerski and the administration concluded that in spite of the services available, treatment remained inadequate. They recognized that there was a need for intensive treatment after drying out or detoxification where patients could learn new ways of coping with frustration from whatever sources, rather than by escaping into the euphoria of alcohol or drugs. Many patients had relapses in between the in-patient and out-patient phase. Physicians occasionally referred some patients to a facility three hundred miles away in the eastern part of the state. It was decided that a new facility was necessary. No grants were available for a treatment facility, but there was a provision that a federal bureau could underwrite a loan to construct a 'nursing' home for alcoholics. Sister Adele and Dr. Twerski, although they considered their idea to be a 'pipe dream' in light of the financial uncertainties, pursued the project. Pennsylvania would issue a nursing home license only if special equipment was installed and a minimum number of registered nurses were hired. These were not necessary, and only raised the cost. Pennsylvania fully agreed to issue a mental health facility license, but then Washington would not underwrite the loan. Fortunately, Harrisburg created a new entity called an intermediate nursing home without construction or staffing standards. St. Francis was, therefore, able to get their license from the state and a construction loan from the federal government. Additional grants totaling $215,000.00 were received from the R. K. Mellon Foundation, Westinghouse Electric Corporation, Sara Mellon Scaife Foundation, the Diocese of Pittsburgh, U.S. Steel Foundation, Pittsburgh Foundation and the Alcoa Foundation. St. Francis Hospital loaned $200,000.00, which was to be repaid in eight annual payments.[146]

---

[145] "Varied Drug Abuse: Additional Services," *Community MH/MR Center Bulletin* 1 (July 1972); SFGH *Community Mental Health Mental Retardation Center Newsletter* 2 (March 1974).

[146] *Welcome to the Tenth Anniversary of Gateway Rehabilitation Center,* 1/17/82, brochure, St. Francis Hospital Archives; Abraham J. Twerski, Article VII, manuscript, St. Francis Hospital Archives; Additional minutes of the board, August–October 1969.

Gateway Rehabilitation Center, located in Center Township, outside of Aliquippa, opened in January 1972. The original plans called for the new facility to be a "private institution unrelated to but controlled by St. Francis Hospital." The board of directors were all members of the St. Francis board, except for Dr. Twerski and Mrs. Carl Kirschler, whose husband was president of the hospital board. Gateway provided the missing link, then, between detoxification and out-patient clinics. The establishment of the facility allowed two goals to be realized. Continuity of care was provided, and involvement of the family in the recovery process was implemented. Dr. Twerski was the institution's new medical director, and subsequently left his position at St. Francis Hospital.[147] Although Gateway Rehabilitation Center is no longer officially affiliated with St. Francis Hospital, it remains as a legacy of the hospital's initiatives.

Conclusion

During the first four decades of the twentieth century, the Sisters of St. Francis of Millvale established the basis for what has become one of the largest and most influential of the region's psychiatric facilities. The sisters decided very early to remain abreast of prevailing theories and current trends in the field, and to implement the most up-to-date programs. In addition, during this period, the foundation was laid for specific programs which were expanded upon many decades later. The sisters' tradition of innovations is exemplified by the early treatment of substance abuse and venereal disease. Although service was always the first priority, education and research were not neglected.

After World War II, the Sisters of St. Francis expanded the existing services with a greater focus on the wider community, and not just the hospital itself. They made commitments to serve residents of the surrounding communities whose needs were not being met either by St. Francis Hospital or other agencies. Not only were they interested in patients, but they also sought to offer educational experience and training for myriad health care professionals. Importantly, but not surprisingly, the sisters' awareness of the community was established before the government mandated services because they sensed a profound need for additional forms of psychiatric care.

One of the controversial issues surrounding the debate regarding mental

---

[147] Abraham J. Twerski, Article VII, manuscript, St. Francis Hospital Archives; *Welcome to the Tenth Anniversary of Gateway Rehabilitation Center, 1/17/82*, brochure, St. Francis Hospital Archives.

health policy today is its impact on the community, family and those suffering from psychiatric illnesses. Historians' accounts have focused on the concerns of psychiatrists, other mental health care personnel, theory regarding etiology, new treatment modalities and changes in funding. Mental health policies designed to encourage the deinstitutionalization process were partially due to the stigma associated with those facilities which housed the mentally ill over long periods of time. The literature pays little attention to the chronically ill patient, their needs or the uncertainty regarding how they would benefit from new policies removing them from the institution. The Sisters of St. Francis, cognizant that many individuals needed care which community mental health facilities could not provide, did function as advocates for the chronically mentally ill. The sisters supported the new mental health policies, indeed perceiving the great service which they could provide, but they did not overlook those whose needs were unmet by those policies. The history of the hospital, therefore, demonstrates an interesting interplay between hospital initiative and government policy.

As a result of government legislation, St. Francis, although still one of the leaders in the field of psychiatry, no longer offers services which are unique to the community, but does continue to serve as a model for other agencies. In 1965, St. Francis Hospital and St. John's hospital, established in 1896 by Protestant deaconesses, were still the only hospitals other than Mayview to offer treatment for alcoholics. Several small facilities for recovering alcoholics existed in low income areas of the city, but they did not provide detoxification services. Although there were several information and referral agencies and out-patient clinics, including Dr. Browne's clinic at Arsenal Health Center, there is no evidence to suggest that any other facility had taken the initiative to treat alcoholics. Only a handful of hospitals, in addition to St. Francis, offered general psychiatric out-patient services, including Allegheny General Hospital, Montefiore Hospital, Shadyside, Western Psychiatric (WPIC), West Penn and the Veterans Administration. In addition, several facilities offered out-patient services to children. Interestingly, the hospitals which offered in-patient treatment were not those that provided out-patient services. Homestead, Suburban, WPIC, Veterans Administration and the state hospitals provided in-patient care. The other Catholic hospitals in the area evidently did not endeavor to provide services for psychiatric patients or addicts at that time. Clearly, St. Francis was one of the few hospitals to offer comprehensive services. Three years later, by 1968, mental health services in the community had expanded somewhat with the addition of several more hospitals offering in-patient and out-patient services. Programs to deal with alcoholism and substance abuse were still limited, although two other hospitals, including Mercy Hospital, had developed services by that time. St. Francis Hospital had remained a leader in the field of chemical abuse.[148]

By 1971, because of government mandates and county and state funding, comprehensive services were offered throughout the county, diminishing St. Francis Hospital's role as the only provider of extensive psychiatric care. Significantly, this relieved the problem of over crowding within the facility, partially alleviating the tension between administration, medical staff and other institutions. The most important change during this short period is the widespread development of chemical abuse programs which demonstrates recognition of, and response to, a problem which the sisters of St. Francis had been aware of for a century.[149]

Throughout the twentieth century, the sisters struggled with a conflicting set of goals and objectives in the psychiatric area. They were adamant that the hospital provide care to any individual in need of medical or psychiatric services, and they had a very broad definition of the hospital's purpose. It is because of the sisters' mission to serve the afflicted that St. Francis Hospital developed programs in substance abuse long before other institutions would handle such concerns. Spiritual beliefs also encouraged the sisters to maintain the tradition of simply providing care, even when treatment was impossible. However, conflict arose when the psychiatric department became overcrowded and was incapable of providing adequate services, reflecting the tension between maintaining a modern psychiatric facility and meeting the administration's spiritual goals. Because the sisters never relinquished their authority, however, they did indeed continue in their mission to serve the neglected, fulfilling needs which otherwise would have been unmet. As the century comes to a close, the hospital's psychiatric division stands as a major psychiatric facility, having been built on a long established foundation; and the sisters' goal of healing the body, mind, and spirit continues.

[148]*Pittsburgh's Fortresses of Health, 200 Years of Hospital Progress, 1758–1958*, 1959, brochure, p. 15; *Directory of Health and Welfare Services in Allegheny County* (Pittsburgh: Health and Welfare Association of Allegheny County, 1965 and 1968).

[149]*Where to Turn, Directory of Health and Welfare and Community Services for Residents of Allegheny County*, (Pittsburgh: Information and Volunteer Services of Allegheny County, 1971).

Chapter Five

Community Service

Hospitals clearly are institutions designed to offer the highest standards of care within the framework of medical technology, but historically, they also have been perceived as institutions providing for the social welfare of the community. This has often resulted in struggles for the individual hospitals, communities, medical schools and third party payment providers. St. Francis, like many other hospitals, has offered the best in medical care while maintaining its concern for the community welfare. The Sisters of St. Francis Hospital set their priorities from the outset, and have not altered their course. Their efforts to develop modern, new equipment and facilities attests to the fact that they have successfully competed with the most up-to-date institutions. However, St. Francis has differed from many other hospitals in its unusual emphasis on service. Its leaders have never criticized the focus of other facilities, for they have always recognized the need for research and extensive education, but because of their intent to meet spiritual needs, the sisters directed their hospital to address social and community problems in greater depth than many other hospitals. This commitment to the community seems typical of religious institutions, but St. Francis may have carried it out with particular fervor.

St. Francis Hospital's commitment to the community manifested itself in several ways. The establishment of a social service department, discussed previously, and several educational programs exemplified the sisters' goal to reach out beyond the hospital plant as many institutions attempted to do. The establishment of nurse training schools, internships and residencies in hospitals was standard procedure for many health care facilities during the early twentieth century. What is interesting, however, is the sisters' attitudes regarding education. Not only were they augmenting their staff, but by training nurses and doctors, they provided educated personnel for other hospitals as well, extending their influence well beyond St. Francis Hospital.

The sisters' commitment to the community expanded a great deal in the latter half of the century, reflecting and building upon a trend that was established when the sisters first opened their doors in the nineteenth century. The sisters always welcomed neighbors, offering advice, friendship and hospitality, and never neglected to respond to a crisis or tragedy in the community, offering emergency medical services whenever called upon. The notable change during the post World War II era, however, was the sisters' efforts to seek out the residents of the community in order to understand and respond to their needs. It was the extent of the larger community commitment on the part of the sisters that was particularly unusual.

Education

Characteristic of the entire pre-World War II period was the development of educational programs designed to increase the expertise of nurses, physicians and other personnel, providing educational experience for citizens of the community. The sisters, while adamant that they be adequately prepared to perform their duties, also provided educational experiences for others in order that the hospital continue to be progressive. This, too, reflects the fulfillment of the mission of the sisters to extend care to the community. Not only did they provide care directly to individuals in their own hospital, but they educated physicians and nurses who left St. Francis and went on to provide care in other institutions, thus carrying the mission of the hospital much further. Sister Adele recalled how it bothered her at first when she realized that many of the St. Francis nurses and physicians were leaving the hospital to practice elsewhere. She was especially disturbed when she was aware that many of the psychiatric nurses left to work at the university. They held higher positions there than they could ever attain at St. Francis because the administrative positions were always held by sisters. Her distress, however, turned to pride when she realized how well educated and prepared they were. As she noted, the Lord said, "Go ye therefore, and teach all nations."[1]

The hospital's major educational focus was on the development of nurses and physicians for obvious reasons, but very early the sisters developed educational programs for other employees as well. In 1917, a vocational school

---

[1] Interview with Sister M. Adele Meiser, 1993, quote from Matthew 28:19.

for disabled veterans was established, but little is known of this project. At the same time, an occupational school within the psychiatric department was also developed.[2]

Other educational programs were also implemented at the hospital in the years following World War II in order to provide qualified personnel capable of functioning in the expanding medical technological environment. In the fall of 1953, for example, a school for X-ray technicians was opened,[3] and in the mid-50's, the hospital participated in a program for foreign students in hospital administration.[4]

Not only was the administration interested in providing educational experience for their employees, but they also attended various meetings and seminars as participants and as educators in the field. Sister Adele recalled a fire prevention seminar for hospital administrators which she attended in Milwaukee. She was to be a member of a panel discussion, but when she arrived at the auditorium, her name did not appear on the program and she was told not to participate. The fire department members, experts in the field, were unable to comprehend that the sister knew anything about fire safety. Sister Adele sat herself on the stage uninvited, knowing the host would be forced to introduce her, and when he did, it was by saying, "she doesn't know anything about it." It was to Sister's credit that she was merely amused, not angry or frustrated. After she presented her paper, other participants commented in surprise that "she does know something." The men insisted that she have lunch with them and made her an honorary member of the Milwaukee fire department. They noted, "that little sister knows how to handle herself." It is worth mentioning that Sister's topic differed somewhat from all of the others because she was the only one to discuss 'prevention.' This anecdote serves to emphasize the administrators' interest in remaining current as well as their assertive nature which served them well in the face of adversity.[5]

St. Francis Hospital functioned as a teaching facility for physicians for many years. The sisters were adamant in their belief that the hospital and its patients would benefit by being associated with a medical school. Sister M. Thomasine Diemer, OSF, noted that "medical school affiliation is of considerable importance to a hospital as it relates to the staff, since the latter as professors or instructors in their respective branches must keep pace with modern methods and modern literature. A teaching staff entails a better and more progressive type of men, and invites a more ready association with them

[2]History, n.d. but c. 1965–1980, manuscript in the Lawrenceville branch of the Carnegie Library.
[3]*St. Francis,* (Autumn 1953).
[4]Minutes, Board of Managers, 4/26/54, reference to letter from Surgeon General Dr. Leonard A Scheele.
[5]Interview with Sister M. Adele Meiser, 1993.

of the ambitious younger men. Furthermore, the teaching hospital must not lag behind in progress. All the new diagnostic methods and treatment must be supplied if the students are to receive good medical training. The training school profits also by association with a medical school."[6]

Although the University of Pittsburgh School of Medicine had been sending medical students to St. Francis Hospital for several years, at least since 1910, when seniors in the medical school began training at St. Francis, by 1912, a formal alliance was forged. The university had the power to nominate the members of the medical staff of the hospital and its dispensary. The university's associate professors of surgery and gynecology became heads of those departments in the hospital, and they had access to all medical cases in the wards and complete control of all teaching except nursing education, although they would assist there if requested. Chancellor McCormick and Dean Arbuthnot chose to affiliate only with St. Francis and Mercy hospitals.[7] Although the hospital board and administration were pleased to be affiliated with the University of Pittsburgh, they were very careful to preserve their authority and autonomy in the arrangement. As far as the hospital was concerned, there was no financial obligation, and the board of managers had the power to veto any staff nominations of which they disapproved. The affiliation was not to interfere with the "individuality of the hospital; nor make any change whatever in the character of the altruistic or charitable work which the hospital is now doing or may desire to do in the future, and that it shall not interfere with the hospital administration, the board of managers of the hospital remaining in absolute control thereof." The agreement took effect September 1, 1912, and was to continue indefinitely unless either party terminated the agreement on July first of any year with six months notice before that date. In 1927, of the sixty-one doctors on staff, nearly every one was a member of the medical school faculty of the University of Pittsburgh.[8]

St. Francis also accepted interns and residents early in its history. By the

---

[6]Sister M. Thomasine Diemer, "The Material Welfare of the Hospital," manuscript, 1923, St. Francis Hospital Archives.

[7]Barbara I. Paull, *A Century of Medical Excellence, The History of the University of Pittsburgh School of Medicine*, (Pittsburgh: University of Pittsburgh Medical Alumni Association, 1986), p. 66.; Ruth C. Maszkiewicz, *The Presbyterian Hospital of Pittsburgh*, (Pittsburgh: Presbyterian-University Hospital, 1977), p. 48.

[8]Letter from the University of Pittsburgh to Sister M. Baptiste, August 8, 1912, which included copy of affiliation agreement between the School of Medicine and St. Francis Hospital; *Weighing the Evidence*, 1927 building campaign brochure, St. Francis Hospital Archives; *Uniting the Armies of Health and Industry*, published for Industrial Pittsburgh by St. Francis Hospital, c. 1927, St. Francis Hospital Archives; Sister M. Adele Meiser, "Care of the Mentally Ill in the General Hospital," *Hospitals* (September 1951); *Report of the St. Francis Hospital*, 1911 and June 1, 1921 to May 31, 1923; Barbara I. Paull, *A Century of Medical Excellence, The History of the University of Pittsburgh School of Medicine*, (Pittsburgh: University of Pittsburgh Medical Alumni Association, 1986), p. 66.

1920s, it had a well established internship program, which had a widespread excellent reputation. The number of interns had increased yearly since 1900, when there were five. There were eight in 1910, nine in 1916 and by 1921, there were fifteen interns. At least 148 students from nineteen different states sought one of the sixteen internships available at St. Francis in the twenties. The hospital had also decided, long before the existence of specialty boards, that approved residency programs would be provided. In 1911, residents were hired in the pathology, surgical and psychiatric departments. By 1923, a resident bacteriologist, resident cardiographer, resident dentist and two resident gynecologists were also working in the hospital. Two individuals known only as resident physicians were also hired, probably for the department of medicine.[9] By 1936, approved internship and residency programs were firmly established. The American Medical Association approved fourteen rotating internships, two psychiatric residencies, three pathology residencies, one medicine residency, one surgery residency, one cardiology residency and one residency program in obstetrics and gynecology.[10] The sisters were proud of the interns' and residents' achievements after they had finished their training, expressing gratitude to them for "the splendid spirit of cooperation shown during their internship and also for their continued evidence of loyalty and interest."[11]

The physicians and the sisters had established a good rapport very early in the history of the hospital. One of Sister Adele's favorite stories reflects the nature of those relationships. In the 1920s, Sister M. Basil Burns, OSF, was in charge of the doctor's quarters. Sister Basil owned a pet parrot of which she was very fond. When the hospital was having a fund-raising bazaar one year, the physicians raffled off her cherished bird. Not surprisingly, the highest bidder was Dr. J. Huber Wagner, who promptly returned the parrot to Sister Basil after having a few good laughs. There have been other stories, too. Sister Adele recalled that the medical students, who often enjoyed chatting with her, frequently requested that she pray for the University of Pittsburgh football team. She willingly obliged, especially since she considered it to be such a dangerous sport. The fact that these stories were passed on throughout

[9]*Weighing the Evidence*, 1927 building campaign brochure, St. Francis Hospital Archives; *Uniting the Armies of Health and Industry*, published for Industrial Pittsburgh by St. Francis Hospital, c. 1927, St. Francis Hospital Archives; Sister M. Adele Meiser, "Care of the Mentally Ill in the General Hospital," Hospitals (September 1951); *Report of the St. Francis Hospital*, 1911 and June 1, 1921 to May 31, 1923; Barbara I. Paull, A Century of Medical Excellence, The History of the University of Pittsburgh School of Medicine, (Pittsburgh: University of Pittsburgh Medical Alumni Association, 1986), p. 66; Report of the St. Francis Hospital, June 1, 1921 to May 31, 1923, pp. 5, 7, 93.

[10]Letter from the American Medical Association to St. Thomasine, January 6, 1936, St. Francis Hospital Archives.

[11]*Report of the St. Francis Hospital*, June 1, 1921 to May 31, 1923, pp. 5, 7, 93.

the years is testament to the favorable on-going relationships between the sisters and medical staff.[12]

Duties of residents and interns and the organization of physicians varied depending on the department. The department of medicine, one of the largest departments, serves as a good example of the organization of physicians in a teaching facility in the twenties. The department was divided into four services, each under the direction of a Staff physician. An associate physician and one or more assistant physicians worked with him. A resident physician was responsible for the direct care of all medical patients and supervised the work of the interns. When patients were admitted, they were assigned in rotation to one of the four services. All ward patients were available for clinical instruction of medical students, and all staff members were engaged in teaching.[13]

The internship positions offered at St. Francis Hospital were known as rotating internships, meaning that the physician would rotate through a variety of services. In 1936, the hospital's goal was to provide one intern for every twenty-five patients. The duration of the internship was twelve months, during which time the intern rotated through fourteen different services of approximately twenty-five days each. Two of those services, Medicine I and II, offered experience in internal medicine, pediatrics, dermatology and oncology. Another service required the intern to spend time at the Municipal Hospital for Contagious Diseases, which was operated by the city. Four different surgery services provided the intern with experience in emergency treatment, out-patient care, genito-urinary diseases, orthopedics, proctology, plastic surgery, ophthalmology and ear, nose and throat disorders. The intern also participated in three separate laboratory rotations. The obstetrics, anesthesia and gynecology services provided him with experience in those areas. The fourteenth service required that the intern serve the entire hospital during the night.[14] The program for interns did not remain exactly the same throughout the years, changing in response to hospital or community needs. For example, during World War II, in order to compensate for the shortage of physicians, who were desperately needed in the military, the internships were temporarily shortened from twelve months to nine, relieving new physicians for active duty, but also taking them away from the hospital.[15] The various residency and internship training programs, as

[12] Sister M. Adele Meiser, manuscript, St. Francis Hospital Archives; Interview with Sister M. Adele Meiser, 1993.

[13] Report of the St. Francis Hospital, June 1, 1921 to May 31, 1923, p. 17.

[14] Letter from the American Medical Association, William D. Cutter, to Sister M. Thomasine, January 6, 1936, St. Francis Hospital Archives.

well as the affiliation with the University of Pittsburgh School of Medicine, changed over the years, but clearly the hospital administration was dedicated to the education of physicians very early in the institution's development.

Although the administration of the hospital was clearly committed to providing educational programs for physicians, recognizing the importance of serving as a teaching hospital, they were unable to maintain that goal in the fullest sense without sacrificing their autonomy. The University of Pittsburgh School of Medicine, in fact, bemoaned the fact that it was unable to convince their affiliated hospitals to become true teaching institutions during the first two decades of the century. In the early 1920s, when the medical school began to search for a general hospital willing to relocate to Oakland and become the central facility of a new medical center, St. Francis Hospital, as well as several other Pittsburgh hospitals were "too powerful and too independent to cede authority to the university." The St. Francis administration, a decade earlier, had been very careful to maintain their autonomy when affiliating with the university. The university did formalize a relationship with the Presbyterian Hospital, which became a member of the proposed medical center in 1927. After Presbyterian relocated and opened its doors in Oakland, St. Francis clearly was forced into downplaying their role in educating medical students. It is important to note that the university and hospital continued to collaborate in teaching medical students for decades, but with the establishment of the medical center, St. Francis could no longer play a central role.[16]

St. Francis Hospital's dedication to the education of physicians was more typical of Catholic hospitals of the period than of other institutions, but teaching hospitals were clearly the exception. By 1930, only 4.6 percent of the hospitals in the nation were designated as 'teaching hospitals', as they were either affiliated with, or integrated into the life of a medical school as a university hospital. More significant, however, is the fact that of the 641 Catholic hospitals, fifty-four, or 8.4 percent were teaching institutions. That number represented a full 17 percent of all of the teaching hospitals in the country. In the list of hospitals approved for internships by the Council on Medical Education and Hospitals of the American Medical Association, 26 percent of all hospitals approved were Catholic institutions. This is astound-

[15]Sister M. Adele Meiser, "Points for 'On Location' TV Interview," n.d. but c. 1986, St. Francis Hospital Archives.

[16]Kenneth M. Ludmerer, *Learning to Heal, The Development of American Medical Education*, (New York: Basic Books, Inc., 1985), pp. 159–160; Barbara I. Paull, *A Century of Medical Excellence, The History of the University of Pittsburgh School of Medicine*, (Pittsburgh: University of Pittsburgh Medical Alumni Association, 1986), p. 127.

ing when recalling that Catholic hospitals constituted only 9.4 percent of all of the hospitals in the country by 1930. Of all of the internship positions offered in 1928 (5,148), Catholic hospitals provided 19.7 percent of the total. St. Francis, however, was once again the exception within the Catholic pattern in that of all of the Catholic hospitals, only 25.1 percent were approved for internship.[17]

Although Catholic hospitals were not leaders in providing residency programs as they were in providing internships, St. Francis stands out as an outstanding example of the teaching institutions in the United States at the end of the 1920s. The Council on Medical Education and Hospitals of the American Medical Association only approved 294 hospitals, or 4.3 percent, of all hospitals for residencies in the specialties. Only sixteen Catholic hospitals were approved, representing 5.0 percent of the total number of hospitals approved, or 2.5 percent of the total number of Catholic hospitals. At that time, St. Francis and Charity Hospital in New Orleans ranked as the two hospitals offering the highest number of residency positions among Catholic hospitals. Although each offered ten positions, Charity Hospital offered those positions in only five specialties, whereas St. Francis had eight approved residency programs: gynecology, obstetrics, medicine, neuropsychiatry, pathology, radiology, surgery and cardiography. They were the only Catholic hospital in Pittsburgh to have been approved by the AMA for residency specialty programs.[18]

St. Francis Hospital continued to offer numerous residency programs for graduate physicians throughout the years. Generally, they favored their own interns, but they recognized the need for interns from other institutions as well. By 1955, the hospital provided residencies in internal medicine, cardiovascular disease, psychiatry and neurology, general surgery, orthopedic surgery, obstetrics, gynecology, neurosurgery, pathology, radiology, anesthesia and dentistry. Clearly, physicians who trained at St. Francis were pleased with their experiences, for a great many of them remained. In 1955, thirty-nine percent of the physicians on staff had interned and done their residency there. St. Francis, however, also recognized the influence of those who trained elsewhere, for in the same year, twenty-nine percent of staff physicians received their internship training at other institutions.[19]

[17]Alphonse M. Schwitalla, S.J., and M. R. Kneifl, "A Survey of the Catholic Hospitals of the United States and Canada," Hospital Progress (March 1930), pp. 112, 113.
[18]Alphonse M. Schwitalla, S.J., and M. R. Kneifl, "A Survey of the Catholic Hospitals of the United States and Canada," Hospital Progress (March 1930), p. 112.
[19]"1955 Statistics and Information Pertaining to Medical Staff," St. Francis Hospital Archives; Minutes, Board of Managers, 6/7/48.

St. Francis Hospital, unfortunately, did endure periods when attracting interns was difficult, in spite of its reputation. In 1948, the hospital was unable to fill its quota of interns, possibly reflecting a noted shortage of interns nationwide. The medical staff, however, was concerned that the hospital was having difficulty attracting interns because the living quarters were less than adequate, and below the standard of other hospitals in the city. The facilities for interns were poorly lit and lacked adequate telephone equipment. One physician noted that if the hospital "had comparable living quarters, I feel that we could very easily have the pick of the Pitt students, because they fully realize the standard of the work that is done at St. Francis."[20] This reflects the financial struggles which the administrators had to constantly deal with, neglecting the physical plant in order that they might admit and cover the costs of caring for the indigent. St. Francis also had to compete with attractive internships being offered by the Army and Navy, as well as smaller hospitals which paid salaries. The staff at St. Francis disapproved of the recommendation that the interns be paid in order to compete, but by 1950, the board resolved to pay interns fifty dollars per month in order to attract more of them.[21]

St. Francis Hospital was not the only hospital to have a problem finding enough interns to fill its positions. Mercy Hospital also had difficulties finding interns during the same time period due to a national shortage. They, too, noted that other area hospitals were filling their quota because they paid salaries to their interns, or provided living quarters for married interns.[22]

St. Francis Hospital never discriminated against internship and residency applicants based on gender. Dr. Margaret Mary Nicholson, who interned at St. Francis in 1926, was given the Award of Merit of George Washington University School of Medicine Medical Society in 1953. She was the first woman to receive the award for outstanding scientific accomplishment, academic attainment and service to the society and the community.[23] She was an example of Sister Adele's philosophy that teaching physicians to serve elsewhere was fulfilling their mission.

Not only did the hospital teach new graduates from medical school, but they also provided for continuing education of their medical staff and alumni.

[20]Minutes, Board of Managers, 3/21/45, reference to letter from Dr. Glenn H. Davison to the board.

[21]Minutes, Board of Managers, 6/14/48, Report of Intern committee; Minutes, Medical staff, 5/9/49; Minutes, Board of Managers, 3/13/50.

[22]*Pillar of Pittsburgh, The History of Mercy Hospital and The City It Serves*, (Pittsburgh: McCullough communications, 1990), pp. 121–122.

[23]*St. Francis*, Spring–Summer 1953.

St. Francis Hospital Day was a tradition established prior to the 1950s as a day set apart every April for medical alumni to attend clinics, exhibits, demonstrations and lectures. Supervised by the medical staff, the mornings were filled with surgical clinics, clinics in industrial surgery, anesthesia demonstrations, X-ray exhibits and clinicopathological conferences. Demonstrations continued into the afternoon with the presentation of scientific papers. The attendance totaled several hundred every year.[24]

Within the various departments, St. Francis Hospital administrators and physicians also strove to provide for continuing education. The Tumor Clinic was established partially to allow for increased understanding on the part of physicians. In the year ending May 31, 1948, forty-three meetings were held with an average of ten physicians present at any one meeting. Patients were examined, discussed and treatment was recommended. During that year, eighty-one new patients and fifty-three old patients were seen.[25] Also in 1948, after a year of planning, the Research and Publication Committee was established. The hospital held monthly clinical-pathological meetings. Each month, assignments were made to different groups. The staff physician, with the help of residents, provided a presentation. Following the meeting, the sisters served dinner for the doctors, reflecting the ongoing rapport and collaboration established between the sisters and physicians.[26]

Nursing

The sisters recognized at the turn of the century that it was imperative to have trained, educated nurses to care for the patients within the hospital. Aware also of the need to enhance their nursing staff, the sisters established a nurse training school in the spring of 1901. Interestingly, of the approximately 393 nursing schools in the United States in the early 1900s, fifty-nine, or 15 percent, were owned and operated by women religious.[27] One third of the Catholic schools of nursing which existed by 1930 in the United States had been established during the decade 1900 to 1909, also the period during

---

[24] _Hospital Progress_, October 1954.

[25] Minutes, Board of Managers, 6/14/48, Tumor clinic report.

[26] Minutes, Board of Managers, 6/7/48.

[27] Mary Carol Conroy, SCL, "The Transition Years," in _Pioneer Healers: The History of Women Religious in American Health Care_ eds. Ursula Stepsis, CSA, and Dolores Liptak, RSM, (New York: Crossroad Publishing Co., 1989), p. 148.

which the greatest increase in the number of the Catholic hospitals took place.[28]

The St. Francis Hospital Nurse Training School held their first commencement exercises on May 3, 1904, for fourteen nurses, seven lay women and seven sisters.[29] Nursing students at that time were housed on the fourth floor of the Sisters' residence.[30] Within the first nine years of the school's existence, there were forty-nine graduates, thirty-one of whom were lay nurses.[31] According to historian, Mary Carol Conroy, SCL, admission to most nursing schools which were established at the turn of the century was limited to members of the respective religious congregations. St. Francis, once again,

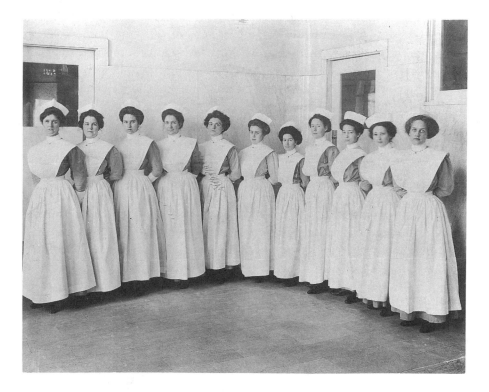

Nurses' Training School Graduating Class, 1913

[28] Alphonse M. Schwitalla, S.J., and M. R. Kneifl, "A Survey of the Catholic Hospitals of the United States and Canada," *Hospital Progress* (March 1930), p. 126.

[29] Sister M. Clarissa Popp, *History of the Sisters of St. Francis of the Diocese of Pittsburgh, 1868–1938,* (Millvale: Sisters of St. Francis, 1939), p. 138; "St. Francis Hospital," manuscript, c. 1940, St. Francis Hospital Archives, p. 10.

[30] Sister Mary Bertin Paulus, *Seventy-Fifth Anniversary 1901–1976,* (Pittsburgh: St. Francis General) Hospital, 1976), p. 8.

[31] *Report of the St. Francis Hospital,* 1911, p. 9.

displayed their practical approach to problems, regardless of the trends within Catholic schools at the time.[32]

The three year program, in 1911, under the direction of Edna R. Sparey, R.N., included numerous lectures given primarily by physicians. It was customary at that time for members of the medical staff to give most of the lectures, whereas the superintendent of nurses provided demonstrations of actual nursing practice and hospital housekeeping.[33] The juniors, or first year students, studied elementary nursing, anatomy and physiology, dietetics, bandaging, materia medica, bacteriology, surgery, urinalysis, hygiene and nursing ethics. The intermediates studied obstetrics, gynecology, infectious disease, medical nursing, general surgery, massage and Swedish movements and surgical technique in their second year. Seniors studied pediatrics, psychiatry, nursing of the insane, orthopedics and diseases of the skin, ear, eye, nose, and throat. If they passed their examinations and behaved satisfactorily, they received their diploma.[34] In the 1920s, curriculum was planned in accordance with the syllabus of the American Nursing Association, and included practice and theory in all branches of medicine, occupational therapy and physiotherapy.[35] The curriculum changed as necessary over the years in order to remain current. One of the major changes, however, was to condense the three year program into two years. In 1966, the School of Nursing admitted their first class under a new two-year curriculum.[36]

It is important to note that the student nurses were a major part of the hospital's nursing staff. In 1910, of the forty-two nurses on staff, twenty-six were students. The staff grew considerably, and in the following year, there were sixty-two staff nurses, which included forty-four student nurses.[37] Hospitals simply could not afford to hire their staff and, as a result, depended upon students to provide care. It was not unusual for graduate nurses to function only in a supervisory capacity. The following chart illustrates that St. Francis, then, serves as an example of how hospitals were staffed at the time.[38]

[32] Mary Carol Conroy, SCL, "The Transition Years," in *Pioneer Healers: The History of 'Women Religious in American Health Care*, eds. Ursula Stepsis, CSA, and Dolores Liptak, RSM, (New York: Crossroad Publishing Co., 1989), p. 148.

[33] Ann Doyle, R.N., "Nursing by Religious Orders in the United States," *American Journal of Nursing* 29 (September 1929), p. 1088.

[34] *Report of the St. Francis Hospital*, 1911, pp. 9–10.

[35] *Report of the St. Francis Hospital*, June 1, 1921–May 31, 1923.

[36] Sister Mary Bertin Paulus, *Seventy-Fifth Anniversary 1901–1976*, (Pittsburgh: St. Francis General Hospital, 1976), p. 9.

[37] *Report of the St. Francis Hospital*, 1911, pp. 9–10.

[38] *Report of the St. Francis Hospital*, June 1, 1921–May 31, 1923, pp. 7, 49–50.

Nursing Staff—1923[39]

superintendent of nurses	1
asst. superintendent of nurses	1
instructor (full time)	1
night supervisors	2
graduate head nurses—lay	9
graduate head nurses—sisters	24
student nurses	130
affiliate student nurses	15
probationers	34

By 1923, the nursing school had expanded. Applicants for either the March or September class were required to have completed high school, and "must give evidence of a fine spirit for the work, and produce sufficient recommendations to establish fitness in health and character." They were to be between the ages of eighteen and thirty-five. Requiring students to have completed high school was typical of Catholic schools, but the nation's non-Catholic nursing schools did not adhere to such strict admission policies. Of the 429 nursing schools connected with Catholic hospitals in 1928, 54.1 percent required four years of high school for admission. However, of the 1,827 schools listed by the American Nurses' Association in "A List of Schools of Nursing Accredited by the State Board of Nurse Examiners, 1928," only 28.8 percent of the schools enforced the four-year entrance requirement.[40]

As early as 1921, nursing students from other schools spent time at St. Francis in order to study fields not offered at their home schools. The affiliates from the Elizabeth Steel Magee Hospital in Pittsburgh, the New Castle Hospital, Mercy Hospital in DuBois and the Pittsburgh City Hospital in Mayview, studied medical nursing, operating room nursing, pediatrics, dietetics, psychiatry and physiotherapy.[41] A special three-month course in psychiatry was begun in April of 1936 for students affiliated with other schools, including St. John's, Mercy, Ohio Valley, Latrobe, New Castle, St. Joseph's of Reading,

[39]*Report of the St. Francis Hospital,* June 1, 1921–May 31, 1923, p. 49.

[40]*Report of the St. Francis Hospital,* June 1, 1921–May 31, 1923, pp. 49–50; Alphonse M. Schwitalla, S.J., and M. R. Kneifl, "A Survey of the Catholic Hospitals of the United States and Canada," *Hospital Progress* (March 1930), p. 129.

[41]*Report of the St. Francis Hospital,* June 1, 1921–May 31, 1923, pp. 49–50; Sister Mary Bertin Paulus, *Seventy-Fifth Anniversary 1901–1976,* (Pittsburgh: St. Francis General Hospital, 1976), p. 8.

and the Pennsylvania Hospital.[42] By 1953, nineteen other schools sent their nursing students to St. Francis to study psychiatry.[43]

The sisters directing the School of Nursing were also well aware that they were not always able to provide for their own students' educational needs. In 1944, they established affiliation with the University of Pittsburgh for nurse experience in communicable disease at Municipal Hospital. Seven years later, they affiliated with the Veterans Administration for students' experience in tuberculosis nursing at the Deshon Hospital in Butler.[44]

The sisters were not only concerned about their students' educational needs, but their recreational and spiritual ones as well. Social activities were organized for the nursing students. In the 1930s, for example, the students participated in a small orchestra, choral singing, dramatics, dancing, singing, sewing, cards, swimming, story telling, reading, tennis, mush-ball, basketball and weekly 'moving pictures.'[45] The administration also carefully planned for the spiritual development of the student nurses, as well as their educational training. In 1916, they held the first retreat for the nurses at the hospital. The retreats were held annually until 1928, when they were held at Mt. Alvernia. "Rest, quiet and spiritual inspiration were here assured to all."[46]

Not only did the sisters take the religious needs of their nurses into account, but, not surprisingly, the spiritual needs of patients were incorporated into every aspect of the curriculum in the school. St. Francis of Assisi, the Patron Saint of the Sisters of St. Francis of Millvale, led a life of humility and self-denial, a life based on the Beatitudes, which are the "blueprint for the Christian way of life. At St. Francis General Hospital School of Nursing, his spirit has been perpetuated in the philosophy of the education of nurses and in their administration of health care."[47] During the transitional period of nursing education, after World War II, as many schools adapted to changes in medical technology by expanding and specializing curriculum, and as nursing education entered into the educational mainstream, the philosophy and objectives of Catholic-sponsored nursing schools lost some of their religious significance. By the 1980s, the educational and professional practice of nurs-

[42]Minutes, Board of Managers, 12/13/37.

[43]Sister Mary Bertin Paulus, Seventy-Fifth Anniversary 1901–1976, (Pittsburgh: St. Francis General Hospital, 1976), p. 8.

[44]Sister Mary Bertin Paulus, Seventy-Fifth Anniversary 1901–1976, (Pittsburgh: St. Francis General Hospital, 1976), p. 9.

[45]Minutes, Board of Managers, 12/14/37.

[46]Popp, p. 140.

[47]Sister Mary Bertin Paulus, Seventy-Fifth Anniversary 1901–1976, (Pittsburgh: St. Francis General Hospital, 1976), p. 2.

ing had assumed a much more secular and scientific base.[48] The Sisters of St. Francis Hospital, however, clearly adapted to these changes in medicine without relinquishing their belief that religious foundations were necessary to the development of fundamental nursing skills.

Although the Sisters of St. Francis clearly believed that members of their own religious congregation should be in positions of authority, this belief did not take precedence over the practical realization that it was imperative that those in charge of various departments be adequately prepared to meet the required tasks. It is probably for this reason that throughout the school's early years, several of the directors of nursing or school superintendents were lay women. In fact, the first director, Catherine Hickey, held that position for the first four years when another lay woman, Ellen Mullet, took her place for another year. Sister M. Cadsilda Rueve, OSF, was the first sister director but served only for one year. Four different lay superintendents directed the school from 1907 until 1912, when Sister M. Laurentine Harrington, OSF, held the position. Since that time, the school has primarily been under the direction of one of the Sisters of St. Francis. It was not unusual for many of the early sisters' training schools to be conducted by lay superintendents, reflecting the belief on the part of many congregations that prepared leadership was essential in order to provide nursing students with the best in education in order to prepare them to function in the changing medical system.[49] Sister nurse educators, in fact, advocated the utilization of lay superintendents whenever necessary, and promoted their views in national publications. Sister Immaculata of New York noted in 1925 in the official organ of the Catholic Hospital Association, *Hospital Progress*, that "unless the Sister supervisor has a thorough professional knowledge of what she proposes to teach, it will be utterly impossible for her to fulfill the obligations of her position.... When we undertake to meet our obligations in this respect [training school], it is absolutely essential that we comply with the requirements outlined by the educational department of the state in which the school is located."[50]

Throughout its history, the school readily received any necessary accreditation, and in addition, graduated women competent to pass any necessary

[48]Mary Carol Conroy, SCL, "The Transition Years," in *Pioneer Healers: The History of Women Religious in American Health Care* eds. Ursula Stepsis, CSA, and Dolores Liptak, RSM, (New York: Crossroad Publishing Co., 1989), pp. 150–151.

[49]Sister Mary Bertin Paulus, *Seventy-Fifth Anniversary 1901–1976* (Pittsburgh: St. Francis General Hospital, 1976), p. 10; Ann Doyle, R.N., "Nursing by Religious Orders in the United States," *American Journal of Nursing* 29 (September 1929), p. 1086.

[50]Ann Doyle, R.N., "Nursing by Religious Orders in the United States," *American Journal of Nursing* 29 (September 1929), pp. 1090–1091.

licensing examination. In 1912, the Pennsylvania State Board of Examiners for Registration of Nurses required graduates to pass an examination in order to be granted an R.N., or registered nurse certification. Prior to this period, graduates merely paid a five dollar fee, and demonstrated proof of graduation from a school in order to become a registered nurse. Records suggest that the early graduates from the St. Francis nursing school were successful in passing the state examination.[51] The school itself was approved by the Pennsylvania State Board of Nurse Examiners in 1918.[52] In 1941, the nursing school was accredited by the National League of Nursing Education, included in the first listing of schools which they accredited.[53] Also at that time, the hospital was able to proudly boast that the nursing school ranked with those schools having no graduates failing the State Boards, whereas the State Board of Nurse Examiners had noted during the same period that there was an increase in the number of graduates failing state boards state-wide.[54]

The Sisters of St. Francis, as noted earlier, valued education, and strove to remain current as they developed every aspect of their hospital, including the nurse training school. Sister M. Laurentine favored on-going education for both doctors and nurses, and membership in national associations. Sister Adele gave her much credit for emphasizing the value of education in the early years of the century. In 1934, Sister M.Laurentine, then Director of the School of Nursing, served on the State Committee, and won recognition state-wide for her work in insuring that nurses work only eight-hour days. She also served as a member and chairman of the Pennsylvania State Board of Nurse Examiners from 1936 until 1942. Sister Adele remembered that she always attended the Catholic Hospital Association meetings herself, often being quite outspoken there. Apparently, she was not always fond of the priest who presided over the meetings, who referred to the CHA members as "poor little sisters."[55] Sister Mary John Evans, who directed the school from 1935 until 1946, was appointed a member of the Accrediting Committee, National League of Nursing Education in 1939. The Director of Nursing Education in 1956 was appointed to the same position. Other faculty members served on an assortment of local and district committees. Students also were involved

[51]Sister Mary Bertin Paulus, *Seventy-Fifth Anniversary 1901–1976*, (Pittsburgh: St. Francis General Hospital, 1976), p. 8.

[52]Sister M. Adele Meiser, manuscript, history of St. Francis Hospital, paper given at Lawrenceville Historical meeting, June 1985, St. Francis Hospital Archives; "Manpower Training Program," manuscript, c. 1968, St. Francis Hospital Archives.

[53]Sister M. Adele Meiser, manuscript, history of St. Francis Hospital, paper given at Lawrenceville Historical meeting, June 1985, St. Francis Hospital Archives.

[54]Minutes, Medical Staff, 6/4/45.

[55]Interview with Sister M. Adele Meiser, 1993.

with state and national nursing organizations, representing the school at state and national conventions throughout the school's history.[56]

The St. Francis Hospital Nurse Training School serves as a good example of other nurse training schools of the period. During the late nineteenth and early twentieth centuries, since hospitals relied primarily on student nurses to staff their facilities, graduate nurses worked as nursing school or hospital superintendents. Until the 1930s, many graduates worked as private duty nurses or in the area of public health. Hospitals were unable to afford a full-time staff of graduate nurses. St. Francis' admission and graduation requirements were similar to those of other schools as well. The essential element which differentiated the trained nurse from her untrained predecessors, with the exception of the sisters, was her character. The trained nurse was to have all of the attributes that defined the gentlewoman of middle and upper class America. Acceptance to a school was often dependent upon a woman's class, upbringing, education, health and character. Age requirements generally were similar to those at St. Francis, as it was generally thought that training was too difficult for an older women, for she would be too set in her ways to be malleable.[57] The St. Francis Nurse Training School not only reflects nursing education in America at that time, but also illustrates the willingness of the sisters to maintain an institution staffed with educated and well-prepared individuals.

St. Francis not only represents other hospital schools of nursing, but also serves to emphasize the role played by schools affiliated with Catholic hospitals. By 1930, only 31.8 percent of the 6,825 hospitals, of all kinds, in the United States had nursing schools. In contrast, 429, or 66.9 percent of the 641 Catholic hospitals, had established schools for nurses' training. In addition, 19.7 percent of all of the schools of nursing in the nation were attached to hospitals under Catholic control. Further, while one of five nursing schools was affiliated with a Catholic hospital, one of every four nursing students was a student in a Catholic institution. In other words, 28.6 percent of all nursing students were enrolled in Catholic controlled nursing schools, as those schools tended to be larger than other schools. Average enrollment in the United States was 35.2 nurses per school, whereas in Catholic nursing schools, the average was 51.7 students per school. This may reflect the fact that hospitals under Catholic control had a greater average bed capacity than either local government hospitals and private hospitals or other church

[56]Sister Mary Bertin Paulus, *Seventy-Fifth Anniversary 1901–1976*, (Pittsburgh: St. Francis General Hospital, 1976), pp. 8–9.

[57]Susan M. Reverby, *Ordered to Care: The Dilemma of American Nursing, 1850–1945*, (Cambridge: Cambridge University Press, 1987), pp. 49–50, 79, 85, 95.

controlled hospitals. Only federal and state hospitals were larger. St. Francis was clearly above average with 165 students enrolled in 1928. Schools with 151 to 200 students represented only 1.8 percent of the Catholic schools of nursing.[58]

Housing accommodations for the students changed over the years to meet the demands of the students, the hospital and national organizations. Soon after the school was opened, a separate residence was purchased in 1906. By the early 1920s, however, the school, under the direction of the superintendent of nurses, Sister M. Claudia Evans OSF, R.N., had grown, and the sisters were cognizant of the need for a new nurses' home. In 1923, the sisters tried in vain to secure additional property adjoining the nurses' cottages so that a new nurses' home could be erected. Without an adequate facility for housing students, they were unable to attract qualified applicants. In addition, they needed more classrooms and 'demonstrating rooms.' They were eventually successful, however, and the new home was dedicated in 1931. The students remained there until 1963, when the facility was renovated to accommodate the department of psychiatry.

The psychiatric patients had been housed in a building which had been erected toward the end of the nineteenth century. It was not fireproof, and the sisters worried endlessly about the patients there. Whenever the sisters in the hospital convent heard the fire trucks' sirens, they became anxious. In the early 1960s, it became imperative that the sisters find new housing for the psychiatric patients and Sister Adele visualized using the nurses' home. The hospital had neither time nor money to erect a new facility. Sister Adele was relieved when the director of nursing was so supportive of the suggestion, noting that it would be difficult to compete with other educational institutions who had begun to condone changes in housing policies, such as the establishment of coeducational dormitories, and other policies which conflicted with the sisters' beliefs. They felt they did not want to be responsible for eighteen year old girls in light of the newer, more liberal views held and practiced by so many young women. In addition, the school no longer had affiliates from other institutions coming for psychiatric experience because by the 1960s, so many other hospitals had established their own psychiatric departments. Utilizing the nurses' residence for the psychiatric department was, therefore, beneficial in more ways than one.[59] Many other hospitals wanted to utilize their nurses' residences for patients, but were forbidden to do so on the grounds that they did not meet required safety standards for patients. St. Francis Hospital, how-

[58] Alphonse M. Schwitalla, S.J., and M. R. Kneifl, "A Survey of the Catholic Hospitals of the United States and Canada," *Hospital Progress* (March 1930), pp. 104, 125, 132, 162.
[59] Interview with Sister M. Adele Meiser, Fall 1993.

ever, did receive permission. Nursing students commuted to the School of Nursing, since housing was no longer provided. Classrooms and offices had been moved to the old psychiatric building, which was deemed safe for any activity but sleeping. In 1974, the School of Nursing was moved to the newly erected medical/parking complex.[60]

World War II created an increased need for hospital personnel to care for wounded soldiers, and the St. Francis nursing school, like many others, participated in the federally sponsored Cadet Nurse Corps.[61] Funded by the federal government, the Cadet Nurse Corps, which was designed in association with the professional associations, offered favorable terms to hospitals and students. The Bolton Act, passed on June 15, 1943, provided that the United States Public Health Service subsidize the entire education of nursing students. Participating hospitals were to have a minimum of fifty patients per day. Students were to have a high school diploma and record of good academic performance. They did not have to prove need of funds, but did have to promise they would engage in essential military or civilian nursing for the duration of the war. Candidates were to be in good health and between the ages of seventeen and thirty-five. In return, they received free training, uniforms, books and a small stipend. Programs were designed as thirty month accelerated programs offering theory and practice. Most students worked an additional six month stint on the ward to meet state requirements for three years of training. Quite often, however, students undertook an important practice assignment in another civilian, military or government institution to meet the requirements.[62]

In order to help the war effort and alleviate their own shortages, the St. Francis Hospital implemented the Cadet Nurse Corps and a school of anesthesia. The Cadet Nurse Corps, under the auspices of the training school, admitted four classes every year instead of just one, following the recommendation of Surgeon General Dr. Thomas Parran, who urged the hospital to take as many Cadet nurses as possible and to increase classes to the limit. Ninety percent of the student nurses at that time had joined the United States Cadet Nurse corps.[63] In 1944, the nurse training school had 261 students, 231 of which were part of the United States Cadet Nurse Corps. The hospital was unable to admit larger classes due to limited housing. The original three-year

[60]Report of the St. Francis Hospital, June 1, 1921–May 31, 1923, pp. 7, 49–50; Sister Mary Bertin Paulus, Seventy-Fifth Anniversary 1901–1976, (Pittsburgh: St. Francis General Hospital, 1976), pp. 8–9.

[61]Minutes, Board of Managers, 12/14/42.

[62]Barbara Melosh, "The Physician's Hand," Work Culture and Conflict in American Nursing, (Philadelphia: Temple University Press, 1982), p. 45; Beatrice J. Kalisch and Philip A. Kalisch, The Advance of American Nursing, (Boston: Little, Brown and Co., 1986), pp. 529–530.

[63]Minutes, Board of Managers, 12/13/43.

program had been condensed into thirty months. The United States Public Health service required that the hospital release 50 percent of those cadets during the last six months for service elsewhere, such as in a government or military hospital.[64] By the fall of 1945, the nursing school ended their Cadet Corps program and resumed the previous program of study. In January 1942, a course in anesthesia was also organized for nurses in order to provide anesthetists for the military, and local hospitals as well. The nurses selected for the course were to "be of good moral character and ethical quality ... pleasant personality, emotional stability and intellectual qualifications." Nurses were not required to pay tuition, as the hospital furnished housing, meals, laundry service for uniforms and also a stipend.[65] The hospital was clearly willing to offer extended services to assist the wider medical community.

During the war, and the years immediately following World War II, many hospitals nationwide experienced a shortage of nurses, and, in addition, those nurses who did remain at the bedside were burdened with tasks previously performed by others. In 1938, most of the bedside care was provided by graduate or student nurses. By 1943, however, nonprofessional personnel had assumed an appreciable part of this burden, reflecting a decline in the quality of care in the nation's hospitals. The shortage of physicians forced nurses to perform duties formerly performed by doctors. In addition, a shortage of auxiliary personnel, such as ward clerks and kitchen maids, compelled the bedside nurse to carry out activities for which these workers had formerly been responsible. Many nurses left hospitals to assist the war effort directly, but many left nursing for better paying war industry jobs. Some left the hospital to join their husbands, who were in military service. Following the war, many women married and joined the "forced exodus of white women to hearth and home."[66] By 1944–1945, the nursing shortage had become an acute problem. A survey conducted by the American Hospital Association noted that beds, wards and operating rooms in 23 percent of the nation's hospitals were not being utilized because of insufficient personnel.[67] Training schools were not receiving enough applicants to fill their quotas. A survey of graduating classes conducted in 1947 showed a 30 percent withdrawal rate of student nurses.[68]

St. Francis, like other institutions, suffered from a shortage of nurses at

[64]Minutes, Medical Staff, 6/6/44.

[65]*Course in Anesthesia for Nurses*, booklet, n.d. but c. late 1940's, St. Francis Hospital Archives.

[66]Susan M. Reverby, *Ordered to Care, The Dilemma of American Nursing, 1850–1945*, (Cambridge: Cambridge University Press, 1987), p. 196; Beatrice J. Kalisch and Philip A. Kalisch, *The Advance of American Nursing*, (Boston: Little, Brown and Co., 1986), pp. 526–527.

[67]Beatrice J. Kalisch and Philip A. Kalisch, *The Advance of American Nursing*, (Boston: Little, Brown and Co., 1986), pp. 534–535; Minutes, Board of Managers, 6/11/45.

[68]Beatrice J. Kalisch and Philip A. Kalisch, *The Advance of American Nursing*, (Boston: Little, Brown and Co., 1986), p. 553.

the beginning of the war, and then shortly thereafter as well. In June of 1946, the hospital bemoaned the fact that they were unable to secure the quota of nursing school applicants.[69] They noted late in 1946 that, although they had a quota of sixty nursing students, they admitted only forty-one and nine of those had dropped out. The board was especially concerned because other local area hospitals were filling their quotas. There was some thought that, perhaps, St. Francis school's regulations were too stringent and out of line with modern youth. In order to combat the nurse shortage, the medical staff, wanting to assist in remedying the situation, gave an annual cash prize to the most efficient nurse in the graduating class with the hope of attracting more applicants to the school.[70] In the 1950s, the board agreed to give nursing scholarships to worthy applicants, refusing to deny admission to anyone because of financial hardships.[71]

In order to deal with the shortage of nurses, the hospital developed new educational programs and created new positions for auxiliary personnel. The sisters endeavored to keep the general duty nurse as close to the patient as possible, allowing her to provide direct patient care and freeing her from other responsibilities, making every effort to assign non-nursing duties to auxiliary help, such as the Red Cross volunteer Nurses Aides.[72] In 1940, the hospital established the Central Supply department, which relieved nurses of the task of sterilizing equipment. A messenger service was later established to provide transportation of patients, drugs and supplies, allowing nurses to remain in their departments. In 1945, the hospital developed a program to train male volunteer aides. The first class of ten men graduated in June of that year. The hospital also began training operating room technicians. The twenty week course, first established by Sister Mary Carmen Puhl, OSF, in 1951, lasted twenty weeks. The first students were those selected from a group of auxiliary workers who were already known to the hospital operating room staff. In addition, ward clerks and nurses aides were hired.[73]

Just as the hospital developed programs to train auxiliary personnel, many hospitals in America developed their own. As a result, new categories of nursing workers were established, such as the practical or vocational nurse or nurses aides.[74] In August 1941, New York Mayor LaGuardia, director of civilian de-

[69]Minutes, Board of Managers, 9/10/45, 6/10/46.

[70]Minutes, Board of Managers, 12/16/46; Minutes, Medical staff, 3/3/47.

[71]Minutes, Board of Managers, 6/24/57.

[72]Minutes, Board of Managers, 12/14/42.

[73]Sister M. Adele Meiser, "Auxiliary Personnel Ease Critical Nurse Shortage," *Hospital Progress* (September 1954); Minutes, Board of Managers, 6/11/45.

[74]Susan M. Reverby, *Ordered to Care, The Dilemma of American Nursing, 1850–1945,* (Cambridge: Cambridge University Press, 1987), p. 196.

fense, invited 800 nursing schools to participate in a nationwide program to augment the nursing services of hospitals, clinics, public health and field nursing agencies. He urged these institutions to cooperate with the American Red Cross and the Office of Civilian Defense in training 100,000 volunteer nurses' aids. During the war, approximately 150,000 volunteer nurses' aides had been trained and had served in wartime hospitals.[75]

Nursing shortages continued occasionally in subsequent years, and the board of managers and the sisters always seemed to find ways to resolve problems. In 1960, the board of managers, concerned because of the scarcity of nurses, thought due to the difficulty in finding housing at reasonable rents, decided to investigate the development of a practical nurse course; and in September of that year, the board resolved to open a practical nursing school.[76] St. Francis' Alvernia School of Practical Nursing was recognized in Great Britain as being representative of American practical nursing schools. It was chosen by the Royal College of Nursing as a site for visitation by Irene Kirkham for three days during her tour of American and Canadian hospitals.[77] St. Francis Hospital was the first general hospital in Pennsylvania to offer professional and practical nursing at the same time.[78]

The Sisters of St. Francis proudly boast that their nurses have influenced health care delivery throughout the world. Sister Adele noted that, "the graduates who today are serving the sick, injured and the needy attest to the influence they and their alumni members have had in other States of the Union, extending as far as Alaska and Hawaii." Graduates of the program, as of 1976, served in every state, including the District of Colombia, except for Arkansas, Nebraska, Vermont and Wyoming. During the war, St. Francis nurses were active in North Africa, Normandy, India, China, Iceland, New Guinea and many other foreign countries. Graduates have also served in Canada, Mexico, Australia and the Netherlands.[79]

Following the second world war, the number of Catholic nursing schools decreased. Extensive curriculum changes, consolidation of the small schools and efforts to achieve national accreditation are all factors which, combined, led to the decline in the number of schools. By 1968, there were only 308 diploma programs in Catholic institutions. It is to the St. Francis Hospital

[75]Beatrice J. Kalisch and Philip A. Kalisch, *The Advance of American Nursing,* (Boston: Little, Brown and Co., 1986), pp. 503–504, 557.

[76]Minutes, Board of Managers, 7/25/60, 9/26/60.

[77]"English Nurse Visits St. Francis General Hospital," article, n.d., St. Francis Hospital Archives; Sister M. Adele Meiser, manuscript, history of St. Francis Hospital, paper given at Lawrenceville Historical meeting, June 1985, St. Francis Hospital Archives.

[78]"Manpower Training Program," c. late 1960's, St. Francis Hospital Archives.

[79]Sister Mary Bertin Paulus, *Seventy-Fifth Anniversary 1901–1976,* (Pittsburgh: St. Francis General Hospital, 1976), pp. 3, 20; Minutes, Board of Managers, 6/11/45.

sisters' credit that they were able to maintain their schools in the wake of significant changes in the field of nursing education.[80]

Community

Residents of the Lawrenceville community had developed a good rapport with the hospital sisters early in their history. During the first half of the century, the St. Francis sisters were directly involved with the people of the community, knowing most of their neighbors. They would often sit out on the porch talking with neighbors. Neighborhood boys served mass for the sisters.[81] Sister Adele remembered how previous patients would come back to the hospital just to visit with a particular sister. In the early days when the hospital lacked an extensive telephone or intercom system, Sister Adele would race up several floors to find the sister whom the patient requested to see. Patients usually came just to chat, and she did everything in her power to help the visitor locate a particular sister.[82]

Sister Adele recalled elderly neighbors complaining because some of the local boys were vandalizing the hospital. She talked to the boys, stressing that St. Francis was "their hospital" and they should be proud of it and take care of it. Sister Adele told the boys she would pay them each ten cents per week if they would please keep an eye on the institution for her. They agreed, but when she went to pay them they refused any money because their mothers would not allow them to take money from the sisters. Sister's ability to handle the boys so astutely paid off, however. The vandalism problem ceased.[83] These anecdotes serve as examples of how the sisters related to their neighbors and, as a result, were able to determine needs of the community and serve the people.

The St. Francis Hospital, not unlike many other institutions, has a history of providing for the sick and injured during times of great epidemics or local disasters. In 1918, the Spanish influenza epidemic strained hospitals, many already without adequate nursing personnel or physicians because of the world war. Half a million Americans died in the epidemic of 1918–1919, five times

[80]Mary Carol Conroy, SCL, "The Transition Years," in *Pioneer Healers: The History of Women Religious in American Health Care* eds. Ursula Stepsis, CSA, and Dolores Liptak, RSM, (New York: Crossroad Publishing Co., 1989), p. 149.

[81]Manuscript of talk given by Sister Adele Meiser, n.d., St. Francis Hospital Archives.

[82]Interview with Sister M. Adele Meiser, 1993.

[83]Interview with Sister M. Adele Meiser, 1993.

greater than total World War I American military deaths.[84] Just as they served victims of smallpox in the nineteenth century, the sisters responded to the needs of influenza victims. In addition, one of the medical wards was reserved for soldiers. Sister M. Laurentine Harrington, OSF, received a commission from the U.S. Army to administer this service.[85] St. Francis, like many other facilities, was pressed into greater service.

The hospital was always eager to serve the community in times of crisis. On March 17, 1936, Pittsburgh's rivers overflowed, resulting in a deluge unprecedented in the city's history. The Pittsburgh *Sun-Telegraph* reported, "deaths mounted every hour. Houses were swept loose from their foundations. Power went off.... Phone lines went down. Fires broke out all over the district.... " Many people died in the flood, and approximately 3,000 had been injured.[86] Sister Adele remembered that St.Francis was the only hospital in the city to have light because they manufactured their own steam electricity and were, therefore, able to provide services to those injured in the flood. Sister Adele noted that "with the grace of God we had light."[87]

On November 11, 1940, a tragedy occurred at the Salvation Army Men's Social Center in Lawrenceville. Roach poisoning had accidentally been added to the pancake flour, poisoning the men who had had breakfast at the center. One of the interns from St. Francis went directly to the center to administer to the men. Others were sent to the hospital. Forty-five men were cared for, and an additional twelve men died.[88] These anecdotes are not unusual, but do serve to emphasize the hospital's commitment to the community.

World War II introduced new problems to the hospital, as previously noted, encouraging greater participation in the community at large. The hospital serves as a striking example of how a facility, already beset with financial difficulties, was able to continue serving the community during stressful periods and also share in the war effort. For example, St. Francis offered their facilities to Local Board #6, which requested the use of the Out-Patient Department for examining men for selective service.[89] The hospital administrators, concerned about community welfare during the war years, explored the possibilities of a Civilian Defense Program designed to protect the hospital

[84]Beatrice J. Kalisch and Philip A. Kalisch, *The Advance of American Nursing*, (Boston: Little, Brown and Co., 1986), pp. 360–361.

[85]Sister M. Adele Meiser, "History of St. Francis Medical Center," paper given at the Lawrenceville Historical Meeting, manuscript, June 1985, St.Francis Hospital Archives; Rosemary Stevens, *In Sickness and In Wealth, American Hospitals in the Twentieth Century*, (New York: Basic Books, Inc., 1989), p. 101.

[86]Stefan Lorant, *Pittsburgh, The Story of an American City*, (Lenox, Massachusetts: Authors Edition, Inc., 1975), pp. 355, 370.

[87]Interview with Sister M. Adele Meiser, 9/25/92.

[88]*Pittsburgh Sun-Telegraph* 11 November 1940.

[89]Minutes, Board of Managers, 12/8/41.

against a possible interruption of service if light, power, water and electricity services were curtailed. A committee was appointed to make a study of a defense program for protection of the hospital against such contingencies. A National Defense Committee was also established within the medical staff to make preparations for action in the event of a disaster.[90] The Hospital Council of Western Pennsylvania recommended that each hospital in Allegheny County reserve a private unlisted telephone line to be used only for receipt of air raid alarms from the appropriate Civilian Defense body and for communication from the Central Medical control room at the time of an accident. They also suggested, in accordance with the Office of Civilian Defense in Washington, D.C., that the hospital organize two large squads, each consisting of eight teams made up of doctors, nurses and auxiliary personnel.[91]

The hospital also assisted the federal government during the Vietnam years. In order to meet the need for trained personnel to care for wounded soldiers from Vietnam, the hospital made facilities available to members of the 339th General Hospital, United States Army Reserve Unit. This selected Reserve Force unit was one of one thousand combat support, technical and administrative units of the Army Reserve and National Guard selected for accelerated on-the-job training. The program was authorized in November 1965 by Secretary of Defense Robert McNamara. The 339th was capable of taking over and operating a one thousand bed general hospital within seven days notice. Commanded by Colonel George R. Gallagher, the 339th was the first Reserve unit in Western Pennsylvania to seek on-the-job training in civilian hospitals. The reservists received training in numerous departments, supplemented by electives and demonstrations provided by St. Francis doctors and nurses, and other trained personnel. Areas of training included admissions and disposition, central supply, inhalation therapy, laboratory, maintenance, neuropsychiatry, nursing service, pharmacy and radiology.[92]

The sisters' mission to maintain a very strong commitment to the community is one of the hospital's most interesting aspects. The sisters had always had a powerful link to the Lawrenceville and Bloomfield-Garfield areas, but they widened their focus to include the Homewood-Brushton and East End areas as well. The hospital was the epitome of a community institution, and this was manifested in several different ways. The community thought of St. Francis as the city hospital. Although prior to the second world war a

[90]Minutes, Board of Managers, 12/8/41.

[91]Minutes, Board of Managers, 3/9/42.

[92]"Army Reservists Receive Training at St. Francis General Hospital," n.d., St. Francis Hospital Archives; "Fact Sheet—United States Army reserve On-the-Job Training Program," manuscript, St. Francis Hospital Archives.

city hospital existed at Mayview, it was geographically inaccessible to local city residents. As noted, St. Francis accepted any patient, regardless of their ability to pay. Sister Adele noted, "we wanted to take care of the poor," and "we're always going to take care of the poor."[93] Robert M. Sigmond, noted health economist, notes that "community programs generally involve an in-equitably large contribution of time and money, by the most interested and fortunate, to assure some minimum (not equal) benefit to the less fortunate. That is the essence of a community program, as contrasted with a government program."[94] St. Francis Hospital, then, served the community by functioning as a municipal hospital, in the absence of one in the city, but unlike the other community facilities described by Sigmond, it assured maximum benefit to the less fortunate.

The Sisters of St. Francis committed themselves to the surrounding com-munity in ways unsurpassed by other community hospitals.[95] The unique strength of the community hospital, notes Sigmond, was its pluralistic fi-nancing, its control by community leadership, its commitment to the disad-vantaged, its shared responsibility among the medical practitioners for quality, a close linkage of the hospital with the community's physicians and a com-mitment to take care of community crises and disasters such as epidemics and natural disasters. In addition, an informal process of regionalization, reflect-ing a willingness to share medical staff members and other services on an ad hoc basis also existed.[96] At St. Francis, it went much further. It did not just focus on providing services, but the sisters were committed to the social welfare of the surrounding community in ways not noted by other institu-tions. It has been suggested that the ideas about 'community' worked best in small or mid-sized hospitals in areas where the population was relatively small, homogeneous and stable.[97] The characteristics of small community hospitals were often in stark contrast to the large teaching hospitals in the city. St. Francis, however, reflects another category of hospital, the teaching hospital whose emphasis is, in fact, on community and service. St. Francis functions as a community hospital within an urban area that is not homoge-neous and has not been stable throughout the century, experiencing drastic

---

[93] Interview with Sister M. Adele Meiser, 1993.

[94] Rosemary Stevens, *In Sickness and In Wealth, American Hospitals in the Twentieth Century*, (New York: Basic Books, Inc., 1989), p. 233.

[95] The literature suggests that the St. Francis Hospital commitment was unusual. Refer to Diana Elizabeth Long and Janet Golden, *The American General Hospital, Communities and Social Contexts*, (Ithaca: Cornell University Press, 1989).

[96] Rosemary Stevens, *In Sickness and In Wealth, American Hospitals in the Twentieth Century*, (New York: Basic Books, Inc., 1989), p. 233.

[97] Rosemary Stevens, *In Sickness and In Wealth, American Hospitals in the Twentieth Century*, (New York: Basic Books, Inc., 1989), pp. 233, 235.

demographic changes. The sisters' increasing involvement with the people of the community is characteristic of the period following the second world war.

St. Francis was committed to community service and to using its position of influence in the community for the benefit of all citizens. It "cannot help but recognize that one of the most important needs in its community today is that of curing the disease of social injustice—an illness that can no longer remain ignored or tolerated. St. Francis' adherence to good human relations principles in relationship to its patients and employees predates by many, many years recent civil rights legislation and community focus on social injustice." By the late 1960s, St. Francis had developed programs and policies in four different broad areas, all designed to give positive leadership and set good examples. They offered improved and expanded health services. Secondly, they had a history of hiring and training minorities and other disadvantaged individuals. Thirdly, St. Francis endeavored to extend its influence outside of the immediate environment and further into the community. Finally, and most specifically, it established a human relations committee.[98]

The hospital's community health services have already been noted as they had an active out-patient department for many years. In addition, their community mental health programs and out-patient alcoholic clinics, for example, provided care for members of the community outside of the immediate hospital setting. By the late sixties, the hospital served the following areas as part of their community mental health program: Lawrenceville, Bloomfield, Garfield, East Liberty, Homewood, Brushton, Stanton Heights, Morningside, Sharpsburg, Etna, Millvale and Shaler Township.[99]

Several programs serve as examples of the hospital's community commitment. In 1966, the hospital was awarded a grant to establish a hospital based Cancer Detection Program in conjunction with the United States Public Health Service. The program, which provided free pap smears for all indigent and low income group women, was viewed as an "important contribution to the health care of the people of the community."[100] In 1958, St. Francis Hospital established a Home Health Services division, although the Social Security Administration didn't accept it as a Home Health Agency until August 1966. Its primary purpose was to give home health services to those over sixty-five, but it made services available to younger patients, too, who would have been charged for services. "By making it available to younger patients, it is hoped that better utilization of hospital beds will be accomplished." The

[98]"Human Relations Report," manuscript, 10/23/68, St. Francis Hospital Archives.
[99]"Human Relations Report," manuscript, 10/23/68, St. Francis Hospital Archives.
[100]*Probe* 3 (January 1967); *Signs of Life* 3 (Autumn 1966).

Home Health Service planned to offer numerous services including nursing care; physical, speech and occupational therapies; nutritional guidance; appliances and equipment service; vocational guidance; and resident service where indicated in conjunction with the Visiting Nurses Association and the Public Health Nurse Service. This was not intended to be a service for patients requiring twenty-four hour custodial care.[101] Clearly, the hospital provided numerous health care services to community residents.

Not only did the hospital endeavor to provide health care, but it intentionally developed programs to assist ethnic and racial minority individuals within the community. Although the St. Francis Hospital sisters had always been non-discriminatory in their hiring practices, after World War II they became even more actively involved in programs specifically designed to upgrade members of minority, ethnic and other disadvantaged groups. In the late sixties, they committed themselves to train forty practical nurses in one and a half years in cooperation with the Manpower Division of the Mayors Committee on Human Resources (MCHR). There were nine students in the 1968 class. Also in cooperation with MCHR, St. Francis Hospital trained and hired twenty-two psychiatric aids. The program was a continuing one. In 1967, the hospital trained and hired fifty-two disadvantaged citizens as nursing assistants in cooperation with the Hospital Educational and Research Foundation of Pennsylvania (HERF) and the Bureau of Employment Security (BES). In addition, in cooperation with the same two groups, the hospital provided additional training to fourteen underemployed nursing assistants from disadvantaged groups and upgraded them to senior nursing assistants. Another program, begun in 1963, also in cooperation with BES, trained disadvantaged individuals to be Operating Room Technicians. Inhalation therapists, certified laboratory assistants and medical records technicians, in cooperation with BES, were also trained. The Personnel Training Center, one of the more influential programs, established with the cooperation of the Bureau of Vocational Rehabilitation, trained and placed over two hundred handicapped persons, the majority of whom represented minority, ethnic and other social disadvantaged groups.[102]

On November 29, 1965, St. Francis Hospital opened the Personnel Training Center (PTC), which was designed to train nursing and dietary assistants. The purpose of the program was two-fold. It served the hospitals of Western Pennsylvania by answering the chronic need for trained personnel. In addi-

---

[101] Minutes, Board of Managers, Medical Director's Report, 5/19/66; Minutes, Executive committee, 9/26/66; Sister M. Adele Meiser, "Points for 'On Location' TV Interview," n.d. but c. 1986, St. Francis Hospital Archives.

[102] "Human Relations Report," manuscript, 10/23/68, St. Francis Hospital Archives.

tion, the program aided those individuals who, because of physical, mental, emotional, cultural, educational or economic problems, were not able to benefit from existing programs. This program was the result of joint planning of St. Francis Hospital and the Pennsylvania State Bureau of Vocational Rehabilitation (BVR).[103] In June 1966, the PTC added the housekeeping assistant program, a twelve week program which provided ninety percent of the graduates with jobs after training.[104]

The housekeeping aide and dietary assistant programs were discontinued in 1972, but the nursing aide program continued. Thirty to thirty-five nursing assistants graduated every year. The program was committed to serving the clients of the Bureau of Vocational Rehabilitation as well as other agencies. The nursing assistant program provided clinical and classroom experience, vocational and personal counseling services and job placement.[105]

Admission requirements were such that many educationally disadvantaged individuals would qualify for the program. An applicant was to have sixth grade reading skills, fourth grade mathematics skills and physical and emotional capabilities. The sponsoring agency was to provide transportation via the Port Authority Transit, three uniforms, one pair of shoes, one watch and one textbook. The agency was to financially sponsor the trainee as well.[106] Unfortunately, the hospital was unable to continue the program because the administration had increasing difficulty locating positions for the graduates of the program, but clearly the program was effective and beneficial for many individuals while it existed, and reflected the hospital's larger commitment.[107]

Although the hospital sisters were interested in extending their role into the community, helping the community meet its needs, it was imperative to them that they not be paternalistic and determine those needs themselves. They responded to community needs as defined by the community. As noted earlier, one of those ways was in establishing mental health clinics at the request of leaders in Homewood-Brushton and Sharpsburg. Also at the request of Homewood-Brushton leadership, they assisted in the planning and developing of a narcotics treatment program. Hospital personnel worked with the East Liberty/Garfield Office of Economic Opportunity and the United Health Services to organize the Citizens Mental Health Council, whose function was

[103]"Manpower Training Program," manuscript, n.d. but c. 1968, St. Francis Hospital Archives; *Probe* 2, #1.

[104]"Personnel Training Center," manuscript, n.d., St. Francis Hospital Archives.

[105]"Personnel Training Center—Policies and Procedures," manuscript, 6/66, revised 2/27/79, St. Francis Hospital Archives.

[106]"Personnel Training Center—Policies and Procedures," manuscript, 6/66, revised 2/27/79, St. Francis Hospital Archives.

[107]Interview with Sister M. Adele Meiser, 1993.

to advise the hospital regarding mental health needs of their neighborhood. In addition, the hospital created the position of 'health care expediter' to provide a liaison between the hospital and the community. The expediter was to offer home and hospital visits, meeting patients in the clinic, emergency room and clinical areas. The expediter was to attend civic meetings and functions that furthered health education and welfare needs of the patient, but the key role of the expediter was to inform hospital officials of community needs.[108]

The hospital offered numerous other services as they expanded their focus to include the general welfare of the community at large. In 1966, it agreed to participate with the Pittsburgh Public Schools under the Manpower Development and Training Act by providing training of medical laboratory assistants in bacteriology. The program, designed by the United States Department of Health, Education and Welfare, began in June.[109] In August 1967, the administration signed an agreement with the school district to train medical records clerks.[110] The hospital implemented a program, known as "Learn to Become a Health Professional," in cooperation with the Pittsburgh Parochial and Public School system and the Pittsburgh Urban League in the same year. The purpose of the project was to motivate and encourage junior high students to become interested in the health professions. Women's auxiliary members conducted tours for nine hundred students.[111]

As the hospital widened its focus, no longer providing just educational and medical services, the sisters, cognizant of the turmoil in the city as a result of the Civil Rights Movement, extended their services to ease the tension in the local community. In 1967, the Hospital Council of Western Pennsylvania met to discuss the development of a community wide disaster plan in response to the "recent wide spread riots" which were causing considerable concern. St. Francis was designated as a primary hospital, with a 'hot line' to the Disaster Center, for Homewood-Brushton. Other participating hospitals in the district which were to provide back-up services were West Penn, Pittsburgh Hospital and Columbia Hospital. Central communications were established at the Department of Public Safety, which had communication lines to major emergency centers.[112]

More important than the hospital's willingness to comply with the recommendations of the Hospital Council of Western Pennsylvania was the sisters' intent to deal directly with individuals in the community itself, in order to

[108]"Human Relations Report," manuscript, 10/23/68, St. Francis Hospital Archives.
[109]Minutes, Board of Managers, Executive Committee, 5/23/66; Administrator's report, 6/27/66.
[110]Executive Director's report, August–September 1967; *Probe* 2 (September 1966).
[111]Minutes, Board of Managers, Executive Director's Report, 4/3/67; *Probe* 3 (March 1967).
[112]Executive Director's report, August–September 1967; Minutes, Board of Managers, 10/23/67.

cope with the increasing tension. In fact, the sisters addressed the issues several years before the riots which occurred in other areas of the city. The hospital administration has a history of working closely with the Lawrenceville Economic Action Program, Inc. (LEAP). Funded by the Office of Economic Opportunity, and administered by Community Action Pittsburgh, Inc. (CAP), the city's poverty program, LEAP's purpose was to further the economic development of the second, sixth and 10-A wards of the Lawrenceville area. The objectives of citizen members were to construct new housing, rehabilitate existing structures, develop self-sustaining economic ventures in the area and to involve residents directly in the programs. LEAP also sought to develop a positive learning and working atmosphere for residents, offering the services of professionals such as social workers, physicians and attorneys. Dr. William Mooney recalls providing psychiatric consultation services to the social workers. The hospital offered services as well. In 1967, for example, St. Francis agreed to do physical examinations for 140 children enrolled in the Head Start program. LEAP implemented a Revolving Loan Fund for Housing, designed to provide low-interest rate loans to the elderly and low income families, and the Neighborhood Employment Center, which provided job referral services, on the job training and vocational counseling. The Family Service Unit of LEAP provided counseling services for families suffering from marital problems, difficult parent-child relationships or other family oriented crises. A Neighborhood Legal Services division was established to provide legal counsel for residents unable to afford attorney's fees. In addition, a Department of Public Welfare Consultant and Human Service Aide were housed within the LEAP office in order to advise individuals regarding the state medical program, food stamps, financial assistance, the Home-Maker Service, complete DPW services or services for the blind. Youth and senior citizens groups were developed to provide activities and experiences for those groups. In essence, the organization offered a variety of services designed to aid residents in need.[113]

One of LEAP'S first interests was the implementation of a head start program for neighborhood children. Community social service workers had asked Sister Adele, then the CEO, to attend the organizational meeting. She, along with Sisters M. Sylvia Schuler, OSF, and M. Rosita Wellinger, OSF, attended what was a very rowdy meeting. It became very clear that there was a great deal of racial tension. Sister Adele learned later that police detectives had been assigned to the area, expecting difficulty. The white members of the

[113]*LEAP, Inc.* brochure, Archives of Industrial Society, University of Pittsburgh; Interview with Dr. William Mooney, April 28, 1994; Minutes, Board of Managers, 6/8/67; Executive Director's Report, 4/3/67; Executive director's annual report, 10/23/67.

community, somewhat offended that their community had been designated a poverty area by CAP, were not interested in participating in the program with their African American neighbors. Sister Adele, on her own, approached the stage and addressed the audience. She requested that those who would not vote to implement the head start program kindly leave. There was a mass exodus of most of the white people in attendance. As a result, the LEAP organization was organized and administered by the African Americans of the community, but for a number of years, the sisters were elected to the board and worked for the association. The board of directors was responsible for all policy divisions as well as contracts and proposals submitted by the neighborhood for approval. The sisters, therefore, played a key role in the organization.[114]

Members of the Roman Catholic church hierarchy were well aware of the racial tension and bigotry which had long been present in Lawrenceville, and many leaders within the church attempted to ease that tension. The Rev. Stanley Lubarski, a Capuchin and assistant pastor of St. Augustine's Church, which provided the chaplains for the hospital, was also a member of LEAP. He sought to alleviate tensions inherent in an integrated community fraught with prejudice through that association, and through the sermons he preached every Sunday. Sister Adele, too, was involved directly with community residents in an attempt to improve community relations. She was frequently invited to attend the African American church services and the churches' women's society meetings. She fondly recalled singing familiar hymns and getting down to pray with her friends in the community, noting that she had good relationships with the African American ministers of the area as well.[115]

Historian Rosemary Stevens has noted that community leaders, especially those of minority groups, began to challenge traditional hospital paternalism directly during the 1960s. The St. Francis sisters met these challenges head-on with a sensitivity that compared favorably with other hospitals of the period.[116] The administration at St. Francis Hospital was instrumental in assuaging the tension in the local area surrounding the hospital, becoming directly involved with the African American community.

William 'Bouie' Haden, exemplifying those who challenged hospital pa-

[114]*LEAP, Inc.* brochure, Archives of Industrial Society, University of Pittsburgh; Minutes, Board of Managers, 6/8/67; Executive Director's Report, 4/3/67; Executive director's annual report, 10/23/67; "List of Hospital Services and Departments," manuscript, St. Francis Hospital Archives; Interview with Sister M. Adele Meiser, 1993; Interview with Mrs. Mary Thompson, 5/4/94.

[115]Interview with Sister M. Adele Meiser, 1993; R. F. Karlovits, "Lawrenceville Is His 'Parish,'" *Pittsburgh Press Roto*, 23 April 1972.

[116]Rosemary Stevens, *In Sickness and In Wealth, American Hospitals in the Twentieth Century*, (New York: Basic Books, Inc., 1989), p. 234.

ternalism, was an African American leader in the East End who, Sister Adele remembered, had a propensity for quoting Shakespeare. An active and successful leader during the civil rights era, he worked for equal housing opportunities for the African Americans of the city, and addressed other issues as well. One of his concerns was the small number of African American students admitted to the graduate school of social work at the University of Pittsburgh in the mid-sixties. His demand for greater access for students was met in 1968, when half of the class was comprised of African Americans. He was perceived as someone who was forthright and sincere, but he has also been described as a "gruff, fiery, table-pounding, expletive-uttering Homewood-Brushton grassroots figure." Bouie Haden was very active in the Pittsburgh community, holding positions as chairman of the United Movement for Progress, and member of the board of the Mayor's Commission on Human Resources. Mr. Haden was also chairman of the 9B-1 citizens council, the citizens advisory council which was established within the catchment area. Mr. Haden was concerned that the hospitals in the community were not providing for the care of heroin addicts. Although St. Francis had a history of always admitting addicts for treatment, they did not have a separate unit for them away from the mentally ill patients. He demanded that every hospital provide thirty beds specifically designated for those undergoing heroin detoxification. Other local hospitals ignored his request, but Sister Adele agreed to establish a unit on the top floor of the nurses' residence. Within days of Mr. Haden's request, one of the physicians, Sister Sylvia and Sister Adele set up six beds, for they had room for no more. Although the unit was in operation for only several years, the experience cemented a cordial relationship between the sisters and the local community.[117]

The hospital sisters and Mr. Haden cooperatively altered the staffing within one of the community health centers in order that the center be more receptive to community needs. Mr. Haden had charged that the hospital and the community mental health centers were not responsive enough to the poor and the African Americans of the community. He thought the hospital could be more responsible if the community mental health center had on its staff a representative from the citizens council, whose role was not clearly defined, but who could lobby for the priorities of the citizens of the community. Convinced that Mr. Haden's idea was beneficial, the administration sought funding from the County MH/MR program, wrote the job description and supplied office space in the community mental health center in East Liberty.

---

[117]Interview with Sister M. Adele Meiser, 1993; Interview with Dr. William Mooney, April 28, 1994; Alvin Rosensweet, "Civil Righters Ask Citywide Rent Strike," *Pittsburgh Post-Gazette*, 18 July 1967; "Haden Named to MCHR Board," *Courier* 3 August 1968; Interview with Mrs. Mary Thompson, 5/4/94.

The person presented to the hospital as the citizens council choice for the position was Mr. Haden's daughter, who functioned as a liaison or trouble shooter.[118]

Mr. Haden, a highly respected individual within the community mental health center and St. Francis Hospital, was honored by the citizens council in 1972 at a testimonial dinner. It was noted that "all spoke in honor of Mr. Haden, pointing out the value of this man in the community." He has been given credit for providing the impetus to further a specific drug treatment program within the hospital and community mental health center. Although the heroin detoxification in-patient unit did not continue in its original form, it was, perhaps, the forerunner of the programs that were subsequently established and continue to function currently.[119]

The administration and medical staff, desiring to understand the community needs, did not rely only on liaison personnel, but communicated directly with local area residents. Physicians and sisters attended the citizens council meetings, some of which were held in the meeting room at the East Liberty library as well as on hospital grounds. One of the concerns of the citizens was that the hospital attempt to hire African Americans, and the hospital tried to be receptive to that need, exemplifying the hospital's commitment.[120]

This acceptance by the community cannot be merely due to the fact that St. Francis Hospital is a religious institution. Mercy Hospital, for example, desirous of assisting the African American people in the Hill District, applied for a federal grant in 1964 to improve health services there. Their grant was refused because the Black community had a poor image of Mercy Hospital. One embittered resident noted, "you treated us, but you never accepted us." The Sisters of Mercy, relentless in their work to aid the community, continued to attend neighborhood meetings where they were screamed at with foul language. To their credit, the Sisters of Mercy pursued their goal, and eventually were able to establish neighborhood health care facilities to aid the African American community.[121]

Other individuals employed at St. Francis Hospital have also been active in community organizations and social agencies. Many of the sisters of the Order were working with Opportunities Industrialization Center as volunteer tutors to help school drop-outs achieve their high school diplomas. Other employees and sisters were also involved in the organization and establishment

[118]Interview with Dr. William Mooney, April 28, 1994.
[119]*SFGH Community Mental Health Mental Retardation Center Newsletter* 1 (December 1972).
[120]Interview with Dr. William Mooney, April 28, 1994.
[121]*Pillar of Pittsburgh, The History of Mercy Hospital and The City It Serves*, (Pittsburgh: McCullough Communications, 1990), pp. 156–157.

of LEAP. Many of the sisters were members of the Urban League, and have worked with its Educational and Medical Program to help teenage unwed mothers obtain employment. Other employees, sisters and physicians have been active in numerous programs throughout the city.[122]

In 1967, a hospital human relations committee was established to act as an advisory body to the executive director. It was endowed with educational, investigative, judicial and public relations powers. Designated responsibilities were varied. Members were to review all existing policies for inequities with regard to race. The committee was to investigate all complaints of employees, and was to establish mechanisms to educate staff, patients and community in sound human relations principles. In addition, they were to represent the hospital to the community on such matters as fell within its jurisdiction.[123]

Conclusion

St. Francis was not only interested in serving the surrounding community, but it endeavored to extend its influence internationally. The Foundation for World Health, which serves as an example of this commitment, was established in the early 1980s to eliminate tuberculosis in India.[124] Every year, one of the staff physicians traveled to India to teach medical personnel there how to administer medication to combat the disease. They would use some of their own funds to have medications sent from the United States, and were instrumental in establishing clinics in India.[125] The foundation's main objectives were to assist and encourage health care providers to establish themselves in rural and poverty areas throughout the world by offering assistance with health services, research and the award of grants. The eradication of tuberculosis in India was the foundation's first area of focus.[126]

From the era when sisters counseled neighbors on the convent porch to providing for tuberculosis victims on the other side of the world, the Sisters of St. Francis have clearly made a commitment to the community at large. One of those commitments has been expressed through education. They have established training schools for registered nurses, practical nurses and other health care technicians. In addition, they provided for the education of medi-

[122]"Human Relations Report," manuscript, 10/23/68, St. Francis Hospital Archives.
[123]"Human Relations Report," manuscript, 10/23/68, St. Francis Hospital Archives.
[124]"List of Hospital Services and Departments," manuscript, St. Francis Hospital Archives.
[125]Interview with Sister M. Adele Meiser, 1993.
[126]"Foundation for World Health," brochure, St. Francis Hospital Archives.

cal students, interns, residents and medical staff. They have also demonstrated
their eagerness to aid the community in times of disaster whether that be of
a local or global nature.

What is more distinctive about the community commitment of the Sisters of St. Francis of Millvale is its sheer range and extent. Unusual, too, is the
sisters' direct involvement with the local citizenry in their attempt to alleviate problems not always directly related to health care. The sisters' mission
to provide for the healing of the body, mind, and spirit often resulted in a
conflict for them as they were unable, or unwilling, to separate the provision
of health care services from their wider goals. In their attempt to balance the
delivery of health care services with their broader socioeconomic concerns,
the sisters influenced the development of the local community and its citizens profoundly. The sisters' community commitment has helped to define
the nature of the St. Francis Health System at the dawn of the twenty-first
century.

The sisters' involvement with the wider community followed from their
religious values, but other factors played a role, particularly in the more competitive medical atmosphere after World War II. In the sixties, the designation
of the Lawrenceville area as a poverty neighborhood by Community Action
Pittsburgh, Pittsburgh's federally funded poverty agency, may have motivated
the sisters to pay closer attention to local residents. In 1960, the hospital
enlarged and renovated the physical plant, at a significant cost. The price
of new medical technology was soaring and with the enactment of Medicare
and Medicaid in the mid -sixties and the anticipation of reimbursement for
services rendered, the sisters may have been eager to encourage local citizens
to utilize their facility. The enhancement of relationships with community
leaders and agencies might have strengthened the hospital's position as a local
health care provider, especially in light of the competition from surrounding
area hospitals and the changing demographic characteristics of the community itself. Whatever the mix of motives, the sisters' role in the community
must not be undervalued for their influence on the local citizenry and the aid
which they provided are inestimable.

Chapter Six

Conclusion

During the late 1970s, 1980s and early 1990s, St. Francis Hospital has expanded dramatically, emphasizing the strength of the administration, which has remained in authority since the hospital's founding over a century ago. Since Sister Adele resigned from her position as chief executive officer of the hospital in 1977, the physical plant continued to grow, and new programs for the care of the sick were implemented. Clearly, however, nothing completely new developed as the foundation for the St. Francis health center had been firmly laid many years previously. The hospital's history clearly demonstrates its ability to maintain continuity, while being innovative within the face of change in the medical world.

The physical plant expanded to meet the changing needs of the health care industry. A major building and renovation campaign resulted in new facilities, which opened in 1987. The east pavilion was erected for psychiatric patients, and an eleven story wing was added to the South building. A three-story extension on the north side of the hospital between the south building, and the chapel was added to expand the Emergency Room; in addition, a Lobby-Pedestrian bridge was erected between the parking complex and the south building.[1]

The East Pavilion, the new nine-story triangular building at the corner of Forty-fifth and Penn Avenues, housed 228 psychiatric beds. The design was described as being distinctively less institutional, and more homelike, with all patient rooms private with their own baths. The Pavilion housed in-patient adult, adolescent, children and geriatric psychiatric services, as well

---

[1] St. Francis General Hospital—The Groundbreaking 4/5/83, St. Francis Hospital Archives.

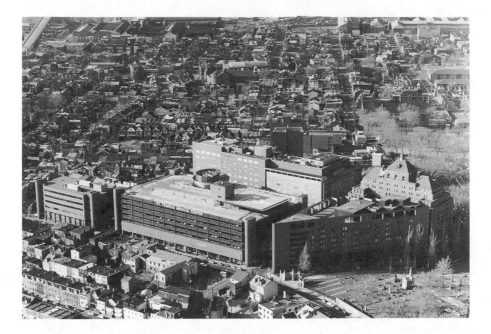

St. Francis Medical Center, 1990s

as an adolescent chemical dependency unit and adult detoxification unit. The building connected at each floor to the East Building, the former nurses' residence, which provided office space for professionals in social work services and the centers for chemical dependency treatment and psychiatric medicine, as well as other out-patient services. The East Pavilion was dedicated to Sister Adele in commemoration of her administration from 1959 to 1977.[2]

The Liberace concourse, the new main entrance to St. Francis, joined the medical/parking complex to the south wing of the medical facility. The new suspended lobby was the largest in Pittsburgh, featuring an atrium-like atmosphere. The concourse was dedicated to pianist and performer Liberace, who was a loyal supporter of the hospital, and credited hospital personnel with saving his life. In November 1963, at the beginning of a two week engagement at the Holiday House, a local supper club in Pittsburgh, Liberace became gravely ill and was taken to St. Francis Hospital. He visited the sisters on several occasions following his recovery. On November 8, 1965, to show his gratitude to the administration and staff of the hospital, he gave a concert sponsored by the women's auxiliary, resulting in a twenty thousand

[2] Program, Dedication of the New Facilities, March 16, 1987.

dollar donation to the hospital. Liberace died February 4, 1987, just six weeks before the dedication of the new facility on March 16, 1987.[3]

Numerous other departments were expanded or remodeled as part of the 1987 building project. An additional parking floor and a helicopter landing site were added to the medical/parking complex, providing additional parking and air access for Angel I, an emergency helicopter transport service. Renovated departments included the Cardiac Catheterization lab, laboratory and pathology services, the dietary department, surgical department, emergency department and the ambulatory care center. The medical surgical addition to the south wing was dedicated to Gurdon F. Flagg, who served as chairman of the board from 1970 until his death on June 13, 1984.[4]

The St. Francis Medical Center continues to provide innovative treatment in a traditional setting, maintaining policies that date back to the 1920s. In 1987, the Pittsburgh Laser Center was established, offering patients a choice when they are faced with the prospect of surgery. With more than one hundred surgeons trained in the latest techniques, using the most-up-to-date equipment, the health care consumer may undergo laser surgery in a number of different specialties. The Center for Cardiac Care, continuing what Dr. D'Zmura began eighty years ago, offers the services of over ninety cardiologists and cardiovascular surgeons. Comprehensive services utilizing modern technology for diagnosis and treatment are incorporated with educational and rehabilitation services all designed to guide patients towards a healthy lifestyle. The Pittsburgh Chest Pain Center at St. Francis, one of the first chest pain emergency treatment centers in the region, and among only a handful in the nation, was established to augment the services of the cardiac center. The Center for Physical Rehabilitation continues what was first established officially in 1960, providing a multidisciplinary team of allied health professionals for patients suffering from disabling illness or injury. The Center for Critical Care offers high technology and specially equipped transportation in conjunction with a specially trained team to provide intensive surgical and medical care.[5] As the dawn of the twenty-first century approaches, the St. Francis Medical Center continues to offer comprehensive services in virtually all areas of medicine.

The Center for Psychiatric Medicine at St. Francis Hospital continued to be very innovative during the eighties, establishing additional psychiatric

[3] Minutes, Board of Managers, January 1966; *Signs of Life* 11 (Fall 1965).

[4] Program, Dedication of New Facilities, March 1987.

[5] *Introducing St. Francis Health System*, (Pittsburgh: SFHS, 3/92); "St. Francis Celebrates 125 Years of Excellence," *Hospital News Pittsburgh*, January 1990, pp. 8–9; *29th Annual Personnel Picnic*, program, 1990, St. Francis Hospital Archives.

programs for those with special needs. Unfortunately, in spite of the fact that the sisters clearly were committed to the citizens of the local community, they were unable to continue to maintain all of the local satellite community mental health centers. By 1994, due to a lack of funding, only the East Liberty center remained. The Garfield program was closed by 1978, and by 1982, the Sharpsburg Satellite Adult and Children Programs had been closed due to a consolidation program. The Homewood program was closed two years later.[6] Other psychiatric services designed to serve special needs of residents of the community were initiated, however, and some of those programs offered an outreach component. Several examples include a second adolescent unit opened in 1980, which was designed to deal with psychosomatic and eating disorder illnesses. In 1985, an outreach project was implemented to provide services to Personal Care Homes and homeless facilities, and in 1991, PATH was established to care for homeless mentally ill patients. Special programs for women were implemented, offering specialized services for those suffering from premenstrual syndrome or other emotional disorders. A sexual dysfunction program had also been developed by that time.[7]

By the 1980s, the Center for Chemical Dependency Treatment had expanded dramatically with the implementation of a variety of programs, which included medically supervised detoxification as well as rehabilitation. In 1980, the hospital established the first comprehensive chemical dependency program in the tri-state region, which was designed specifically for adolescents, and treats adolescent chemical dependency as a primary and separate illness. The program, which has several components, also offers prevention services to the community. Prevention specialists train parents, teachers and counselors how to reach children before the teen years. A comprehensive Student Assistance Program was developed whereby expertise was brought into area school systems.[8] Other addiction programs, including regional programs, had been established by 1985, including a Maternal Addiction program and an Elderly Outreach program[9] The Center for Education and Drug Abuse Research is another component of the program. In addition, workshops for adult children of alcoholics (ACOA) and young children of alcoholics (CAPERS)

---

[6]"County Request for 25th Anniversary Retrospective," manuscript, 1994, Adult Outpatient division of the Community Mental Health Center.

[7]"County Request for 25th Anniversary Retrospective," manuscript, 1994, Adult Outpatient division of the Community Mental Health Center; "St. Francis Medical Center Department of Psychiatry Position Paper," manuscript, 6/25/87, St. Francis Hospital Archives.

[8]"Faces the Facts," *Pittsburgh Press*, ads which ran in 1983–1984; *Twenty-ninth Annual Personnel Picnic*, program, 1990, St. Francis Hospital Archives.

[9]"St. Francis Medical Center Department of Psychiatry Position Paper," manuscript, 6/25/87, St. Francis Hospital Archives; Letter from Alan Jacobson, Manager, St. Francis Community MH/MR Center to Sister Lucene, 4/22/85, St. Francis Hospital Archives.

have been established. The center, treating more than eight hundred people every day, is one of the most comprehensive in the nation, offering a wide array of services to treat chemical dependency.[10] The Chemical Dependency Program established outreach programs in Monroeville, Wilkinsburg, Tarentum, East Liberty and the Hill District as well as the hospital.[11]

It is important to note, however, that although new programs had been continuously implemented, they fit into well established tradition. Even as the staff defined specific programs for target populations and implemented new treatment methods, they built on a concept of treating chemical abuse that had been prevalent for a century.

By 1990, many other agencies had begun to offer psychiatric and substance abuse treatment, but as noted earlier, government mandates and funding, as well as the establishment of several private facilities, have diminished St. Francis Hospital's distinctive role as a provider of psychiatric services. Clearly, the hospital was the first to offer many services, and served as a role model for facilities which developed later, while remaining a leader in the field. To be sure, many of the personnel who trained at St. Francis went on to care for patients in these other institutions. St. Francis remains one of only a handful of facilities equipped to offer detoxification treatment.[12] Further, four catchment areas of the nine within Allegheny County are serviced by St. Francis Medical Center's Alcohol and other Drugs Program, which serves as an example of its widespread influence.[13] St. Francis Hospital, moreover, continues to differ from most of the other general acute care hospitals' psychiatric units in several ways. St. Francis has ten locked units and one unlocked unit, whereas most of the other general hospitals only provide unlocked units. As a result, most of the patients require minimal restrictive care, and are usually only mildly ill. St. Francis, on the other hand, accepts acute, moderately and mildly ill individuals. The restrictive environment is dependent on patient needs. St. Francis has a larger percentage of patients on medical assistance unlike the other hospitals, which admit primarily privately insured patients. Modalities of care at St. Francis are more widely varied because of the nature of patient illnesses. Group therapy is used much more at St. Francis than in most other facilities.[14] Although many other facilities have followed in St.

[10] *Introducing St. Francis Health System,* (Pittsburgh: SFHS, 3/92).

[11] *Where to Call,* brochure, (Pittsburgh: Allegheny County Mental Health/Mental Retardation/Drug and Alcohol/Homeless and Hunger Program, 1994)

[12] *Where to Turn,* (Pittsburgh: United Way, 1990).

[13] *Where to Call,* brochure, (Pittsburgh: Allegheny County Mental Health/Mental Retardation/Drug and Alcohol/Homeless and Hunger Program, 1994).

[14] St. Francis Medical Center Department of Psychiatry Position Paper," manuscript, 6/25/87, St. Francis Hospital Archives.

Francis' footsteps, the hospital remains as one of the few facilities to offer wide ranging comprehensive services.

In July 1985, in a corporate restructuring, St. Francis General Hospital was renamed the St. Francis Medical Center, a subsidiary of the parent corporation, St. Francis Health System. Sister M. Sylvia Schuler served as President and Chief Executive Officer of the health system. Sister M. Rosita Wellinger was Chief Executive Officer of the medical center, and Executive Vice President of the corporation.[15] As of September 1, 1994, Sister M. Sylvia became President Emeritus. Sister M. Rosita Wellinger assumed the position of President and Chief Executive Officer of St. Francis Health System and St. Francis Medical Center. The St. Francis Medical Center includes not only the specialized care centers within the hospital setting in Lawrenceville, but also operates outreach facilities. St. Francis Medical Center-North in Cranberry Township is a freestanding facility offering twenty-four hour emergency and urgent care, emergency helicopter transport to specialty hospitals when necessary as well as medical, diagnostic and ambulatory services. The 150 bed St. Francis Nursing Center-North is a skilled nursing and intermediate care facility. St. Francis Surgery Center-North is a one-day surgery site, and the St. Francis Medical Office Building-North provides physician office space for thirty different groups in most of the specialties. St. Francis Nursing Center-East on Highland Avenue in Pittsburgh is another 150 bed skilled nursing facility.[16]

Two other area hospitals also function under the auspices of the St. Francis Medical Center. The St. Francis Hospital of New Castle was founded by the sisters in 1908. At the turn of the century only one hospital existed in New Castle, Pennsylvania. Under the control of a board of trustees, that hospital neglected the spiritual needs of Roman Catholic patients. "Catholic patients were often deprived of the ministrations of the priest and a number died, without the last sacraments, consequently, the Catholics of the district were eager for a hospital under Catholic control." The Sisters of St. Francis of Millvale, cognizant of the community's needs, purchased and remodeled an eighteen-room building, which opened on November 19, 1908. Ten sisters, who were experienced nurses, cared for the patients there. They subsequently opened their own nurse training school in 1919.[17] By 1994, the St. Francis Hospital of New Castle was a 184 bed community hospital offering comprehensive

[15]*Inspirations* 1 (Fall 1985).

[16]"St. Francis Health System Healthline," supplement to the *Pittsburgh Post-Gazette*, 3 May 1994.

[17]Seniors of 1966, Mt. Alvernia H.S., *100 Years of Franciscan Spirit 1866–1966*, (Pittsburgh 1966), p. 43; Popp, p. 143.

services, including neuropsychiatry, laser surgery, physical rehabilitation and a skilled nursing unit.[18] The St. Francis Central Hospital, formerly Central Medical, is a recently acquired acute care hospital and the newest member to the St. Francis Health System.[19]

Several other branches comprise the St. Francis Health System. The St. Francis Health Foundation is the fund-raising arm of the health system. Advantage Health, another branch of the health system, is a managed care provider developed by St. Francis Health System in 1986.[20]

The Franciscan sisters maintained their mission to care for the indigent, a vital continuity that distinguished their administration from other local institutions. In 1979, Medicaid paid for 12 percent of the total number of in-patient days in the general hospital, and 33 percent of the total number of in-patient days in the psychiatric department.[21] For fiscal year 1985 to 1986, the St. Francis Hospital served a greater percentage of Medicaid patients than any other Pittsburgh area hospital, regardless of the size of the institution.[22]

Percentage of Medicaid Patients, 1985–1986

Hospital	% Medicaid Patients	Average Daily Census
AGH	10.4	540
Mercy	11.0	385
Presbyterian	8.8	444
Shadyside	4.0	351
West Penn	11.6	401
St. Francis	14.3	509

Because of the unusual commitment to the indigent, St. Francis Hospital, even in recent years, has continued to rely on the sisters to help alleviate the financial burdens inherent in serving an indigent population. In 1983, for example, the sisters pledged $200,000.00 a year for five years to the building fund of the hospital.[23] Over the years, various arrangements have been made with the sisters whereby they regularly returned a portion of their salaries to

---

[18]"St. Francis Health System Healthline," supplement to the *Pittsburgh Post-Gazette*, 3 May 1994.

[19]"St. Francis Health System Healthline," supplement to the *Pittsburgh Post-Gazette*, 3 May 1994.

[20]*Pittsburgh Hospital News* 4 (January 1990), pp. 8–10.

[21]Manuscript, St. Francis Hospital Archives.

[22]These hospitals were listed because they are of comparable size. Note, however, that regardless of the size of the hospital, St. Francis still treated a greater percentage of Medicaid patients. Source: Butcher/Singer Study 5/87—St. Francis Hospital Archives.

[23]Letter from the Sisters of St. Francis to the board of directors, August 9, 1983, Motherhouse Archives.

the hospital. Unfortunately, due to the number of aging members and the decline in numbers of new members capable of earning a salary, the sisters were compelled, in 1989, to reduce the percentage of their subsidy to the hospital. As of July 1 that year, they were only able to return 20 percent of their salaries.[24] Catholic hospitals clearly are unique in their traditional reliance on the sisters to serve the institution without the disadvantage of having to pay exorbitant salaries. The implication of the declining numbers of younger sisters, and the rising costs of caring for their aged, pose a threat to the future of Catholic hospitals in America. St. Francis, in spite of these challenges, has been able to maintain its Catholic position within the hospital community. The problem of declining numbers of women entering religious orders reflects a national trend.

By the 1970s, the numbers of women religious active in the hospitals had declined dramatically due to fewer applicants and the increased attrition by death and withdrawals. Hospital sisters, although concerned about the financial ramifications of declining applications, placed more emphasis on the maintenance of their religious values within their institutions. Since the physical presence of the sisters could no longer be relied upon to transmit the culture and ideals of the Order, or the Church at large, the hospitals were forced to rely on legal structures that preserved the Catholic control of the institution.[25] This was common to Catholic hospitals in general, and St. Francis was no exception.

In 1992, due to their diminished physical presence, the by-laws of the St. Francis Medical Center were amended to assure the sisters' position within the organizational structure, in order that the Catholic values be maintained. Article I, Section 1, states plainly that "The Corporation was founded and is operated in affiliation with the Sisters of St. Francis of Millvale, Pennsylvania, a religious congregation of the Roman Catholic Church. As a separate and autonomous entity, the Corporation is dedicated to the continuation of the provision of charitable, health care and community services in the Franciscan tradition."[26] The Board of Directors was to include ex officio members who occupied the position of chief executive officer of the corporation, president of the medical staff of the corporation, president of the auxiliary of the corporation and major superior of the Sisters of St. Francis of Millvale. In addition, if at any time the Board of Directors chose

---

[24]Letter from Sister M. Dolita Kessler, Community Director, to Sister M. Sylvia Schuler, June 12, 1989, Motherhouse Archives.

[25]Margaret John Kelly, D.C., "Toward the Twenty-first Century," in *Pioneer Healers: The History of Women Religious in American Health Care*, eds. Ursula Stepsis, CSA, and Dolores Liptak, RSM, (New York: Crossroad Publishing Co., 1989), p. 172.

[26]Amended and Restated By-Laws of St. Francis Medical Center, October 27, 1992.

to dissolve the corporation, merge the corporation, liquidate the assets of the corporation or transfer effective control over the assets of the corporation, they must have the consent in writing of the Sisters of St. Francis of Millvale.

Further, the members of the Board of Directors are indirectly chosen by the sisters since the nominating committee is comprised entirely of five Sisters of St. Francis of Millvale, three of whom shall be the Major Superior of the Order, the President of the St. Francis Health System and the Chief Executive of the Corporation. All other members of the nominating committee shall be appointed by the Major Superior, and shall be chosen from the Sisters of St. Francis currently serving as board members of the St. Francis Health System or any of its affiliated corporations.[27]

The by-laws assure that the administration of the hospital and the parent body, the St. Francis Health System, remain under the control of the sisters. The Chief Executive officer of the corporation is to be nominated by the president of the St. Francis Health System, and elected by the Board of Directors. The CEO is to be chosen from the Sisters of St. Francis as long as a qualified sister of that order is available. In the event that a qualified sister is not available, the Sisters of the order are to submit the name of a qualified person to the board.[28]

It is interesting that, by 1992, St. Francis had become the exception to the rule regarding sister administrators in Catholic Hospitals. In many facilities, there are no longer qualified sisters available to fill the role. In 1965, only 3.2 percent of the Catholic Hospitals had lay administrators. That figure rose to 23 percent within five years, and by 1975, 38 percent of the CEO's were lay administrators. By 1980, the percentage had increased to 51 percent. By 1985, 70 percent of all Catholic hospitals had lay personnel serving as the chief executives of the hospital. The fact that the Sisters of St. Francis have always emphasized the need for education in order to manage their hospitals helps to explain why the St. Francis Hospital is now the exception to the rule.[29]

Several of the policies regarding medical staff are also rooted in the religious beliefs of the sisters. "By reason of the moral and ethical principles of the

[27] Amended and Restated By-Laws of St. Francis Medical Center, October 27, 1992, Article VI, Sections 1, 2.

[28] Amended and Restated By-Laws of St. Francis Medical Center, October 27, 1992, Article VII, Section 5.

[29] Christopher Kauffman, "The Modern Association; Preserving a Catholic Presence in the United States Healthcare System," *Health Progress* 71, (July–August 1990), p. 36; Margaret John Kelly, D.C., "Toward the Twenty-first Century," in *Pioneer Healers: The History of Women Religious in American Health Care*, eds. Ursula Stepsis, CSA, and Dolores Liptak, RSM, (New York: Crossroad Publishing Co., 1989), p. 177.

Corporation, the Board of Directors/Administration may require a Medical Staff member to comply with certain religious/moral and ethical principles of the Corporation as a condition of membership on the Medical Staff or continuation of membership on the Medical Staff. This proviso may be considered by the Board of Directors as a condition of admission to, renewal, or continuance of a member on the medical staff." The clear implication that the physicians are to submit to the authority of the sisters emphasizes one of the key differences between many Catholic hospitals and other American general hospitals. As noted previously, however, many Catholic institutions are beginning to hire lay administrators as the number of sisters declines, but the Sisters of St. Francis of Millvale have been able to maintain their authority throughout the years.[30]

The authority of the sisters is noted again in the last article of the by-laws, which states that no "amendment may be made to those provisions of these by-laws which affect the rights of the Sisters of St. Francis of Millvale without the written consent of the Sisters of St. Francis.[31] Never before the 1990s did the sisters feel it was necessary to protect their rights within the institution by incorporating them into the institution's by-laws. Throughout the hospital's history, it was always clearly understood that the sisters had complete authority. Board members, medical staff and hospital personnel submitted to that authority. As the number of sisters began to decline, however, they had to resort to other methods in order to continue to administer their hospital within the framework of their own religious values. Only by continuing to dominate the direction of the hospital could they be assured that their spiritual mission would be accomplished, providing comprehensive, holistic care to the hospital patients and community at large.

The historiography has generally neglected the role of Catholic sisters in hospital development, focusing generally on alms houses, facilities created for lying-in women, or teaching hospitals and medical centers commonly located in the larger metropolitan areas. There is a dearth of studies on the role of women religious in the establishment of hospitals in the historical literature, which is surprising considering the involvement of organized religion in the organization of health care institutions. Hospitals founded during the first several hundred years after the birth of Christ were often established by Christians, believing they were commanded to provide charity to the infirm. The first Ecumenical Council of Nicea ordered each bishop to build a hospital

---

[30] Amended and Restated By-Laws of St. Francis Medical Center, October 27, 1992, Article VIII, Section 1.

[31] Amended and Restated By-Laws of St. Francis Medical Center, October 27, 1992, Article XV.

in his diocese.[32] Religious orders of women in America, as previously noted in the first chapter, established numerous hospitals. By 1885, Roman Catholics had established 154 hospitals throughout the country, more than the total number existing in the late 1860s.[33]

The growth of America's hospitals has been shaped by the concerns of the medical profession, developing technology, alterations in community demographics and changes brought on by urbanization and industrialization. This study of the St. Francis Hospital, which in many cases exemplifies many of America's Roman Catholic institutions, illustrates the fact that not all hospitals fit into the model previously created by other medical historians. That model proposes that many conflicts occurred in the development of any medical facility between administration, medical staff and board members, with the physicians ultimately assuming control over the future direction of the hospital.[34] Clearly, this history demonstrates that, although that model explains the development of other institutions, it is not necessarily applicable to all, for in many Catholic facilities, the sisters retained their authority in spite of many conflicts.

Conflict was persistent throughout much of St. Francis Hospital's history. The sisters, desiring to model their facility after the most modern medical centers, utilized the rhetoric of the medical profession, which often conflicted with their own spiritual ideology. Research has shown, for example, that the administration wanted St. Francis to be a major teaching facility, reflecting the views of the medical staff. Another example was the sisters' advocation of the psychopathic hospital, designed to admit only mentally ill patients deemed to be curable. In reality, however, these goals, and others, were not completely met, for the sisters could not jeopardize their religious mission to serve the indigent, regardless of their diagnoses or ability to pay. Reality and ideology, then, were often in conflict in hospitals under the direction of women religious.

The sisters also endured the conflict of maintaining their spiritual goals

[32] Margaret Brindle, "Hospitals," in *Encyclopedia of Social History*, ed. Peter N. Stearns, (New York: Garland, 1994), p. 327.

[33] Charles E. Rosenberg, *The Care of Strangers, The Rise of America's Hospital System*, (New York: Basic Books, Inc., 1987), p. 111.

[34] For a thorough historical analysis of hospital development see the following: Charles E. Rosenberg, *The Care of Strangers, The Rise of America's Hospital System*, (New York: Basic Books, Inc., 1987); David Rosner, *A Once Charitable Enterprise: Hospitals and Health Care in Brooklyn and New York, 1885–1915*, (Princeton: Princeton University Press, 1982); Paul Starr, *The Social Transformation of American Medicine: The Rise of a Sovereign Profession and the Making of a Vast Industry*, (New York: Basic Books, Inc., 1982); Rosemary Stevens, *In Sickness and in Wealth: American Hospitals in the Twentieth Century*, (New York: Basic Books, Inc., 1989); Morris J. Vogel, *The Invention of the Modern Hospital: Boston 1870–1930*, (Chicago: University of Chicago Press, 1980).

while attempting to remain financially solvent. They were forced to make decisions which caused much suffering for them. Historian Joan Lynaugh has noted that institutional leaders frequently made decisions which improved hospital income in order to keep their institutions financially solvent.[35] The Sisters of St. Francis were no different in that regard, but they had their limits. They were willing to remove the crucifixes from the hospital's walls, and freely described the hospital as being non- sectarian in order that they obtain the necessary state appropriation, but they would not compromise on their mission to admit the indigent in spite of monetary shortages. All this was done with the Bishop's approval. Lynaugh has suggested that the effect of such decisions often narrowed the scope of care thought appropriate to hospitals by restricting services to persons with curable health problems. The opposite was true at St. Francis in that people were admitted who often were refused care elsewhere because they were not acutely ill and had a dubious probability of cure. These policies, however, proved to be beneficial. The sisters, cognizant of the unmet needs of many of their patients, developed programs which became the foundation for services which continue to function today. The numerous and highly specialized programs in psychiatry and chemical dependency attest to that fact.

The ultimate conflict, however, was that over authority of the hospital. The sisters had established themselves as owners of the hospital even before the twentieth century began, allowing them to direct policy. They never relinquished that authority, unlike other general hospitals, and even many Catholic institutions. There are numerous examples which illuminate such tensions. The sisters, refusing to deny care, conflicted with the medical staff over such issues as psychiatric admissions. Their authority was sometimes questioned by community leaders, as exemplified by the story of the construction of the tunnel connecting the new garage with the main building. Community members challenged the sisters when health care planners wanted to close the obstetrics department. Board members also infringed on the sisters' authority. As a result, the Order felt it was imperative that it protect its rights in legal documents such as the 1950s agreement and the 1990s by-laws. To be sure, one of the reasons the sisters were able to remain in control of the hospital was due to the deference paid to them by those who challenged them. Because they were sisters, they commanded a certain respect which inadvertently forced adversaries not to push too hard, a trend still apparent in the hospital today.

[35]Joan E. Lynaugh, "Institutionalizing Women's Health Care in Nineteenth and Twentieth Century America," in *Women, Health, and Medicine in America*, ed. Rima D. Apple, (New York: Garland, 1990), p. 267.

Just as conflict was a major aspect of the hospital's history, the study of St. Francis also serves to enhance understanding of community tensions and conflicts. For example, nineteenth-century Pittsburgh was characterized by changing demographics and the resultant ethnic and religious tensions. Individuals of different nationalities, as well as Catholics and Protestants sharing the same ethnicity, were at odds with one another. In the post-World War II period, changing community demographics again resulted in racial tension. This research, too, demonstrates the needs of the surrounding community. Clearly, the residents of the region suffered from mental illness, chemical dependency and, more significantly, alcoholism, throughout the hospital's history. The number of alcoholics treated at St. Francis suggests that this may have been a widespread community problem, which demands additional research. Further, a study such as this not only demonstrates prevailing community issues, but also illuminates the interaction of the religious hospital with the community.

This history illustrates the distinctiveness of hospitals administered by women religious. The conflicts between ideology and reality, spiritual missions and desire for financial solvency, and the struggle to maintain authority in order to preserve Catholic tradition are somewhat unique. The conflicts endured by the sisters strengthened their resolve to remain autonomous and in control of their institutions. It was not, therefore, just the sisters' spiritual beliefs which directed their health care institutions, but the struggles which they had to endure in order to maintain their religious goals. Only by assuring their place in the administration of the health system could they do that. This study emphasizes the need for additional research in this area in order to fully understand the factors which shaped the American health care system and all of its components.

It is difficult to assess the success of any given health care institution. Generally, a hospital's quality is defined by its technological offerings, significant research or the achievements of the affiliated medical school. Rarely do scientific-minded Americans consider a hospital's involvement with the community at large. The St. Francis Hospital's commitment to the community in no way diminishes its success but attests to it. In addition, late twentieth century institutions are generally described as being impersonal and cold despite providing the most modern, scientific care and fostering feelings of hope and faith among its consumers. The history of hospitals under the direction of women religious suggests that hospital development has also been guided by spiritual principles, resulting in facilities which seek to provide a shield against the impersonal care generally associated with today's modern health care providers.

Catholic institutions serve as a stark reminder that hospitals do indeed strive to provide services to the community and a form of care in addition to those typically understood. Although modern diagnostic techniques, preventive methods and curative and palliative treatments are of inestimable value, St. Francis Hospital, in contrast, stresses the importance of spiritual care. The importance of humane care, that aspect of healing so often overshadowed by medical technological accomplishments, continues to be recognized in hospitals under the auspices of religious orders, as exemplified by the St. Francis Medical Center.

Index